Contents

How to use the book   5

Symptoms and Signs   7

Conditions   171

This book is not intended to be a substitute for doctors, nurses or health professionals. Diagnosis of any condition may be very difficult, differentiating the mild from the serious, and self-diagnosis is even more problematic. This is why health professionals spend so long training, and why doctors consult other doctors when they themselves have a health problem.

If in any doubt about the severity of any condition, medical help should be sought. But it should be borne in mind, that time spent attending to trivial conditions is time that doctors or health professionals cannot spend with those individuals who may have serious illnesses.

While every effort has been made to provide accurate information in this book, errors and omissions may have occurred as medical knowledge is constantly changing. The publishers and authors cannot accept liability for any action, lack of action or loss resulting from the use of the material within the book. Information is for guidance only, and a doctor should always be consulted if a health problem is suspected or before beginning any treatment.

How to use the book

This book is divided into two sections.

SECTION ONE: SYMPTOMS AND SIGNS

The first section is an alphabetical listing of common symptoms and signs, and their combinations. Symptoms are what we feel wrong and complain of. Signs are manifestations of illness that can be seen by others, and are looked for by a doctor. The section is arranged alphabetically, either by the part of the body where the symptom is experienced (such as Mouth, Neck or Chest) or by the type of sign (such as Breath, Urine or Vomit). It is extensively cross-referenced.

Each entry in the first section consists of the name of the sign or symptom, a note about what this may mean including its potential severity, and a list of conditions with which this symptom or sign may be associated. This list is extensive but not exhaustive, and many of the conditions are not illnesses as such, including baldness, pregnancy, travel sickness, menstruation. In order to highlight the most likely of these we have preceeded the condition with a bullet point (•). The condition may then be reviewed in more detail in Section Two.

SECTION TWO: CONDITIONS

The second section is an alphabetical listing of conditions, again with extensive cross-referencing. This selection is extensive but not exhaustive, concentrating on a range of conditions from common complaints to serious illnesses.

Each entry consists of the name of the condition, general information about it, a list of bullets of signs and symptoms, a note about treatment and other information, and cross-references.

It should be said that most mild or minor illnesses will resolve by themselves in an otherwise healthy individual. The human body has a great capacity to heal itself. If, however, there is any doubt about the severity of a condition, medical help should be sought.

To get as wide an overview as possible, consult all the relevant sections on a problem, such as all the entries on Diarrhoea, Abdominal Pain or Weight Loss. The severity of symptoms, or the extent to which they may be tolerated, varies from individual to individual. While one person may regard a headache as the most severe symptom of a Migraine, another may experience violent vomiting, while a third may find the aura that proceeds it (where vision and speech may be affected and parts of the body go numb) as the most disturbing.

Diagnosing any illness may be very difficult. Many individuals will suffer from headaches from time to time. To determine what may be causing it on the basis of simply describing the main symptom of the condition as a 'headache' would be impossible. Possibilities range from a simple tension headache to a subarachnoid haemorrhage: one should resolve with rest, relaxation and possibly a mild analgesic; while the other may result in death. Three main questions may be asked in assessing the sign or symptom, (or a combination of them):

1 *Is it new or unusual?*
2 *Does it then persist for some time?*
3 *Is it getting steadily worse?*

Is it new or unusual?

Many individuals may be constipated, in that they may only open their bowels once or twice a week, while other people may do so once or twice a day. If this is part of an established pattern of bowel movements, it is probably nothing to worry about. If, however, somebody who has formerly opened their bowel every day then finds that they suddenly stop for a week, this may be serious. It is the change from what is usual for that individual that may be significant.

Does it then persist for some time?

Most people will have minor problems occasionally, such as colds, flu, headaches and stomach upsets. In most cases, these will resolve by themselves with rest, plenty of fluids, and over-the-counter remedies. If a 'new' serious problem persists for a week or more, however, it may be a sign of a serious illness.

Is it getting steadily worse?

If the symptom or condition is getting markedly worse, either quickly over a few hours or days, or more gradually over a couple of weeks, this may again be a cause for concern. How debilitating the condition is should also be taken into account. Severe toothache can get more and more difficult to cope with over time, and should prompt a visit to the dentist; while a severe headache which persists and worsens over time should prompt the seeking of medical help.

In the end, it may be difficult even for a doctor to diagnose many conditions without diagnostic tests, and even then this will usually take some time. If in doubt, consult a doctor or get medical help, but bear in mind that any wasted trips, tests or time spent on minor compaints are resources taken from somebody who may be suffering from a serious problem.

Sudden collapse or unconsciousness whatever the cause, and particularly if the individual stops breathing, may require emergency procedures, such as cardiopulmonary resuscitation – but these are beyond the scope of this book. There are many courses on these procedures and there are more detailed texts on first aid. In general, however, medical help should be sought as soon as possible, in these emergencies.

Section One: Symptoms and Signs

Severity of signs and symptoms may vary from individual to individual so it may be worthwhile consulting all the sections on a particular indication or part of the body.

In most cases there is a large list of possible conditions. In order to highlight the most likely of these we have preceeded the condition with a bullet point (•).

A—Z

Abdomen, Swollen: Adults

A swollen-looking abdomen can be caused by being overweight, wind or constipation, pregnancy or menstruation. It may also be the sign of a more serious condition.

POSSIBLE CONDITIONS
Cancer of the Colon or Rectum (Bowel)
Cirrhosis of the Liver
•Constipation
Constrictive Pericarditis
Diverticulitis
Fibroids
•Flatulence
Heart Attack and Failure
Hepatitis
Intestinal Obstruction
Irritable Bowel Syndrome
Jejunal Diverticulitis
Malignant Ascites
Meckel's Diverticulum
Mesenteric Vascular Occlusion
Obesity
Ovarian Cyst
Pancreatitis
Perforated Viscus
Pregnancy

Relapsing Fever
Tumour of Kidney, Womb, Ovaries, Bowel
Typhoid Fever
Ulcerative Colitis

Abdomen, Swollen: Children

Children can have a swollen stomach or abdomen for various reasons, not least they are constipated. It may be the indication of serious underlying illness, although this will usually be combined with other signs.

POSSIBLE CONDITIONS
Coeliac Disease
•Constipation
Cystic Fibrosis
Hirschsprung's Disease
Intussusception
Kwashiorkor
Tumour of kidneys or elsewhere
Typhoid Fever

Abdomen: Lump, Mass or Swollen Area

A lump, mass or swelling which can be felt in the stomach or abdomen (apart from Pregnancy) is usually a sign of serious underlying disease.

POSSIBLE CONDITIONS
Aortic Aneurysm
Appendicitis
Cancer of the Bile Ducts
Cancer of the Bladder
Cancer of the Cervix
Cancer of the Colon or Rectum (Bowel)
Cancer of the Gall Bladder
Cancer of the Kidney
Cancer of the Liver
Cancer of the Ovaries
Cancer of the Pancreas
Cancer of the Stomach
Cancer of the Womb
Cirrhosis of the Liver
Diverticulitis
Enlarged Bladder
Gall Bladder Infection
Hepatitis
• Hernia, Inguinal
• Hernia, Umbilical
Injury to the Lower Chest or Pelvis
Jejunal Diverticulitis
Kala-azar
Leukaemia
Malaria
Myelofibrosis
Ovarian Cyst
Pancreatitis
Pregnancy
Tapeworms
Wilms' Tumour

POSSIBLE CONDITIONS
Cancer of Colon or Rectum (Bowel0
Crohn's Disease
Hypercalcaemia
Inflammatory Bowel Disease
Intestinal Obstruction
• Irritable Bowel Syndrome
Peritonitis

Abdomen: Pain and Diarrhoea

Usually an indication of minor food poisoning or Gastroenteritis, but may be a sign of serious disease.

POSSIBLE CONDITIONS
Botulism
Cancer of the Colon or Rectum (Bowel)
Carcinoid Syndrome
Cholera
Crohn's Disease
Dysentery
• Gastroenteritis
Henoch's Purpura
Intestinal Ischaemia
• Irritable Bowel Syndrome
Jejunal Diverticulitis
Pancreatitis
Phaeochromocytoma
Post-Gastrectomy Syndrome
Post-Viral Syndrome
Typhoid Fever
Ulcerative Colitis

Abdomen: Pain and Constipation

A sign of Irritable Bowel Syndrome. Also consult the sections on Constipation and on Abdominal Pain.

Abdomen: Pain and Persistent Weight Loss

Pain in the abdomen and long-term weight loss may

be a sign of serious disease, and medical help should be sought.

POSSIBLE CONDITIONS
Cancer of the Colon or Rectum (Bowel)
Cancer of the Kidney
Cancer of the Liver
Cancer of the Pancreas
Cancer of the Stomach
Coeliac Disease
Crohn's Disease
Diabetes
Pancreatitis
Ulcerative Colitis

Abdomen: Pain and Vomiting

An indication of minor food poisoning or Gastroenteritis, but may be a sign of serious disease.

POSSIBLE CONDITIONS
Appendicitis
Biliary Colic
Cancer of the Stomach
Diabetes
• Gastroenteritis
Hernia, Umbilical
Intestinal Ischaemia
Intestinal Obstruction
Kidney Disease or Failure
Kidney Stones
Meckel's Diverticulum
Mesenteric Adenitis
Ovarian Cyst
Pancreatitis
Peptic Ulcer
Peritonitis

Porphyria
Salpingitis

Abdomen: Pain and Vomiting Blood

A sign of serious underlying disease, and medical help should be sought.

POSSIBLE CONDITIONS
Adverse Drug Reaction
Cancer of the Stomach
Cirrhosis of liver with oesophageal varices
• Gastric or Duodenal Ulcer
• Gastritis
• Hernia, Hiatus
Mallory-Weiss Tear
Oesophagitis
Yellow Fever

Abdomen: Pain, Vomiting and Fever

An indication of food poisoning, Gastroenteritis or Urinary Tract Infection, but may be a sign of serious disease.

POSSIBLE CONDITIONS
Appendicitis
Gall Stones
• Gastroenteritis
Intestinal Obstruction
Meckel's Diverticulum
Pancreatitis
Pelvic Inflammatory Disease
Porphyria
• Urinary Tract Infection

Abdomen: Pain, Vomiting and Jaundice

Combination of symptoms which indicates serious

illness. Medical help should be sought immediately.

POSSIBLE CONDITIONS
• Biliary Colic
Cancer of the Liver
Cancer of the Pancreas
Cancer of the Stomach
Gall Stones
Hepatitis
Pancreatitis
Sickle Cell Anaemia

Abdomen: Prominent Blood Vessels

Prominent blood vessels become apparent on the stomach or abdomen. This may be a sign of serious underlying disease, and medical help should be sought and investigations undertaken.

POSSIBLE CONDITIONS
Cancer of the Bladder
Cancer of the Kidney
• Cirrhosis of the Liver
Malignant Ascites
Ovarian Cyst
Pancreatitis

Abdomen: Rigid

If the abdomen is swollen and rigid to the touch, combined with severe pain and illness, this is a sign of Perforated Viscus. Medical help should be sought immediately.

POSSIBLE CONDITIONS
Abcess of Appendix or Diverticulum
Ectopic Pregnancy
Perforated Viscus
Ruptured Ovarian Cyst

Abdomen: Severe Intermittent Pain

Severe pain in the abdomen which appears to resolve but then recurs. If this goes on for any length of time, particularly if not associated with food poisoning or similar condition, medical help should be sought immediately.

POSSIBLE CONDITIONS
• Biliary Colic
Fibroids
Injury to the Lower Chest or Pelvis
Intestinal Obstruction
Irritable Bladder
Jejunal Diverticulitis
• Kidney Stones
• Urinary Tract Infection

Abdomen: Severe Persistent Pain

Severe and persistent pain in the abdomen is usually a sign of serious disease, and medical help should be sought immediately.

POSSIBLE CONDITIONS
Aortic Aneurysm
Bladder Neck Obstruction
Injury to the Lower Chest or Pelvis
Intestinal Ischaemia
Mesenteric Vascular Occlusion
Pancreatitis
Perforated Viscus
• Peritonitis
Salpingitis
Urethral Stricture

Abdomen: Swollen and Constipation

Many individuals will suffer from bouts of

constipation from time to time, and anyway frequency and consistency of motions varies from person to person. A change in bowel habit may be significant, although this combination of signs may simply be the result of too much refined food, too little fluid or too little roughage. If it persists for a long time, and cannot be related to lifestyle changes, it is possible that this may be an indication of a serious condition.

POSSIBLE CONDITIONS
Cancer of the Colon or Rectum (Bowel)
Constipation
Diverticulitis
Flatulence
Irritable Bowel Syndrome

Abdomen: Swollen and Diarrhoea

Most individuals will suffer from bouts of diarrhoea from time to time, and the frequency and consistency of motions varies from person to person. A change in bowel habit may be significant, although often this is simply the result of too much rich food, alcohol, fruit or roughage, nerves, or minor food poisoning. If it persists for a long time, and cannot be related to lifestyle changes, it is possible that this may be an indication of serious conditions.

POSSIBLE CONDITIONS
Cancer of the Colon or Rectum (Bowel)
Constipation
Crohn's Disease
Diverticulitis
• Flatulence
Gastroenteritis
• Irritable Bowel Syndrome
Laxatives

Ulcerative Colitis

Acne

Most individuals will suffer from spots, pimples and blackheads at some time, especially in their adolescence. Rarely Acne can be a sign of more serious disease.

POSSIBLE CONDITIONS
• Acne Vulgaris
Congenital Adrenal Hyperplasia
Cushing's Syndrome
Polycystic Ovaries

Ankle: Pain and Weak

Pain is experienced in or around the ankle, and the joint is weak or cannot bear weight. This is most likely an indication of injury or fracture of the ankle.
POSSIBLE CONDITIONS
Broken Ankle
Cellulitis
• Injury to the Ankle

Ankle: Swollen

Ankle and/or leg may become swollen, usually from injury, from a build of fluid, or because of Deep Vein Thrombosis (DVT). Swollen ankles may be the result of water retention during Menstruation Cycle, but it may also more unusually be an indication of heart or kidney problems. If one leg suddenly becomes swollen and pale then this may be an indication of DVT.

POSSIBLE CONDITIONS
Anaemia
Cellulitis

Deep Vein Thrombosis
• Fluid Retention
Heart Failure
• Injury to the Ankle
Kidney Disease or Failure
Lymphoedema
Menstruation
Mitral or Aortic Valve Disease
Myocarditis
Myxoedema
Nephrotic Syndrome
Phlegmasia Alba Dolens
Pregnancy
Varicose Veins
Vitamin B1 (Thiamine) Deficiency

Anus: Itching (Rectum and Anus)

It is not unusual for the anus to become itchy, particularly if the individual spends a long time sitting in a sweaty environment, has Piles, Threadworms or an infection. Occasionally it is a sign of more serious illness.

POSSIBLE CONDITIONS
Anal Fissure
Candidiasis
Diabetes
Fistula-In-Ano
• Piles
Pilonidal Sinus
Threadworm

Anus: Pain (Rectum or Anus)

Pain around the rectum or anus can be caused by passing hard faeces or anal intercourse: either of these can damage the wall of the bowel. Piles

(haemorrhoids) may also be extremely painful. This may also be a sign of a more serious underlying condition.

POSSIBLE CONDITIONS
Anal Abscess
• Anal Fissure
Crohn's Disease
Diabetes
Fistula-In-Ano
• Piles

Anxiety

Anxiety is both a medical condition and a state of nerves and tension. Most individuals will experience the latter as part of usual life, and such feelings can be exacerbated by smoking, drinking coffee, missing meals and drinking, but it is possible that this becomes a chronic and debilitating condition. This will usually be caused by psychological or psychiatric problems beyond the control of the individual, rather than by a physical illness, and is often associated with Depression. Anxiety, however, may be an indication of a serious physical condition.

POSSIBLE CONDITIONS
Alcohol or Narcotics
• Anxiety
Caffeine
Cluster Headache
Dementia
Depression and Manic Depression
Hyperthyroidism
Hyperventilation
Low Blood Sugar
Phaeochromocytoma
Post-Viral Syndrome

Schizophrenia
Shock

Appetite: Feeling Full on Eating Little

How much food it takes to make an individual feel full varies from person to person, and their emotional state. Nerves or anxiety can reduce appetite. Surgery to remove part of the stomach will obviously reduce the amount of food that can be consumed. In some cases it may be a sign of serious disease. Also see the other sections on Appetite.

POSSIBLE CONDITIONS
•Anxiety
Cancer of the Stomach
Peptic Ulcer
Post-Gastrectomy Syndrome

Appetite: No Appetite and Weight Loss

Unexplained weight loss combined with a lack of appetite is often a cause for concern, particularly in older individuals. Long-term disease and feverish illness can produce this combination, as can cancer in many parts of the body. Although rare, cancer should be investigated if there are also signs such as tiredness, unexplained pain, lumps or swellings, or blood coming from the mouth, vagina or in phlegm, vomit, faeces or urine.

POSSIBLE CONDITIONS
Alcohol or Narcotics
Anorexia Nervosa
•Anxiety
Brucellosis
Cancer of the Cervix
Cancer of the Ovaries

Cancer of the Pancreas
Cancer of the Spine
Depression and Manic Depression
•Fever
Lung Cancer
Peptic Ulcer
Rheumatic Fever

Appetite: No Appetite, Chest Pain and Weight Loss

Combination of symptoms which often indicates a serious underlying disease.

POSSIBLE CONDITIONS
Cancer of the Stomach
Gall Bladder Infection
Hernia, Hiatus
Lung Cancer
•Oesophagitis
•Peptic Ulcer
Tuberculosis

Appetite: Reduced or Lack of

It is not unusual for individuals to lose their appetite from time to time, particularly if going through periods of emotional turmoil or illnesses such as Colds or Flu. In most cases it is not anything to worry about unless it persists for a long time.

POSSIBLE CONDITIONS
Alcohol or Narcotics
•Anxiety
Appendicitis
Brain Abscess
Brucellosis
Cancer of the Stomach

15

Cancer in the Chest
Cold, Common
Depression and Manic Depression
Dyspepsia, Non-Ulcer
• Fever
Flu
Heart Attack and Failure
Hepatitis
Rheumatic Fever
Wilms' Tumour

Back: Lump or Hump

Range of lumps from the small and numerous to a hump can affect the back. Causes range from Boils, Warts and Acne to more serious illness.

POSSIBLE CONDITIONS
Acne Vulgaris
• Boil
Cancer of the Skin
Carbuncle
Cellulitis
• Kyphosis
Lipoma
Metastasis
Scoliosis
• Sebaceous Cyst
Spina Bifida
Tuberculosis
Warts

Back: Pain

Back pain is very common, but can be very severe in intensity. It may be caused by a huge range of conditions, from simple strain, Slipped Disc or Period Pain to cancer and Tuberculosis. Pain is not always related to severity.

POSSIBLE CONDITIONS
Ankylosing Spondylitis
• Back Strain
Cancer of the Cervix
Cancer of the Ovaries
Cancer of the Spine
Cancer of the Womb
Cauda Equine Syndrome
• Cervical Spondylosis
Coccydynia
Crohn's Disease
• Kyphosis
Menstruation
Osteoarthritis
Osteoporosis
Pancreatitis
Pelvic Inflammatory Disease
Peptic Ulcer
Sciatica
Scoliosis
Shingles
• Slipped Disc
Spinal Cord Injury
Tuberculosis
Ulcerative Colitis
Urinary Tract Infection
• Vertebral Fracture/Collapse
Vitamin D (Calciferol) Deficiency

Baldness and Hair Loss

Hair loss and baldness is a natural occurrence in many men, characterised by male pattern baldness. Hair can also become thinner in women as they grow older. In both cases, this is determined by genes.

Baldness or hair loss may also be an indication of underlying disease.

POSSIBLE CONDITIONS
Adverse Drug Reaction
AIDS
• Alopecia
• Alopecia Areata
Dermatitis
Hypopituitarism
Hyperthyroidism
Hypothyroidism
Kwashiorkor
Menopause
Morphoea
Pregnancy
Psoriasis
Ringworm

Bleeding: Blood Slow to Clot

Bleeding in any area does not stop and the individual is also easily bruised.

POSSIBLE CONDITIONS
• Adverse Drug Reaction
Cirrhosis of the Liver
• Disorders of Blood Clotting
Haemophilia
• Vitamin C (Ascorbic Acid) Deficiency

Bleeding: Unexplained and General

Generalised bleeding from parts of the body such as the nose, gums, rectum or vagina, or blood in urine or faeces. This is usually caused by a disorder of blood clotting.

POSSIBLE CONDITIONS

• Adverse Drug Reaction
Anaemia
Bite, Animal
Cancer of the Bones
Cirrhosis of the Liver
• Disorders of Blood Clotting
Haemophilia
Leukaemia
Malaria
Septicaemia
Typhoid Fever
Vitamin C (Ascorbic Acid) Deficiency
Weil's Disease

Blind Spot

A blind spot or area becomes apparent in the field of vision. This blind spot stays in the same position and does not move across the field of vision. The cause is usually damage to the eye or a blow or trauma to the head, but it may be an indication of problems with the nerves or brain. If a blind spot or reduced field of vision is present, medical help should be sought immediately.

POSSIBLE CONDITIONS
Cancer of the Pituitary
Carotid Aneurysm
Choroiditis
Head Injury
Injury to the Eye
• Macular Degeneration
Poisoning
• Stroke
Vitreous Haemorrhage

Blindness, Colour

Inability to distinguish between different colours, commonly between green and red. This is usually simply because of natural variation between individuals and will be present from birth, but it may be the sign of a serious problem should it develop later in life.

POSSIBLE CONDITIONS
Adverse Drug Reaction
Cataract
• Colour Blindness
Detached Retina
Malnutrition
Poisoning

Blindness, Night

Most individuals see much better in bright daylight than at night. Night blindness or greatly impaired vision in darker conditions will be exacerbated if the individual has poor eyesight. It may also be an indication of a lack of Vitamin A.

POSSIBLE CONDITIONS
Malnutrition
• Poor Eyesight
Retinitis Pigmentosa
• Vitamin A Deficiency

Blindness: Slow Onset

Blindness develops over some time, so slowly that the individual may not be aware it has happened until the blindness is advanced. This is a serious sign, and medical help should be sought.

POSSIBLE CONDITIONS

• Cataract
Choroiditis
• Diabetes
Glaucoma
High Blood Pressure
• Macular Degeneration
Paget's Disease
Retinitis Pigmentosa
Trachoma

Blindness: Sudden

Blindness has a sudden onset. Can affect one or both eyes. This is most usually an indication of serious underlying disease, either with the eye itself or the structures and nerves concerned with vision. It is possible that this may be caused by a Migraine, but if this is the case it should resolve fairly quickly. If Migraine is not suspected, medical help should be sought immediately.

POSSIBLE CONDITIONS
• Central Retinal Artery Blockage
Central Retinal Vein Blockage
Detached Retina
Diabetes
Filariasis
Glaucoma
Head Injury
Hysteria
Methyl Alcohol
• Migraine
Optic Neuritis
Poisoning
Stroke
Syphilis
• Temporal Arteritis

Vitreous Haemorrhage

Blisters

Blisters, fluid filled areas, can develop on the skin, usually caused by burns or injury, skin inflammation or infections.

POSSIBLE CONDITIONS
- Adverse Drug Reaction
- Blisters
- Burns

Chickenpox

Chilblains

Dermatitis

Dermatomyositis

Epidermolysis Bullosa

Erysipelas

Erythema Multiforme

Fungal Infections of the Skin

Herpes Simplex

Impetigo

Molluscum Contagiosum

Pemphigus Vulgaris

Porphyria Cutanea Tarda

Scalded Skin Syndrome

Shingles

Blood Vessels: Prominent on Abdomen

Prominent blood vessels become apparent on the stomach or abdomen. This may be a sign of serious underlying disease, and medical help should be sought and investigations undertaken.

POSSIBLE CONDITIONS
Cancer of the Bladder
Cancer of the Kidney

- Cirrhosis of the Liver
Malignant Ascites
Ovarian Cyst
Pancreatitis

Blood Vessels: Prominent on Head

Most usually an indication of Temporal Arteritis, typically if inflamed and tender.

POSSIBLE CONDITIONS
Temporal Arteritis

Blood Vessels: Prominent on Neck

This is usually a sign of serious underlying disease, and medical help should be sought and investigations undertaken.

POSSIBLE CONDITIONS
Cancer in the Chest
- Chronic Lung Disease incl Chronic Bronchitis
- Constrictive Pericarditis
Heart Attack and Failure
Pericarditis
Suffocation

Blood: Between Periods

Bleeding, beyond what would be expected from periods, is experienced between menstruation. This may be a normal variation, but it may also be an indication of a miscarriage (see Pregnancy), Menopause, use of the Contraceptive Pill, and several other conditions.

POSSIBLE CONDITIONS
Cancer of the Cervix
Cancer of the Ovaries

Cancer of the Womb
Cervical Polyp
• Contraceptive Pill
Erosion of the Cervix
Inflammation of the Vagina
• Menopause
• Menstruation (normal variation)
Pregnancy
Urethral Caruncle

Blood: Bruising and Bleeding Under the Skin

The most common cause of bruising or bleeding under the skin is non-penetrating injury which results in bruising. It may be the sign of a serious condition.

POSSIBLE CONDITIONS
• Adverse Drug Reaction
Anaemia
Bite, Animal
• Bruise
Cushing's Syndrome
• Disorders of Blood Clotting
Haemophilia
Henoch's Purpura
Leukaemia
Meninogococcal Septicaemia
• Senile Purpura
Vitamin C (Ascorbic Acid) Deficiency

Blood: Ear

Blood comes from the ear. This may be caused by infections or injury to the ear. If it is prolonged or the result of severe trauma, medical help should be sought.

POSSIBLE CONDITIONS
Boil
Cancer of the Ear
• Ear Infection
Ear Polyp
Head Injury
Ruptured Eardrum

Blood: Gums

Bleeding gums can be caused by brushing teeth too vigorously, but may be the sign of infection. If bleeding gums persist, consult a dentist.

POSSIBLE CONDITIONS
• Disorders of Blood Clotting
Vitamin C (Ascorbic Acid) Deficiency

Blood: Menopause

Older women who have gone through the Menopause may still experience periods of bleeding. This may also be a sign of an underlying problem.

POSSIBLE CONDITIONS
Cancer of the Cervix
Cancer of the Ovaries
• Cancer of the Womb
Cervical Polyp
• Menopause (normal variation)
Urethral Caruncle

Blood: Nose

Nose bleeds are relatively common, and are rarely a sign of any serious problem. Medical help should be sought if there has been severe trauma to the nose as it may be broken. Prolonged bleeding from the nose for no apparent reason may be a cause for concern.

POSSIBLE CONDITIONS
Adverse Drug Reaction
Cancer of the Nose
Cold, Common
Disorders of Blood Clotting
Foreign Body in Nose
High Blood Pressure
• Injury to the Nose
Nasal Polyps
• Picking Nose
Sinusitis

Blood: Phlegm and Cough

A cough with the production of phlegm, which may be yellow or green in colour, but is also streaked or contains blood. This is most usually the result of a serious problem such as severe Chest Infections, Pneumonia or Lung Cancer. Medical help should be sought as soon as possible.

POSSIBLE CONDITIONS
• Bleeding Disorder
Bronchiectasis
• Chest Infection
Heart Disease
Lung Cancer
Mitral Valve Disease
Pneumonia
Q Fever
Tuberculosis

Blood: Rectum

It is not unusual to get blood coming from the anus if the individual has Piles (haemorrhoids). If this is the case, the blood will be fresh and bright red. It may be an indication of serious underlying disease,

however, particularly if the blood is black, dark or tar-like.

POSSIBLE CONDITIONS
Adverse Drug Reaction
Anal Fissure
Bleeding Disorder
Cancer of the Colon or Rectum (Bowel)
Cirrhosis of the Liver
Disorders of Blood Clotting
Diverticulitis
Dysentery
Henoch's Purpura
Intestinal Polyps
Intussusception
Jejunal Diverticulitis
Mallory-Weiss Tear
Meckel's Diverticulum
Mesenteric Vascular Occlusion
Oesophageal Varices
Peptic Ulcer
• Piles
Pregnancy

Blood: Slow to Clot

Bleeding in any area does not stop and the individual is also easily bruised.

POSSIBLE CONDITIONS
• Adverse Drug Reaction
• Disorders of Blood Clotting
Haemophilia
Vitamin C (Ascorbic Acid) Deficiency

Blood: Unexplained and General

Generalised bleeding from parts of the body such as

the nose, gums, rectum or vagina, or blood in urine or faeces. This is usually caused by a disorder of blood clotting.

POSSIBLE CONDITIONS
• Adverse Drug Reaction
Anaemia
Bite, Animal
Cancer of the Bones
Cirrhosis of the Liver
• Disorders of Blood Clotting
Haemophilia
Leukaemia
Malaria
Septicaemia
Typhoid Fever
Vitamin C (Ascorbic Acid) Deficiency
Weil's Disease

Blood: Urine

Blood passed in urine can look bright red or pink, or it may make urine look cloudy. Blood may also only be passed at the beginning or end of the act of urination. Blood in urine can be caused by relatively mild conditions, such as Cystitis (although it may feel anything but mild), but persistent blood in urine can be a sign of serious underlying illness.

POSSIBLE CONDITIONS
Adverse Drug Reaction
Bilharzia
Bleeding
Cancer of the Bladder
Cancer of the Kidney
Cancer of the Prostate
• Cystitis
Disorders of Blood Clotting

Endocarditis
Enlarged Prostate
Exercise
Henoch's Purpura
Injury to the Lower Chest or Pelvis
Kidney Disease or Failure
Kidney Stones
Prostatitis
• Urinary Tract Infection
Wilms' Tumour
Yellow Fever

Blood: Urine and Pain Urinating

Most likely cause is Cystitis or Urinary Tract Infections, but it may be an indication of more serious illness.

POSSIBLE CONDITIONS
Bilharzia
Cystitis
Kidney Disease or Failure
Kidney Stones
Prostatitis
• Urinary Tract Infection

Blood: Vagina

Blood comes from the vagina, beyond that which would be expected during Menstruation. Heavy bleeding is called menorrhagia. This may have many causes, many of them serious, such as miscarriage (see Pregnancy). If unexpected bleeding from the vagina persists and is heavy medical help should be sought.

POSSIBLE CONDITIONS
Bleeding

Cancer of the Cervix
Cancer of the Ovaries
Cancer of the Womb
Cervical Polyp
Contraceptive Pill
Disorders of Blood Clotting
Endometriosis
• Erosion of the Cervix
• Fibroids
Hypothyroidism
Inflammation of the Vagina
Menopause
• Menstruation
Pelvic Inflammatory Disease
Pregnancy
Urethral Caruncle

Blood: Vomit

Blood can be present in vomit. It may be bright red and fresh, or it may be black and like coffee grounds. Either way, this is usually a sign of a serious underlying problem, and medical help should be sought.

POSSIBLE CONDITIONS
Adverse Drug Reaction
Aortic Aneurysm
Bleeding
Disorders of Blood Clotting
• Gastritis
• Hernia, Hiatus
Intussusception
Mallory-Weiss Tear
Oesophageal Varices
• Peptic Ulcer
Yellow Fever

Blood: Vomit and Abdominal Pain

A sign of serious underlying disease, and medical help should be sought.

POSSIBLE CONDITIONS
Adverse Drug Reaction
Cancer of the Stomach
• Gastritis
Hernia, Hiatus
Mallory-Weiss Tear
Oesophagitis
• Peptic Ulcer
Yellow Fever

Body: Swollen, Generalised

Generalised swelling about several parts of the body, such as the face, wrists, abdomen, legs and ankles. This is usually caused by the retention of fluid, and other than Menstruation and Pregnancy, should be investigated as it may be an indication of heart or kidney disease.

POSSIBLE CONDITIONS
Angioneurotic Oedema
• Cirrohis of the Liver
Coeliac Disease
Heart Failure
Hepatitis
• Hypothyroidism
Kidney Disease or Failure
Malnutrition
Nephrotic Syndrome
Pregnancy
Vitamin B1 (Thiamine) Deficiency

Body: Swollen, Part

Parts of (or part of) the body becomes swollen, in most cases because of injury or insect stings, or rarely because of a serious condition.

POSSIBLE CONDITIONS
Allergic Reaction, Severe
Angioneurotic Oedema
Bite, Insect
• Deep Vein Thrombosis
Filariasis
• Injury
Kwashiorkor
Lymphatic Obstruction of the Breast
Lymphoedema
Malignant Ascites
Mitral Valve Disease
Myocarditis
Myxoedema
Nephrotic Syndrome
Phlegmasia Alba Dolens
Sprue

Bone: Breaks Easily

Bones break very easily with a relatively small amount of force. Although the fracture will need treatment, this may be a sign of an underlying problems with the bones. This is far more common in elderly people.

POSSIBLE CONDITIONS
Bedridden
Brittle Bone Disease
Cancer of the Bones
Osteomyelitis
Osteopetrosis

• Osteoporosis
Paget's Disease

Bone: Misshapen or Swollen

Bones look misshapen, swollen or deformed. This will often be caused by a broken bone, but may also be caused by disease.

POSSIBLE CONDITIONS
Acromegaly
• Broken Bone
• Broken Lower Arm Bones (Radius, Ulna and wrist)
• Broken Upper Arm Bone (Humerus)
Cancer of the Bones
Dislocation of the Knee
• Fractures of the Lower Leg (femur, tibia and fibula)
Gout
Osteomyelitis
Paget's Disease
Sarcoma
Spinal Cord Injury
Tuberculosis
• Vitamin D (Calciferol) Deficiency
Yaws

Bone: Pain

Pain is experienced in bones. The most obvious cause is injury or fracture , although this may be a sign of serious illness such as cancer or Tuberculosis.

POSSIBLE CONDITIONS
Ankylosing Spondylitis
Bedridden
• Broken Collarbone
• Broken Bone
• Broken Lower Arm Bones (Radius, Ulna and wrist)

- Broken Upper Arm Bone (Humerus)
Cancer of the Bones (primary or secondary spread)
Cushing's Syndrome
Dengue
Hypercalcaemia
Metastasis
Osteoarthritis
Osteomyelitis
Osteoporosis
Rheumatoid Arthritis
Tuberculosis
Vitamin D (Calciferol) Deficiency

Breast: Change in Breast Size

Breasts may vary in size during a woman's menstrual cycle, and during pregnancy they will usually get larger. It may unusually be a sign of an underlying condition, especially if only one breast changes in size.

POSSIBLE CONDITIONS
Cancer of the Breast
- Change in Breast Size
- Contraceptive Pill
Lymphatic Obstruction of the Breast
- Menstruation (normal variation during cycle)
Pregnancy

Breast: Discharge from Nipple

Discharge from the nipple. This may be caused by several conditions, and medical help should be sought unless the woman is pregnant or has a young baby. A discharge of milk from the breast is possible before giving birth.

POSSIBLE CONDITIONS

Breast Abscess
Cancer of Ducts in the Breast
Cancer of the Breast
Duct Ectasia
Duct Papilloma
Excess of Prolactin
- Fibrocystic Disease of Breasts
Paget's Disease of the Nipple
- Pregnancy

Breast: Lump

Lump develops in the breast. Although this may often may be a harmless lump, medical help should be sought immediately to exclude serious disease.

POSSIBLE CONDITIONS
Cancer of the Breast
Duct Papilloma
Fat Necrosis in Breast
- Fibroadenoma
- Fibrocystic Disease
Mastitis
Metastasis

Breast: Pain

Pain is experienced in or around the breast. This will usually be because of changes during a woman's menstrual cycle or Pregnancy, but may be a sign of an underlying condition.

POSSIBLE CONDITIONS
Breast Abscess
Fibrocystic Disease
Mastitis
- Menstruation (normal variation)
Pregnancy

Breast: Retraction of Nipple

Nipple is retracted. This may be a normal variation if present from birth, and should cause no problems except possibly for breast feeding. If a nipple becomes retracted in later life, this may be a sign of Breast Cancer.

POSSIBLE CONDITIONS
Cancer of the Breast
• Retraction of the Nipple (normal variation if always present)

Breath: Bad and Halitosis

Bad or foul-smelling breath is usually caused either by the consumption of spiced foods or alcohol, indigestion, or by problems with teeth or gums. It may, however, be associated with more serious disease, although it is unlikely that Halitosis is going to be one of the most significant symptoms.

POSSIBLE CONDITIONS
Adverse Drug Reaction
Appendicitis
Bronchiectasis
Bronchitis
Cancer of the Larynx
Cancer of the Mouth
Cancer of the Nose
Cancer of the Oesophagus
Cancer of the Stomach
Cancer in the Chest
Chest Infection
Cirrhosis of the Liver
Cold, Common
Cystic Fibrosis
• Dental Infections
Dentures
Diabetes
Emphysema
Food and Drink
Hay Fever
Hepatitis
Kidney Disease or Failure
Laryngitis
Ludwig's Angina
Lung Abscess
Lung Cancer
Mouth Breathing
Nasal Polyps
Pharyngitis
Poisoning
• Poor Oral Hygiene
Pyorrhoea Alveolaris
Rhinitis
Sinusitis
Sjogren's Syndrome
Smoking
Tonsillitis
• Tooth Decay and Abscess
Tuberculosis

Breath: Bad, Halitosis and Cough

Bad or foul-smelling breath is usually caused either by the consumption of spiced foods or alcohol, indigestion or by problems with teeth or gums. When combined with a persistent cough, however, it may be a sign of Bronchitis, cancer or other lung problems.

POSSIBLE CONDITIONS
• Bronchiectasis
• Bronchitis

Cystic Fibrosis
Hay Fever
Lung Abscess
Lung Cancer
Rhinitis
• Tracheitis
Tuberculosis

Breath: Breathlessness and Cough

A relatively common combination of symptoms, and is usually caused by Chest Infections or problems. This may vary from the relatively mild in a fit and otherwise healthy individual to serious and life-threatening disease in the elderly or those with a pre-existing heart or respiratory condition.

POSSIBLE CONDITIONS
Aspergillosis
Bronchiectasis
• Bronchitis
• Chest Infection
Chest Injury
Emphysema
Lung Cancer
Pneumonia
Tuberculosis
Whooping Cough

Breath: Breathlessness and Fatigue or Exhaustion

A sign, particularly if it is persistent and prolonged, which may indicate serious underlying illness, such as Heart Failure or Anaemia.

POSSIBLE CONDITIONS
• Anaemia

Aortic Stenosis
Cardiomyopathy
Chest Infection
Diabetes
Guillain-Barre Syndrome
• Heart Failure
Heart Disease
Kidney Disease or Failure
Post-Viral Syndrome
Sickle Cell Anaemia

Breath: Breathlessness and Wheezing

This combination of symptoms is not uncommon, and is caused by conditions which result in a narrowing of airways, either from infection or allergy.

POSSIBLE CONDITIONS
Adverse Drug Reaction
Allergic Alveolitis
Allergic Reaction, Severe
Aspergillosis
Asthma
Bronchiolitis
• Bronchitis
Carcinoid Syndrome
• Chest Infection
• Emphysema
Extrinsic Allergic Alveolitis
Hay Fever
Hyperventilation
Myocarditis
Poisoning

Breath: Breathlessness with Chest Pain

A combination of symptoms which may indicate a

serious or even life-threatening condition, such as a Heart Attack, Pleurisy or Lung Cancer.

POSSIBLE CONDITIONS
Aortic Aneurysm
Aortic Stenosis
• Chest Infection
Heart Attack and Failure
Heart Disease
Lung Abscess
Lung Cancer
Pericarditis
Pleurisy
• Pneumonia
Pneumothorax
• Pulmonary Embolism

Breath: Breathlessness, Slower Onset

Slower onset of breathlessness, which may remain unnoticed for some time. The most obvious cause is a general lack of fitness, from lack of vigorous exercise, which may not become apparent until some strenuous activity is attempted. Apparent breathlessness may also be a result of long-term stress or anxiety, and is caused by hyperventilation. In less usual cases, it may be a sign of Heart Failure, Anaemia or cancer.

POSSIBLE CONDITIONS
• Anaemia
Anxiety
Aortic Stenosis
Botulism
• Bronchitis
Diphtheria
Emphysema
Fibrosing Alveolitis

Heart Failure
Lung Cancer
Mountain Sickness
Nephrotic Syndrome
Pneumoconiosis
Pregnancy

Breath: Breathlessness, Sudden Onset

Sudden onset of breathlessness for which there is no obvious cause (such as normal breathlessness from vigorous exercise or anxiety). The breathlessness is not as serious as suffocation, which is covered in a separate section. This may be a sign of a serious condition.

POSSIBLE CONDITIONS
Allergic Alveolitis
• Asthma
Bite, Insect with allergic reaction
Bronchiolitis
Bronchitis
• Chest Infection
Extrinsic Allergic Alveolitis
Heart Attack and Failure
Hyperventilation
Pneumonia
Pulmonary Embolism
Spinal Cord Injury
Suffocation

Breath: Cough and Bloody Phlegm

A cough with the production of phlegm, which may be yellow or green in colour, but is also streaked or contains blood. This is most usually the result of a serious problem such as severe Chest Infections, Pneumonia or Lung Cancer. Medical help should be sought as soon as possible.

POSSIBLE CONDITIONS
Bleeding Disorders
Bronchiectasis
• Chest Infection
Heart Disease
Lung Cancer
Mitral Valve Disease
Pneumonia
Q Fever
Tuberculosis

Breath: Cough and Phlegm

A cough with the production of phlegm, which may be yellow or green in colour. This is most usually the result of infections such as Colds or Chest Infections, although it may be a sign of more serious illness, particularly if it lasts for a long time and is very productive.

POSSIBLE CONDITIONS
AIDS
Bronchiectasis
• Bronchitis
• Chest Infection
Choking
Cold, Common
Cystic Fibrosis
• Emphysema
Flu
Lung Abscess
Pneumonia
Q Fever
Tuberculosis
Whooping Cough

Breath: Cough, Bloody Phlegm and Chest Pain

Chest pain combined with a cough, which also produces phlegm, which may be yellow or green in colour, but is also streaked or contains blood. This is most usually the result of a serious problem such as severe and prolonged Chest Infections, Pneumonia or Lung Cancer. Medical help should be sought as soon as possible.

POSSIBLE CONDITIONS
• Chest Infection
Chest Injury
Lung Cancer
Pneumonia
Pulmonary Embolism
Q Fever

Breath: Cough, Dry

A dry or unproductive cough (one without the production of phlegm) is most usually caused by environmental factors (such as a dry or dusty atmosphere) or Chest Infections. Unusually it is a sign of serious underlying problems.

POSSIBLE CONDITIONS
Adenoids
Adverse Drug Reaction
Allergic Alveolitis
• Asthma
Cancer of the Larynx
Cold, Common
Croup
Hay Fever
Laryngitis
Lung Cancer

Pneumoconiosis
Sinusitis
• Tracheitis
Whooping Cough

Breath: Rasping Breathing and Snoring

Snoring may be extremely tiresome, particularly for a snorer's partner, but it is not usually a sign of underlying disease. Sometimes it may be a cause for concern.

POSSIBLE CONDITIONS
Adenoids
Alcohol or Narcotics
Coma
Sleep Apnoea Syndrome
• Snoring
Stroke

Breath: Smells of Urine

Most usually a sign of Kidney Failure, and medical help should be sought immediately. This is not likely to be the most significant symptom, but it can aid in diagnosis.
POSSIBLE CONDITIONS
Kidney Disease or Failure
Uraemia

Breath: Smells Sweet

Most usually a sign of Diabetes or Liver Failure, and medical help should be sought immediately. This is not likely to be the most significant symptom, but it can aid in diagnosis.

POSSIBLE CONDITIONS

Cirrhosis of the Liver
Diabetes
Hepatitis

Breath: Suffocation

Feelings of suffocation are usually caused by blockage of the airways, either caused by a physical problem such as piece of food, allergic reactions or Epiglottitis. It is also possible that a Heart Attack might have similar symptoms. This is a serious symptom and medical help should be sought immediately. The Heimlich manoeuvre may be needed to dislodge a piece of food or other item from the windpipe.

POSSIBLE CONDITIONS
Allergic Reaction, Severe
Angioneurotic Oedema
Bite, Insect
Chest Injury
• Choking
Croup
Diphtheria
Drowning
• Epiglottitis
Heart Failure
Laryngeal Oedema
Laryngitis
Pneumoconiosis
• Pneumothorax
Poisoning
Pulmonary Embolism
• Suffocation
Tracheitis

Breath: Wheezing

Wheezing is most likely to be caused by Asthma, a Foreign Body being in the gullet and blocking or partially blocking the windpipe, or a Chest Infection.

POSSIBLE CONDITIONS
- Asthma
Choking
Hay Fever
Heart Failure
Laryngeal Oedema
Poisoning

Bruising

Discoloration of the skin, caused by damage or injury. In most cases bruises will resolve themselves, although severe and unexplained bruising may indicate a serious problem. Children who are constantly bruised, particularly in places which would not be expected, may be the victims of abuse.

POSSIBLE CONDITIONS
Anaemia
- Disorders of Blood Clotting
Haemophilia
- Injury/trauma
Suffocation
Vitamin C (Ascorbic Acid) Deficiency

Bruising and Bleeding Under the Skin

The most common cause of bruising or bleeding under the skin is non-penetrating injury which results in bruising. It may be the sign of a serious condition.

POSSIBLE CONDITIONS
Adverse Drug Reaction
Anaemia
Bite, Animal
- Bruise
Cushing's Syndrome
- Disorders of Blood Clotting
Haemophilia
Henoch's Purpura
Leukaemia
Meninogococcal Septicaemia
- Senile Purpura
Vitamin C (Ascorbic Acid) Deficiency

Cataract

A sign as well as a condition. Cornea or lens of the eye is white, cloudy or opaque.

POSSIBLE CONDITIONS
Adverse Drug Reaction
- Cataract
Diabetes
Injury to the Eye
Rubella
Trachoma

Chest: Pain and Breathlessness

A combination of symptoms which may indicate a serious or even life-threatening condition, such as a Heart Attack, Pleurisy or Lung Cancer.

POSSIBLE CONDITIONS
Aortic Aneurysm
Aortic Stenosis
- Chest Infection
Heart Attack and Failure

Heart Disease
Lung Abscess
Lung Cancer
Pericarditis
Pleurisy
• Pneumonia
Pneumothorax
• Pulmonary Embolism

Chest: Pain, No Appetite and Weight Loss

Combination of symptoms which often indicates a serious underlying disease.

POSSIBLE CONDITIONS
Cancer of the Stomach
Gall Bladder Infection
Hernia, Hiatus
Lung Cancer
Oesophagitis
• Peptic Ulcer
• Pneumonia
Tuberculosis

Chest: Pain, Sudden Onset

The sudden onset of severe pain, particularly if concentrated in the centre of the chest but radiates into the left arm or jaw, may be the sign of a Heart Attack. Other problems, some milder, some as severe, can also cause sudden chest pain.

POSSIBLE CONDITIONS
Aortic Aneurysm
• Chest Injury
• Heart Attack
Nerve Irritation in Chest

• Oesophagitis
Pancreatitis
• Peptic Ulcer
Pericarditis
• Pleurisy
Pneumothorax
Pulmonary Embolism

Chest: Persistent or Recurrent Pain

Persistent or recurrent pain, which may be severe, but varies in intensity over a prolonged period. This may be mild, but it can also be the indication of serious underlying problems.

POSSIBLE CONDITIONS
Anaemia
• Angina
Aortic Aneurysm
Aortic Stenosis
Chest Infection
• Chest Injury
• Chondritis
Gall Bladder Infection
Gall Stones
Heart Attack and Failure
Heart Disease
Hernia, Hiatus
Lung Abscess
Lung Cancer
• Oesophagitis
• Peptic Ulcer
Pericarditis
Pleurisy
Pneumonia

Cleft Lip or Palate

Birth defect resulting in a cleft lip and palate when tissues have not formed properly.

POSSIBLE CONDITIONS
• Cleft Lip and Palate

Cold: Sensitivity to

Many individuals are more sensitive to the cold than others, and may find that their extremities become cold quickly or even that they get bluish fingers. It may also take them much longer to warm up than others. This is generally just natural variation between individuals, but a few conditions may cause sensitivity to the cold.

POSSIBLE CONDITIONS
• Hypothyroidism
• Raynaud's Phenomenon

Collapse

The individual deteriorates to the point of collapse with crippling weakness, sweating, confusion, weak pulse and pallor. This can occur very suddenly or may take some time. In either case, this is virtually never a trivial collection of symptoms, and medical help should be sought as soon as possible.

POSSIBLE CONDITIONS
Addison's Disease
Adverse Drug Reaction
Alcohol or Narcotics
Atrial Fibrillation or other Abnormal Heart Rhythm
Botulism
Burns
Crohn's Disease

Dehydration
• Faint
Heart Attack
Heat Exhaustion
Heat Stroke
Hypothyroidism
• Low Blood Pressure
Peritonitis
Pneumothorax
Pulmonary Embolism
Septicaemia
Shock
Sick Sinus Syndrome

Collapse: Abdominal Pain

Collapse in any individual is a serious condition, and combined with abdominal pain can indicate a variety of conditions. Also see the sections on Collapse, Fever and Abdominal Pain. Some of the conditions which can cause collapse are listed below.

POSSIBLE CONDITIONS
Botulism
Crohn's Disease
Gall Bladder Infection
• Gastroenteritis
Intestinal Ischaemia
Intestinal Obstruction
Pancreatitis
• Peptic Ulcer
Pregnancy
Ulcerative Colitis

Collapse: Shock or Coma

Serious combination of symptoms and should be treated as a medical emergency. The individual is pale, has clammy skin, weak pulse and a blue tinge because of a lack of oxygen getting to tissues. This then progresses to shock, unconsciousness or coma. See other sections on Collapse and on Coma. Causes of collapse progressing to unconsciousness include severe pain or infection, while others are listed below.

Possible Conditions
Alcohol or Narcotics
Allergic Reaction, Severe
Aortic Aneurysm
• Bleeding/Blood Loss from Stomach, Bowel, Lungs, Kidneys and Bladder
Burns
Coma
• Dehydration
Diabetes
• Heart Attack and Failure
Heart Disease
Septicaemia
Stroke

Colour Blindness

Inability to distinguish between different colours, commonly between green and red. This is usually simply because of natural variation between individuals and will be present from birth, but it may be the sign of a serious problem should it develop later in life.

Possible Conditions
Adverse Drug Reaction
Cataract
• Colour Blindness
Detached Retina
Malnutrition
Poisoning

Coma

Deep unconscious state, when the individual does not respond to stimuli such as pain, speech or movement. Only included are some of the more common causes; many illnesses may lead to coma and death but these will usually already have been diagnosed from other symptoms. Serious infections and metabolic disease can also lead to coma, which are too numerous to list here, but this will not usually be the first symptom.

Possible Conditions
• Alcohol or Narcotics
Aortic Aneurysm
Bleeding
Botulism
Burns
Carbon Monoxide Poisoning
Chest Injury
• Coma
Dehydration
Diabetes
Drowning
• Epilepsy
Head Injury
Heart Attack and Failure
Hepatitis
Hypothermia
Kidney Disease or Failure
Meningitis
Mountain Sickness
Narcolepsy
Poisoning
Rabies
Septicaemia
Shock

• Stroke
• Subarachnoid Haemorrhage
Subdural Haemorrhage
Suffocation

Coma: Collapse or Shock

Serious combination of symptoms and should be treated as a medical emergency. The individual is pale, has clammy skin, weak pulse and a blue tinge because of a lack of oxygen getting to tissues. This then progresses to shock, unconsciousness or coma. See other sections on Collapse and on Coma. Causes of collapse progressing to unconsciousness include severe pain or infection, while others are listed below.

POSSIBLE CONDITIONS
• Alcohol or Narcotics
Allergic Reaction, Severe
Aortic Aneurysm
• Bleeding
Burns
Coma
• Dehydration
Diabetes
• Heart Attack and Failure
Heart Disease
• Septicaemia
Stroke

Confusion and Delirium

Mixture of distress and disorientation, which is not always easy to define, more extreme in the case of delirium. It can occur in any individual, but is most likely in children and elderly people. Triggers may be emotional upheaval or a break in routine, but infections and more serious disease can also provoke confusion.

POSSIBLE CONDITIONS
• Adverse Drug Reaction
• Alcohol or Narcotics
Bronchitis
Chest Injury
Dehydration
• Dementia (worsened by other illness such as infection)
Diabetes
Emphysema
Epilepsy
Fever
Head Injury
Heart Attack and Failure
Heat Stroke
Hepatitis
Hyperventilation
Hypothermia
Hypothyroidism
Kidney Disease or Failure
Measles
Meningitis
Mountain Sickness
Plague
• Pneumonia
Poisoning
Polio
Relapsing Fever
Shock
Sleeping Sickness
Stroke
Subarachnoid Haemorrhage
Subdural Haemorrhage
Typhus Fever
• Urinary Tract Infection

35

Constipation

The frequency and consistency of faeces or motions varies from individual to individual. Constipation is a usually a harder motion than normal, and usually the individual passes motions less frequently than normal. Constipation will usually be only an indication of a diet too low in roughage or fluid, but may be a sign of a serious underlying condition.

POSSIBLE CONDITIONS
• Adverse Drug Reaction
Anal Fissure
Appendicitis
• Constipation
Crohn's Disease
Diuretics
Diverticulitis
Hernia, Inguinal
Hirschsprung's Disease
Hypercalcaemia
Intestinal Obstruction
Irritable Bowel Syndrome
Porphyria
Porphyria Cutanea Tarda
Potassium Deficiency
Pregnancy
Sarcoidosis

Constipation: Abdominal Pain

A sign of inflammatory bowel disease or Irritable Bowel Syndrome. Also consult the sections on Constipation and on Abdominal Pain.

POSSIBLE CONDITIONS
Crohn's Disease
Hypercalcaemia

Intestinal Obstruction
• Irritable Bowel Syndrome
Peritonitis

Constipation: Combined with Diarrhoea

Periods of diarrhoea, followed by periods of constipation, associated with bowel disease.

POSSIBLE CONDITIONS
Adverse Drug Reaction
Cancer of the Colon (rectum)
Coeliac Disease
Crohn's Disease
Diverticulitis
• Irritable Bowel Syndrome
Ulcerative Colitis

Constipation: Swollen Abdomen

Many individuals will suffer from bouts of constipation from time to time, and anyway frequency and consistency of motions varies from person to person. A change in bowel habit may be significant, although this combination of signs may simply be the result of too much refined food, too little fluid or too little roughage. If it persists for a long time, and cannot be related to lifestyle changes, it is possible that this may be an indication of a serious condition.

POSSIBLE CONDITIONS
Adverse Drug Reaction
Cancer of the Colon or Rectum (Bowel)
• Constipation
Diverticulitis
• Flatulence
• Irritable Bowel Syndrome

Convulsions or Fit

Often heralded by an aura or feeling something is about to happen, followed by unconsciousness and twitching movements of the limbs, and possibly urinary incontinence. Usually the individual will regain consciousness although there will be a period of drowsiness and confusion. It may be a sign of serious underlying disease, and medical help should be sought if there is not a history of Epilepsy.

POSSIBLE CONDITIONS
•Alcohol or Narcotics
Brain Abscess
•Epilepsy
Fever
Hepatitis
Huntington's Chorea
Hydrocephalus
Kidney Disease or Failure
Meningitis
Pregnancy
Rabies
Sleeping Sickness
Stroke
Subarachnoid Haemorrhage
Subdural Haemorrhage
Toxoplasmosis

Cough: Bloody Phlegm

A cough with the production of phlegm, which may be yellow or green in colour, but is also streaked or contains blood. This is most usually the result of a serious problem such as severe Chest Infections, Pneumonia or Lung Cancer. Medical help should be sought as soon as possible.

POSSIBLE CONDITIONS
•Bleeding Disorder
Bronchiectasis
•Chest Infection
Heart Disease
Lung Cancer
Mitral Valve Disease
•Pneumonia
Q Fever
Tuberculosis

Cough: Bloody Phlegm and Chest Pain

Chest pain combined with a cough, which also produces phlegm, which may be yellow or green in colour, but is also streaked or contains blood. This is most usually the result of a serious problem such as severe and prolonged Chest Infections, Pneumonia or Lung Cancer. Medical help should be sought as soon as possible.

POSSIBLE CONDITIONS
•Chest Infection
Chest Injury
•Pneumonia
Pulmonary Embolism
Q Fever

Cough: Breathlessness

A relatively common combination of symptoms, and is usually caused by Chest Infections or problems. This may vary from the relatively mild in a fit and otherwise healthy individual to serious and life-threatening disease in the elderly or those with a pre-existing heart or respiratory condition.

POSSIBLE CONDITIONS
Aspergillosis
Bronchiectasis
• Bronchitis
• Chest Infection
Chest Injury
Emphysema
Lung Cancer
Pneumonia
Tuberculosis
Whooping Cough

Cough: Combined with Halitosis

Bad or foul-smelling breath is usually caused either by the consumption of spiced foods or alcohol, indigestion or by problems with teeth or gums. When combined with a persistent cough, however, it may be a sign of Bronchitis, cancer or other lung problems.

POSSIBLE CONDITIONS
• Bronchiectasis
• Bronchitis
Cystic Fibrosis
Hay Fever
Lung Abscess
Lung Cancer
Rhinitis
• Tracheitis
Tuberculosis

Cough: Dry

A dry or unproductive cough (one without the production of phlegm) is most usually caused by environmental factors (such as a dry or dusty atmosphere) or Chest Infections. Unusually it is a

sign of serious underlying problems.

POSSIBLE CONDITIONS
Adenoids
Adverse Drug Reaction
Allergic Alveolitis
• Asthma
Cancer of the Larynx
Cold, Common
Croup
Hay Fever
Laryngitis
Lung Cancer
Pneumoconiosis
Sinusitis
• Tracheitis
Whooping Cough

Cough: Phlegm

A cough with the production of phlegm, which may be yellow or green in colour. This is most usually the result of infections such as Colds or Chest Infections, although it may be a sign of more serious illness, particularly if it lasts for a long time and is very productive.

POSSIBLE CONDITIONS
AIDS
Bronchiectasis
• Bronchitis
• Chest Infection
Choking
Cold, Common
Cystic Fibrosis
Emphysema
Flu
Lung Abscess

Pneumonia
Q Fever
Tuberculosis
Whooping Cough

Deafness and Hearing Problems (Adults)

Deafness may be from birth or acquired during life, and it is normal for older individuals to have some degree of hearing impairment. Many conditions can make an individual temporarily deaf or deafer, even Ear Wax, but it may also be a sign of a serious condition.

POSSIBLE CONDITIONS
Acoustic Neuroma
Adverse Drug Reaction
Artery Disease
Brittle Bone Disease
Cholesteamota
• Ear Wax
Head Injury
Inner Ear Infection
• Loud Noises (exposure)
Meniere's Disease
Meningitis
Mumps
• Otosclerosis
Paget's Disease
• Presbyacusis
Rubella
Syphilis
Turner's Syndrome

Deafness and Hearing Problems (Children)

Deafness may be from birth or acquired during early life. Many conditions can make an individual temporarily deaf or deafer, even Ear Wax, but it may also be a sign of a serious condition.

POSSIBLE CONDITIONS
Adverse Drug Reaction
Brittle Bone Disease
• Ear Wax
Hypothyroidism
• Inner Ear Infection
Meningitis
Mumps
Rubella
Turner's Syndrome

Dehydration: Combined with Excessive Thirst

This combination of symptoms tends to suggest any condition which more fluid is lost from the body than replaced, such as vomiting, diarrhoea, sweating including fevers, blood loss and haemorrhaging, and even from breathing from asthma. Symptoms of dehydration include thirst, urine being dark and smelly, dry skin, and even confusion and collapse. Babies and elderly people can become dehydrated very quickly, and extra care should be taken if suspected in these groups.

POSSIBLE CONDITIONS
Asthma
Bleeding
• Diabetes Mellitus
Diabetes Insipidus
• Diuretics
Exercise
• Gastroenteritis

Heat Exhaustion
Heat Stroke
• Hypercalcaemia
Kidney Disease or Failure
Rabies
Sarcoidosis

Delirium and Confusion

Mixture of distress and disorientation, which is not always easy to define, more extreme in the case of delirium. It can occur in any individual, but is most likely in children and elderly people. Triggers may be emotional upheaval or a break in routine, but infections and more serious disease can also provoke confusion.

POSSIBLE CONDITIONS
• Alcohol or Narcotics
Bronchitis
• Chest Infection
Chest Injury
Dehydration
Dementia
Diabetes
Emphysema
Epilepsy
Fever
Head Injury
Heart Attack and Failure
Heat Stroke
Hepatitis
Hyperventilation
Hypothermia
Hypothyroidism
Kidney Disease or Failure
Measles

Meningitis
Mountain Sickness
Plague
• Pneumonia
Poisoning
Polio
Relapsing Fever
Shock
Sleeping Sickness
Stroke
Subarachnoid Haemorrhage
Subdural Haemorrhage
Typhus Fever
• Urinary Tract Infection

Delusions

Belief or belief systems which are disturbing, disruptive or damaging to the individual or those around them.

POSSIBLE CONDITIONS
• Adverse Drug Reaction
• Dementia
Depression and Manic Depression
Schizophrenia

Dementia

Progressive but slow memory loss and disintegration of the mind, often accompanied with change in personality, depression, anxiety and a loss of self. Memories of early events such as childhood are often preserved, while day to day events are not remembered.

POSSIBLE CONDITIONS
Adverse Drug Reaction

AIDS
Alcohol or Narcotics
•Alzheimer's Disease
Brain Tumours
•Dementia
Head Injury
Hepatitis
Huntington's Chorea
Hydrocephalus
Hypothyroidism
Stroke
Syphilis
Vitamin B1 (Thiamine) Deficiency
Vitamin B12 (Cyanocobalamin) Deficiency
Vitamin B3 (Niacin) deficiency

Depression

A symptom as well as a condition. More information about Depression and Manic Depression is in the relevant section in the Conditions part of this book.

POSSIBLE CONDITIONS
Adverse Drug Reaction
Dementia
•Depression and Manic Depression
Hypercalcaemia
Hypothyroidism
Parkinson's Disease
•Post-Viral Syndrome
Pregnancy
Schizophrenia

Diarrhoea

The frequency and consistency of faeces or motions varies from individual to individual. Diarrhoea is a looser motion than normal, and usually the individual passes motions more frequently than normal. Diarrhoea may be watery; brown, green, yellow or black; streaked with blood; containing mucus or slimy. Diarrhoea is usually an indication of minor problems such as an upset stomach. If bowel habit does not return back to normal quite quickly, or if faeces are black or very pale, it may be a sign of serious underlying disease.

POSSIBLE CONDITIONS
•Adverse Drug Reaction
Addison's Disease
AIDS
Alcohol or Narcotics
Bilharzia
Botulism
Cancer of the Colon or Rectum (Bowel)
Carcinoid Syndrome
Cholera
Coeliac Disease
Crohn's Disease
Cystic Fibrosis
Diverticulitis
Dysentery
•Gastroenteritis
Henoch's Purpura
Hepatitis
Hookworms (human)
Hyperthyroidism
Intestinal Ischaemia
Intussusception
•Irritable Bowel Syndrome
Jejunal Diverticulitis
Kwashiorkor
•Laxatives
Meckel's Diverticulum
Menstruation

Pancreatitis
Phaeochromocytoma
Post-Gastrectomy Syndrome
Potassium Deficiency
Sprue
Typhoid Fever
Ulcerative Colitis
Vitamin B3 (Niacin) deficiency

Diarrhoea: Abdominal Pain

Usually an indication of minor food poisoning or Gastroenteritis, but may be a sign of serious disease.

POSSIBLE CONDITIONS
Botulism
Cancer of the Colon or Rectum (Bowel)
Carcinoid Syndrome
Cholera
Crohn's Disease
Dysentery
• Gastroenteritis
Henoch's Purpura
Intestinal Ischaemia
• Irritable Bowel Syndrome
Jejunal Diverticulitis
Pancreatitis
Phaeochromocytoma
Post-Gastrectomy Syndrome
Post-Viral Syndrome
Typhoid Fever
Ulcerative Colitis

Diarrhoea: Combined with Constipation

Periods of diarrhoea, followed by periods of constipation, associated with bowel disease.

POSSIBLE CONDITIONS
Cancer of the Colon (rectum)
Crohn's Disease
Diverticulitis
• Irritable Bowel Syndrome

Diarrhoea: Swollen Abdomen

Most individuals will suffer from bouts of diarrhoea from time to time, and the frequency and consistency of motions varies from person to person. A change in bowel habit may be significant, although often this is simply the result of too much rich food, alcohol, fruit or roughage, nerves, or minor food poisoning. If it persists for a long time, and cannot be related to lifestyle changes, it is possible that this may be an indication of serious conditions.

POSSIBLE CONDITIONS
Cancer of the Colon or Rectum (Bowel)
• Constipation
Crohn's Disease
Diverticulitis
Flatulence
• Gastroenteritis
• Irritable Bowel Syndrome
• Laxatives
Ulcerative Colitis

Discharge: Ear

Discharge comes from the ear, usually as a result of infection. The discharge may be clear, yellow or green. Medical help should be sought if this persists, and it is highly coloured or blood stained.

POSSIBLE CONDITIONS
Cancer of the Ear
Cholesteamota
• Ear Infection
Ear Polyp
Head Injury
Inner Ear Infection
Mastoiditis
• Otitis Externa
Ruptured Eardrum

Discharge: Eye

Eye discharges clear fluid or pus, usually as a result of allergies or infections.

POSSIBLE CONDITIONS
Behcet's Syndrome
Blocked Tear Duct
• Conjunctivitis
Dacryocystitis
Ectropion
Gonorrhoea
Hay Fever
Keratitis
Reddened Eyes
Reiter's Disease
Stye

Discharge: Nipple

Discharge from the nipple. This may be caused by several conditions, and medical help should be sought unless the woman is pregnant or has a young baby. A discharge of milk from the breast is possible before giving birth.

POSSIBLE CONDITIONS
Breast Abscess
Cancer of Ducts in the Breast
Cancer of the Breast
Duct Ectasia
Duct Papilloma
Excess of Prolactin
• Fibrocystic Disease of the Breast
Paget's Disease of the Nipple
• Pregnancy

Discharge: Penis

It is not normal for the penis to have a discharge other than sperm, seminal fluid or urine. Residual fluid can occur some time after sex or ejaculation, and it is possible for a man to have some seminal fluid without ejaculating. Any persistent clear or coloured discharge, however, not occurring because of sexual activity is probably from a sexually transmitted disease.

POSSIBLE CONDITIONS
Balanitis
Cancer of the Penis
Chlamydia
Epididymitis
Gonorrhoea
• Non-Specific Urethritis
Trichomonas
Urinary Tract Infection

Discharge: Vagina

Discharge from the vagina, beyond that which would be expected from a normal menstrual cycle. The consistency and odour of discharge does vary. If discharge is particularly profuse, coloured or smells

SYMPTOMS SIGNS AND CONDITIONS

unpleasant, medical help should be sought.

POSSIBLE CONDITIONS
Cancer of the Cervix
Cancer of the Colon or Rectum (Bowel)
Cancer of the Ovaries
Cancer of the Vagina
Cancer of the Womb
Candidiasis
Cervical Polyp
Chlamydia
Erosion of the Cervix
Foreign Body in Vagina
Gardnerella
Gonorrhoea
Inflammation of the Vagina
Menopause
• Menstruation (normal variation through cycle)
Non-Specific Urethritis
Pelvic Inflammatory Disease
Salpingitis
Sexual Abuse
Trichomonas
Womb Prolapse

Dizziness: No Vertigo

This is hard to define. A feeling of dizziness or giddiness, but during which the world does not spin. Often as important is when it happens, is in what circumstances, and how the individual is before and after. Some possible causes are listed, but this remains quite an elusive symptom. In most cases, there will be no obvious cause and no underlying disease.

POSSIBLE CONDITIONS
• Anaemia

Anxiety
Bronchitis
Constrictive Pericarditis
Diabetes
Emphysema
Heart Attack and Failure
Heart Disease
Heat Exhaustion
Heat Stroke
Hyperventilation
• Low Blood Pressure
Low Blood Sugar
Pernicious Anaemia
Polycythaemia
Sick Sinus Syndrome
Temporal Lobe Epilepsy
Travel Sickness

Dizziness: Vertigo

Feeling of dizziness and giddiness with a spinning or falling sensation when the head is turned. Most usually a problem with the ear.

POSSIBLE CONDITIONS
Botulism
Cerebellar Disease
Inner Ear Infection
• Meniere's Disease
Travel Sickness
• Vertebrobasilar Insufficiency
Vestibulitis

Double Vision

Double vision is usually a serious sign, and should not be ignored. The most common cause will be a blow or injury to the head, but it may also be an indication of nerve or neurological problems or infection.

POSSIBLE CONDITIONS
Botulism
Cancer of the Eye
Head Injury
• Hyperthyroidism
Intracranial Aneurysm
Meningitis
Multiple Sclerosis
Myasthenia Gravis
• Stroke
• Vasculitis including temporal arteritis

Drowsiness

Feelings of tiredness and lethargy, beyond what would normally be expected from simple lack of sleep. It can be caused by sleeping pills, and if a problem the dose may need adjusted. It may also herald the onset of an infection, particularly viral. This may be an important symptom in children.

POSSIBLE CONDITIONS
• Alcohol or Narcotics
Brain Abscess
Brain Tumours
Encephalitis
Fever
• Head Injury
Hypercalcaemia
Hypothalmic Disease
Hypothyrodism
Meningitis
Narcolepsy
Sleep Apnoea Syndrome
Sleeping Sickness

Stroke
Subdural Haemotoma
Temporal Lobe Epilepsy

Dyspepsia, Indigestion or Heartburn

A range of symptoms associated with the upper part of the gastrointestinal tract, such as burning pain in the gullet, nausea, belching, flatulence and acid from the stomach being regurgitated into the mouth. If there are only occasional bouts which can be linked to eating certain foods or drinking too much alcohol, then this is nothing to worry about. If pain or discomfort are experienced often or persistently, it may be the sign of a serious underlying condition.

POSSIBLE CONDITIONS
Achalasia
Cancer of the Oesophagus
Cancer of the Stomach
Dyspepsia, Non-Ulcer
Gall Stones
Gastritis
Gastroenteritis
• Hernia, Hiatus
• Oesophagitis
Pancreatitis
• Peptic Ulcer
Pregnancy

Ear: Bleeding from

Blood comes from the ear. This may be caused by infections or injury to the ear. If it is prolonged or the result of severe trauma, medical help should be sought.

POSSIBLE CONDITIONS
Boil
Cancer of the Ear
• Ear Infection
Ear Polyp
• Head Injury
Ruptured Eardrum

Ear: Boil or Lump in

Lump or boil develops in the ear.
POSSIBLE CONDITIONS
• Boil
Ear Polyp
Herpes Simplex
Ramsay-Hunt Syndrome

Ear: Boil or Lumps on

Lump or boil develops on the outside structure of the ear. Most usually this will be caused by Warts or Boils, but occasionally it may be a sign of serious illness. A very misshapen ear will often have been caused by repeated trauma.

POSSIBLE CONDITIONS
Auricular Appendage
• Boil
Cancer of the Skin
Cauliflower Ear
Gout
Warts

Ear: Deafness and Hearing Problems, Adults

Deafness may be from birth or acquired during life, and it is normal for older individuals to have some degree of hearing impairment. Many conditions can make an individual temporarily deaf or deafer, even Ear Wax, but it may also be a sign of a serious condition.

POSSIBLE CONDITIONS
Acoustic Neuroma
Adverse Drug Reaction
Artery Disease
Brittle Bone Disease
Cholesteamota
• Ear Wax
Head Injury
Inner Ear Infection
• Loud Noises
Meniere's Disease
Meningitis
Mumps
• Otosclerosis
Paget's Disease
• Presbyacusis
Rubella
Syphilis
Turner's Syndrome

Ear: Deafness and Hearing Problems, Children

Deafness may be from birth or acquired during early life. Many conditions can make an individual temporarily deaf or deafer, even Ear Wax, but it may also be a sign of a serious condition.

POSSIBLE CONDITIONS
Adverse Drug Reaction
Brittle Bone Disease
• Ear Wax
Hypothyroidism

• Inner Ear Infection
Meningitis
Mumps
Rubella
Turner's Syndrome

Ear: Discharge From

Discharge comes from the ear, usually as a result of infection. The discharge may be clear, yellow or green. Medical help should be sought if this persists, and it is highly coloured or blood stained.

POSSIBLE CONDITIONS
Cancer of the Ear
Cholesteamota
• Ear Infection
Ear Polyp
Head Injury
Inner Ear Infection
Mastoiditis
• Otitis Externa
Ruptured Eardrum

Ear: Giddiness and Vertigo

The ears are also involved with balance and the concept of position, and consequently infections and other problems with the ear will affect balance as well as hearing.

POSSIBLE CONDITIONS
Acoustic Neuroma
Cholesteamota
Cold, Common
• Ear Wax
• Inner Ear Infection
• Meniere's Disease

Otosclerosis
• Vestibulitis

Ear: Itching

Ear feels extremely itchy. Most usually this will resolve in a short time, but it may be the sign of an infection or other condition.

POSSIBLE CONDITIONS
• Eczema
• Otitis Externa

Ear: Pain from and Earache

Earache and pain, experienced in or around the ear. This may be caused by conditions ranging from relatively mild to very severe, and pain may be referred from the teeth or mouth. Severe and prolonged pain should prompt a visit to the doctor or dentist.

POSSIBLE CONDITIONS
• Boil
Cancer of the Ear
Cancer of the Mouth
Cold, Common
Dental Infections
• Ear Infection
Ear Wax
Eustachian Catarrh
Inner Ear Infection
Mastoiditis
Perichondritis
Ramsay-Hunt Syndrome
Rodent Ulcer
Teething Pain
Tonsillitis

Tooth Decay and Abscess
Trigeminal Neuralgia

Ear: Pressure in

Pressure builds with in the ear, and it may feel as it is completely 'full'. This may simply be accumulation of ear wax, but may also be a sign of infection.

POSSIBLE CONDITIONS
- Ear Infection
- Ear Wax
Eustachian Catarrh
Hay Fever
Inner Ear Infection
Otitis Externa

Ear: Ringing, Crackling or Other Noises

Noises are heard in the ear, such as ringing, singing or crackling. If the individual has been exposed to very loud noises, the ears may ring afterwards for a few days, but this will usually resolve. Long-term exposure to loud noises may cause hearing damage. This sign can also be caused by infections and more serious conditions.

POSSIBLE CONDITIONS
Acoustic Neuroma
Adverse Drug Reaction
Anaemia
Artery Disease
- Ear Wax
Eustachian Catarrh
Heart Attack and Failure
Heart Disease
Inner Ear Infection

- Loud Noise Exposure
- Meniere's Disease
Mitral Valve Disease
Otosclerosis
Paget's Disease
Presbyacusis

Ear: Tenderness Behind

Area behind the ear feels very tender to the touch, usually an indication of an infection. Mastoiditis, although unusual, should be excluded should the tenderness last.

POSSIBLE CONDITIONS
- Ear Infection
- Mastoiditis

Earache

Earache and pain, experienced in or around the ear. This may be caused by conditions ranging from relatively mild to very severe, and pain may be referred from the teeth or mouth. Severe and prolonged pain should prompt a visit to the doctor or dentist.

POSSIBLE CONDITIONS
- Boil
Cancer of the Ear
Cancer of the Mouth
Cold, Common
Dental Infections
- Ear Infection
Ear Wax
Eustachian Catarrh
Inner Ear Infection
Mastoiditis

Perichondritis
Ramsay-Hunt Syndrome
Rodent Ulcer
Teething Pain
Tonsillitis
Tooth Decay and Abscess
Trigeminal Neuralgia

Elbow: Pain

Pain is experienced in or around the elbow. This will usually be caused either by an injury, arthritis or fracture, or damage to nerves.

POSSIBLE CONDITIONS
• Arthritis
Broken Lower Arm Bones (Radius, Ulna and wrist)
Broken Upper Arm Bone (Humerus)
Bursitis
Gout
• Injury
Osteoarthritis
Rheumatoid Arthritis
• Tennis Elbow
Ulnar Nerve

Emotional Instability and Irritability

Varies greatly from individual to individual, and many people can be very highly strung without suffering from any underlying disease. More importantly are changes in an individual, such as more pronounced irritability and mood swings, which are out of character.

POSSIBLE CONDITIONS
Adverse Drug Reaction
Alcohol or Narcotics

• Anxiety
Brain Tumours
Dementia
Depression and Manic Depression
Head Injury
Meningitis
• Menopause
Polio
• Premenstrual Tension
Rabies
Schizophrenia
Syphilis
Vitamin B12 (Cyanocobalamin) Deficiency

Exhaustion: Breathlessness

A sign, particularly if it is persistent and prolonged, which may indicate serious underlying illness, such as Heart Failure or Anaemia.

POSSIBLE CONDITIONS
• Anaemia
Aortic Stenosis
• Bronchitis
Cardiomyopathy
• Chest Infection
Diabetes
• Emphysema
Guillain-Barre Syndrome
• Heart Failure
Heart Disease
Kidney Disease or Failure
Pneumonia
Post-Viral Syndrome
Sickle Cell Anaemia

Eye: Blind Spot

A blind spot or area becomes apparent in the field of vision. This blind spot stays in the same position and does not move across the field of vision. The cause is usually damage to the eye or a blow or trauma to the head, but it may be an indication of problems with the nerves or brain. If a blind spot or reduced field of vision is present, medical help should be sought immediately.

POSSIBLE CONDITIONS
Carotid Aneurysm
Choroiditis
Diabetes
Head Injury
Injury to the Eye
• Macular Degeneration
Pituitary Tumour
Poisoning
Stroke
Vitreous Haemorrhage

Eye: Blindness, Colour

Inability to distinguish between different colours, commonly between green and red. This is usually simply because of natural variation between individuals and will be present from birth, but it may be the sign of a serious problem should it develop later in life.

POSSIBLE CONDITIONS
Adverse Drug Reaction
Cataract
• Colour Blindness
Detached Retina
Malnutrition

Poisoning

Eye: Blindness, Gradual Onset

Blindness develops over some time, so slowly that the individual may not be aware it has happened until the blindness is advanced. This is a serious sign, and medical help should be sought.

POSSIBLE CONDITIONS
• Cataract
Choroiditis
Diabetes
Glaucoma
High Blood Pressure
• Macular Degeneration
Paget's Disease
Retinitis Pigmentosa
Trachoma

Eye: Blindness, Night

Most individuals see much better in bright daylight than at night. Night blindness or greatly impaired vision in darker conditions will be exacerbated if the individual has poor eyesight. It may also be an indication of a lack of Vitamin A.

POSSIBLE CONDITIONS
Mascular Degeneration
Malnutrition
• Poor Eyesight
Retinitis Pigmentosa
• Vitamin A Deficiency

Eye: Blindness, Sudden

Blindness has a sudden onset. This is most usually an indication of serious underlying disease, either with the eye itself or the structures and nerves concerned with vision. It is possible that this may be caused by a Migraine, but if this is the case it should resolve fairly quickly. If Migraine is not suspected, medical help should be sought immediately.

POSSIBLE CONDITIONS
Central Retinal Artery Blockage
Central Retinal Vein Blockage
• Detached Retina
Diabetes
Filariasis
Glaucoma
Head Injury
Hysteria
Methyl Alcohol
Migraine
Optic Neuritis
Poisoning
Stroke
Syphilis
• Temporal Arteritis
• Vitreous Haemorrhage

Eye: Blurred Vision

Vision becomes blurred, meaning that it is difficult or impossible to focus. The most common causes are poor eyesight (a visit to an optician is advisable), focusing for long periods on objects such as a computer screen, and excess alcohol consumption or drugs. Individuals who have problems with eyesight may find these are worse at night or when they are tired. This sign may also more unusually be an indication of a serious problem.

POSSIBLE CONDITIONS
Adverse Drug Reaction

Alcohol or Narcotics
Cataract
Detached Retina
Diabetes
Iritis
Macular Degeneration
• Poor Eyesight

Eye: Cataract

A sign as well as a condition. Cornea or lens of the eye is white, cloudy or opaque.

POSSIBLE CONDITIONS
• Adverse Drug Reaction (typically steroids)
• Cataract
Diabetes
Injury to the Eye
Rubella
Trachoma

Eye: Coloured Patches On

Coloured or discoloured patches can develop on the eyeball or eye, including Moles and Warts.

POSSIBLE CONDITIONS
Brittle Bone Disease
Cancer of the Skin
Mole
Pinquecula
• Pterygium
Warts

Eye: Discharge From

Eye discharges clear fluid or pus, usually as a result of allergies or infections.

POSSIBLE CONDITIONS
Behcet's Syndrome
Blocked Tear Duct
• Conjunctivitis
Dacryocystitis
Ectropion
Gonorrhoea
Hay Fever
Keratitis
Reddened Eyes
Reiter's Disease
Stye

Eye: Double Vision

Double vision is usually a serious sign, and should not be ignored. The most common cause will be a blow or injury to the head, but it may also be an indication of nerve or neurological problems or infection.

POSSIBLE CONDITIONS
Botulism
Cancer of the Eye
Head Injury
• Hyperthyroidism
Meningitis
Multiple Sclerosis
Myasthenia Gravis
• Stroke
Temporal Arteritis
Vasculitis eg lupus

Eye: Drooping Eyelid

The eyelid droops, often an indication of Bell's Palsy, or nerve or neurological damage or problems.

POSSIBLE CONDITIONS
Bell's Palsy
Brain Tumours
Ectropion
• Horner's Syndrome
Injury to Eye
• Myasthenia Gravis
Nerve Palsies of the Eye
Syphilis
• Third Nerve Palsy

Eye: Dry

Eyes feel dry and possibly itchy. The most common cause is being in a dry atmosphere, such as an office with many computers.

POSSIBLE CONDITIONS
• Sjogren's Syndrome

Eye: Enlarged or Protruding Eyeball

Eyeballs noticeably protrude from the sockets, although some individuals have naturally bulging eyes. This may also be the sign of several conditions.

POSSIBLE CONDITIONS
Cancer of the Eye
• Hyperthyroidism
Tumour behind the Eye

Eye: Feeling Something is in Eye

There is a distinct feeling that something, such as a foreign body, is in the eye. This is, of course, often the case, and similar feelings can be caused by Styes, Hay Fever and ingrown eyelashes. If there is a foreign body stuck in the eye, great care must be taken in trying to remove it. If in doubt seek medical help.

POSSIBLE CONDITIONS
• Conjunctivitis
Corneal Ulcer
Dermatitis
• Foreign Body in Eye
Hay Fever
Ingrown Eyelash
Reddened Eyes
Stye

Eye: Flashing Lights

The individual experiences flashing lights before their eyes. Common causes are rising too quickly from sitting, a blow or injury to the head or eye, or the aura which heralds a Migraine.

POSSIBLE CONDITIONS
Detached Retina
Flashing Lights
Head Injury
Injury to the Eye
• Migraine
Temporal Lobe Epilepsy

Eye: Floaters

Floaters in the eye are brown or black patches or lines in the field of vision. These move across the vision as the individual looks in different directions or focuses on different objects. They may have no serious cause, although poor eyesight and damage to the eye can both cause floaters. This sign may also be an indication of serious damage to the eye, such as a Detached Retina. If the individual experiences a spot affecting the vision which retains the same position, then this is probably a 'Blind Spot': see the relevant section.

POSSIBLE CONDITIONS
Detached Retina
• Floaters
Injury to the Eye
Poor Eyesight
Vitreous Haemorrhage

Eye: Haloes Around Lights

When the individual looks at lights, there appear to be haloes around them. This may be a result of poor eyesight, but can also be caused by Cataracts or Glaucoma. These are both serious problems.

POSSIBLE CONDITIONS
• Adverse Drug Reaction
• Cataract
• Glaucoma
Poor Eyesight

Eye: Irregular Pupil

Pupils of the eyes are irregularly shaped. This is an unusual sign, and is an indication of a serious underlying condition.

POSSIBLE CONDITIONS
Brain Tumours
• Injury to Eye (or previous surgery)
Iritis
Multiple Sclerosis
Syphilis

Eye: Itchy or Inflamed Eyelid

The eyelid(s) become itchy and inflamed, usually caused by skin problems, bites or infestations.

POSSIBLE CONDITIONS
Bite, Insect
• Blepharitis
• Dermatitis
Lice
Reddened Eyes
Trachoma

Eye: Lens or Cornea is Cloudy

Cornea or lens of the eye is white, cloudy or opaque, often caused by Cataracts.

POSSIBLE CONDITIONS
Blindness
Cancer of the Eye
• Cataract
Glaucoma
Gonorrhoea
Injury to the Eye
Syphilis
Trachoma
Vitamin A Deficiency

Eye: Lump on Eyelid

Various types of lumps can develop on the eyelid. The most common are Styes or Warts, but there may be more serious problems.

POSSIBLE CONDITIONS
Dacryocystitis
Infected Meibomian Cyst
Rodent Ulcer

• Stye
Warts

Eye: Mild Pain

Mild pain in the eye is not uncommon, and may have innocent causes, such as rubbing the eye too much or being in a very dry atmosphere. Flu, Colds, infections or feverish illness will also make the eyes sore. This may also be the sign of serious illness.

POSSIBLE CONDITIONS
Cancer of the Eye
Cold, Common
• Conjunctivitis
Dacryocystitis
Eye Strain
Fever
Flu
Glaucoma
Iritis
Optic Neuritis
Sinusitis

Eye: More Severe Pain

Severe pain in the eye or eyes should not be ignored as it may be the sign of a serious problem. A foreign body in or injury to the eye can cause pain, and there are also several conditions causing the same sign, including Glaucoma and Iritis.

POSSIBLE CONDITIONS
• Conjunctivitis
• Corneal Ulcer
Foreign Body in Eye
Glaucoma
• Injury to the Eye

• Iritis
Multiple Sclerosis
Retrobulbar Neuritis
Shingles

Eye: Red and Pain

Eye (or eyes) become red and painful, the most common cause being Conjunctivitis. It may be a sign of serious eye problems.

POSSIBLE CONDITIONS
• Conjunctivitis
• Glaucoma
Infected Meibomian Cyst
• Iritis
Keratitis
Rubella
• Shingles

Eye: Reddened but No Pain

The eyes becomes red but there is no pain, usually caused by an allergic reaction such as Hay Fever, soap or shampoo getting in eyes, or by Conjunctivitis. Unusually this is a sign of serious disease.

POSSIBLE CONDITIONS
Conjunctivitis
Fever
• Hay Fever
Measles
Meningitis
Reddened Eyes
Rubella
• Subconjuctival Haemorrhage
Typhus Fever

Weil's Disease

Eye: Ring Around Cornea

Some conditions can cause a coloured or noticeable ring to develop around the cornea of the eye.
POSSIBLE CONDITIONS
• Arcus Senilis
Hepatolentricular Degeneration
Iron Ring

Eye: Sensitive to Light

Normal reaction of the pupil of the eye is to constrict in bright light. Going from a dark environment to a very bright one may hurt the eyes until they adjust, but this should be short term. Many infections make the eye especially sensitive to light, including Meningitis, as can injury to and infections of the eye.

POSSIBLE CONDITIONS
Albinism
Conjunctivitis
Corneal Ulcer
Dermatitis
Injury to the Eye
Iritis
Keratitis
Measles
Meningitis
• Migraine
Polio
Reddened Eyes
Subarachnoid Haemorrhage

Eye: Skin Changes Around

The colour or texture of the skin changes in or around

the eye, usually caused by bruising or Dermatitis.

POSSIBLE CONDITIONS
• Black Eye
Dermatitis
Rodent Ulcer
• Xanthomata

Eye: Squint

Eyes appear to look in different directions. Most usually this will be found in children due to natural variation between individuals. It should be corrected, if possible, because it can lead to problems with sight if left untreated. It may also be a sign of serious underlying disease.

POSSIBLE CONDITIONS
Cancer of the Eye
Nerve Palsies of the Eye
• Squint

Eye: Swollen Eyelid

Eyelid may become red and swollen. The most common causes are Styes or skin inflammation, but there may be more serious problems.

POSSIBLE CONDITIONS
• Blepharitis
Dermatitis
Hypothyroidism
Nephrotic Syndrome
Orbital Cellulitis
Reddened Eyes
• Stye

Eye: Tunnel Vision

Field of vision becomes narrower, and seems as if the individual is looking down a tunnel. If the field of vision becomes reduced, this is an indication of a serious problem with the eye or the structures in the brain concerned with vision. Medical help should be sought immediately.

POSSIBLE CONDITIONS
Brain Tumours
Carotid Aneurysm
• Glaucoma
Hypothalmic Disease
Retinitis Pigmentosa
Stroke
Syphilis

Eye: Twitching Movements

The eyes twitch and dart about, most usually found in blind individuals or those with poor eyesight. It may also be a sign of serious disease.

POSSIBLE CONDITIONS
Alcohol or Narcotics
Blindness
Brain Tumours
Cerebellar Disease – including Stroke
Multiple Sclerosis
• Nystagmus
Poor Eyesight
Vestibulitis
Vitamin B1 (Thiamine) Deficiency

Eye: Very Large Pupil

Size of the pupil of the eye varies with the intensity of light, so that in bright light it is very small, in dark conditions it is much larger to let in as much light as possible. Large pupils may also be the sign of several conditions.

POSSIBLE CONDITIONS
Adie's Pupil
•Adverse Drug Reaction
Anxiety
Blindness
Botulism
Coma
Horner's Syndrome
Injury to the Eye
Nerve Palsies of the Eye
Stroke
Third Nerve Palsy

Eye: Very Small Pupil

Size of the pupil of the eye varies with the intensity of light, so that in bright light it is very small, in dark conditions it is much larger to let in as much light as possible. Small pupils may also be the sign of several conditions.

POSSIBLE CONDITIONS
•Adverse Drug Reaction
Brain Tumours
•Horner's Syndrome
Iritis
Longsightedness
Lung Abscess
Lung Cancer
Multiple Sclerosis

Eye: Vision Distorted

Vision is distorted and fractured. This will usually be

because of problems with the retina of the eye, but certain drugs can also cause this sign.

POSSIBLE CONDITIONS
Alcohol or Narcotics
Detached Retina
•Mascular Degeneration

Face: Blisters or Ulcers

Blisters or ulcers, either singly or in groups can develop on the face. These are usually caused by conditions such as Herpes (Cold Sore), Dermatitis, Impetigo or Shingles.

POSSIBLE CONDITIONS
•Dermatitis
Erythema Multiforme
Impetigo
Pemphigus Vulgaris
Rodent Ulcer
•Shingles

Face: Expressionless

Most individuals reflect their mood in their facial expression. An expressionless or emotionless face, however, can be caused by conditions such as Parkinson's Disease, Depression and neurological damage.

POSSIBLE CONDITIONS
Adverse Drug Reaction
•Depression and Manic Depression
Hepatolentricular Degeneration
•Parkinson's Disease
Scleroderma

Face: Grinning

Involuntary grinning, caused by spasms of the face muscles, is a significant symptom of Tetanus (Lock Jaw).

POSSIBLE CONDITIONS
Tetanus

Face: Nodules or Bumps

Nodules or bumps develop on the face, which may be caused by Gout or very rarely Leprosy.

POSSIBLE CONDITIONS
• Acne
Gout
Leprosy
Sarcoma

Face: Pain

Facial pain may be an indication of many conditions, including dental problems, pain referred to the face from other parts of the body, nerve problems or even cancer.

POSSIBLE CONDITIONS
Bell's Palsy
Cancer of the Mouth
Cancer of the Nose
• Dental Infections
Migraine
Paget's Disease
Post-Herpetic Neuralgia
Sinusitis
Temporal Arteritis
• Tooth Decay and Abscess
• Trigeminal Neuralgia

Face: Part Paralysed

Part of face is paralysed and cannot be moved normally. Causes can range from the relatively mild to the severe.

POSSIBLE CONDITIONS
• Bell's Palsy
Brain Tumours
Cancer of the Ear
Guillain-Barre Syndrome
Motor Neurone Disease
Polio
• Stroke

Face: Reddened or Flushed

The most common causes for a face which looks red or flushed are embarrassment, consuming alcohol and being hot or in hot conditions. It may, more rarely, also be the sign of serious underlying disease.

POSSIBLE CONDITIONS
• Acne Rosacea
Alcohol or Narcotics
Carcinoid Syndrome
Heat Stroke
• Menopause
Mitral Valve Disease
Phaeochromocytoma
Polycythaemia
Systemic Lupus Erythematosis (SLE)

Face: Swollen or Puffy Face

The face looks swollen or puffy, either generally or one particular area. This can be caused by allergic reactions, bites or stings, dental problems or build up of fluid.

POSSIBLE CONDITIONS
Acromegaly
Angioneurotic Oedema
Bite, Insect
Cushing's Syndrome
Erysipelas
• Hypothyroidism
Kidney Disease or Failure
Liver Disease or Failure
Kwashiorkor
• Nephrotic Syndrome
Suffocation
Tooth Decay and Abscess

Faeces: Dark or Tar-Like

Dark, black or tar-like faeces are an indication that there is blood coming from somewhere in the gastrointestinal tract. This is usually because of a serious underlying problem, and medical help should be sought immediately.

POSSIBLE CONDITIONS
Adverse Drug Reaction
• Bleeding Disorder
Cancer of the Colon or Rectum (Bowel)
Cirrhosis of the Liver
Disorders of Blood Clotting
Diverticulitis
Dysentery
• Gastritis
Henoch's Purpura
Hookworms (human)
Intestinal Ischaemia
Intestinal Polyps
Intussusception
Jejunal Diverticulitis

Mallory-Weiss Tear
Meckel's Diverticulum
Myxoedema
Oesophageal Varices
• Oesophagitis
• Peptic Ulcer
Ulcerative Colitis

Faeces: Hard

The frequency and consistency of faeces or motions varies from individual to individual. Constipation is a usually a harder motion than normal, and usually the individual passes motions less frequently than normal. Constipation will usually be only an indication of a diet too low in roughage or fluid, but may be a sign of a serious underlying condition.

POSSIBLE CONDITIONS
Adverse Drug Reaction
Anal Fissure
• Constipation
Crohn's Disease
• Diuretics
Diverticulitis
Hirschsprung's Disease
Hypercalcaemia
Intestinal Obstruction
Irritable Bowel Syndrome
Potassium Deficiency
Pregnancy
Sarcoidosis

Faeces: Pale

Faeces can vary in colour, but are usually brown from bile pigments and the action of bacteria during digestion. If they are pale in hue then this may be a sign of serious underlying disease.

POSSIBLE CONDITIONS
Cancer of the Bile Ducts
Cancer of the Gall Bladder
Cancer of the Pancreas
Coeliac Disease
• Gall Stones
Hepatitis
Malabsorption
Pancreatitis
Pregnancy
Sclerosing Cholangitis (Adult)

Fainting

The individual passes out for a short time, caused by flow of blood to the brain being interrupted. This usually has a simple and harmless cause, such as standing for too long, too little food, or not having enough sleep. It may also be a sign of serious underlying disease.

POSSIBLE CONDITIONS
• Anxiety
Aortic Stenosis
Bleeding
Cardiomyopathy
Constrictive Pericarditis
Dehydration
Epilepsy
Heart Attack and Failure
Heart Disease
Heat Exhaustion
• Low Blood Pressure
Mountain Sickness
Paroxysmal Tachycardia
Pregnancy

Sick Sinus Syndrome
Stroke

Fatigue: Breathlessness

A sign, particularly if it is persistent and prolonged, which may indicate serious underlying illness, such as Heart Failure or Anaemia.

POSSIBLE CONDITIONS
• Anaemia
Aortic Stenosis
• Bronchitis
Cardiomyopathy
Diabetes
• Emphysema
Guillain-Barre Syndrome
Heart Failure
Heart Disease
Kidney Disease or Failure
Post-Viral Syndrome
Sickle Cell Anaemia

Feeling Full on Eating Little

How much food it takes to make an individual feel full varies from person to person, and their emotional state. Nerves or anxiety can reduce appetite. Surgery to remove part of the stomach will obviously reduce the amount of food that can be consumed. In some cases it may be a sign of serious disease. Also see the other sections on Appetite.

POSSIBLE CONDITIONS
Anxiety
Cancer of the Stomach
Gastritis
• Peptic Ulcer

Pyloric Stenosis
Post-Gastrectomy Syndrome

Fever: Abdominal Pain and Vomiting

An indication of food poisoning, Gastroenteritis or Urinary Tract Infection, but may be a sign of serious disease.

POSSIBLE CONDITIONS
Appendicitis
Gall Stones
• Gastroenteritis
Intestinal Obstruction
Meckel's Diverticulum
Pancreatitis
Pelvic Inflammatory Disease
Porphyria
Urinary Tract Infection

Fever: Chills, Shivers and Headache

Most usually the symptoms of a viral illness, normally mild but occasionally there may be a serious underlying condition. If there are further symptoms affecting other parts of the body, also consult those sections, as well as tropical fevers and fever.

POSSIBLE CONDITIONS
Chest Infection
• Cold, Common
• Flu
Lung Abscess
Malaria
Meningitis
Mumps
Osteomyelitis

Septicaemia
Typhus Fever
• Viral Infection

Fever: General

Fever is the body's response to infection, and probably aids the ability to fight off the disease. Fever involves a rise in body temperature (which is usually 37 degrees Celsius or 98.4 degrees Fahrenheit). Many illnesses can cause Fever, and it is not necessarily of great concern of itself unless there is a high fever (over 40 degrees C or 104 degrees F). Other factors to take into account is if the individual has returned from travel abroad, particularly if they have visited tropical countries. Cancers may cause fever. There are many illnesses which can cause fever, and a selection is listed below.

POSSIBLE CONDITIONS
Adverse Drug Reaction
AIDS
Allergic Alveolitis
Anal Abscess
Appendicitis
Aspergillosis
Bartholin's Cyst
Biliary Colic
Brain Abscess
Breast Abscess
Bronchiectasis
Brucellosis
Cancer of the Bladder
Cancer of the Kidney
Cancrumoris
Cellulitis

SYMPTOMS SIGNS AND CONDITIONS

Chagas' Disease
Chest Infection
Chickenpox
Cholera
Chondritis
• Cold, Common
Cystitis
Dengue
Dental Infections
Diverticulitis
Dysentery
Ear Infection
Endocarditis
Epididymitis
Epiglottitis
Erysipelas
Erythema Multiforme
Extrinsic Allergic Alveolitis
Fever
Fistula-In-Ano
• Flu
Gall Bladder Infection
Gall Stones
Gastroenteritis
Glandular Fever
Gout
Hepatitis
Hodgkin's Disease
Infective Dislocation of the Hip
Intestinal Obstruction
Jejunal Diverticulitis
Kala-azar
Kidney Disease or Failure
Kidney Stones
Laryngitis
Leukaemia

Ludwig's Angina
Lymphoma
Malaria
Mastoiditis
Measles
Meckel's Diverticulum
Meningitis
Meninogococcal Septicaemia
Menstruation
Mesenteric Adenitis
Mumps
Myocarditis
Orbital Cellulitis
Osteomyelitis
Pancreatitis
Pelvic Inflammatory Disease
Pericarditis
Peritonsillar Abscess
Pernicious Anaemia
Pharyngitis
Plague
Pneumonia
Poisoning
Polio
Polymyalgia Rheumatica
Polymyositis
Porphyria
Prostatitis
Q Fever
Rabies
Relapsing Fever
Rheumatic Fever
Rheumatoid Arthritis
Roseola
Ross River Fever
Rubella

Salpingitis
Scalded Skin Syndrome
Scarlet Fever
Septicaemia
Shingles
Sickle Cell Anaemia
Sinusitis
Sleeping Sickness
Syphilis
Systemic Lupus Erythematosis (SLE)
Tetanus
Tonsillitis
Toxoplasmosis
Tracheitis
Tuberculosis
Typhoid Fever
Typhus Fever
Ulcerative Colitis
Urinary Tract Infection
Vincent's Angina
•Viral Infections
Weil's Disease
Wilms' Tumour
Yellow Fever

Fever: Headache and Pain

Usually will be a sign of viral infection such as a Cold or Flu, but may be an indication of more serious illness.

POSSIBLE CONDITIONS
Brain Abscess
Brucellosis
•Cold, Common
•Flu
Glandular Fever

Malaria
Meningitis
Meninogococcal Septicaemia
Polio
Sinusitis
Temporal Arteritis
Typhus Fever
Weil's Disease

Fever: Recurrent Bouts

Conditions which cause recurrent bouts of fever, apart from Brucellosis, are rare in Britain and developed countries. If the individual has been travelling in or visiting tropical or undeveloped countries, great care should be taken with any fever, and especially one which recurs.

POSSIBLE CONDITIONS
Adverse Drug Reaction
•Brucellosis
Cancer of the Bowel, Stomach, Kidney or Ovaries
Crohn's Disease
Dengue
Gout
Malaria
Rabies
Relapsing Fever
Rhematoid Arthritis
Sleeping Sickness
Temporal Arteritis
Toxoplasmosis
Tuberculosis
Typhoid Fever
Ulcerative colitois
•Vasculitiseg lupus
Yellow Fever

Fever: Sore Throat

Usually an indication of common infections, such as Colds, Tonsillitis or Laryngitis, although occasionally this combination may be associated with more serious conditions.

POSSIBLE CONDITIONS
Adverse Drug Reaction
Cancrumoris
•Cold, Common
Dental Infections
Flu
•Glandular Fever
Laryngitis
Ludwig's Angina
•Pharyngitis
Rabies
Rheumatic Fever
•Tonsillitis
Tracheitis
Vincent's Angina

Fever: Swallowing Problems

This combination of symptoms is usually an indication of infections, such as Tonsillitis and Laryngitis, and rarely will be an indication of serious underlying illness.

POSSIBLE CONDITIONS
Cancer of the Oesophagus
Epiglottitis
Erythema Multiforme
Laryngitis
Ludwig's Angina
•Tonsillitis

Fever: Tiredness

Illnesses which have fever as a symptom will also cause tiredness and fatigue. Any chronic infection will cause fatigue. Also see sections of fever.

POSSIBLE CONDITIONS
Adverse Drug Reaction
Cancer of the Bowel, Stomach, Kidney or Ovaries
•Cold, Common
Crohn's Disease
Endocarditis
•Flu
Glandular Fever
Rheumatic Fever
Rheumatoid Arthritis
Tuberculosis
Ulcerative Colitis
Vasculitis eg Lupus

Fever: Tropical

Infectious illnesses which are rare in Britain and the developed world, but are more common in tropical parts of the world, such as Africa, India, the Near, Middle and Far East, and South America. Any fever occurring after travelling or visiting tropical parts of the world should be taken seriously and medical help should be sought.

POSSIBLE CONDITIONS
Bilharzia
Dengue
Kala-azar
•Malaria
Plague
Relapsing Fever
Sleeping Sickness

Typhus Fever

Yellow Fever

Finger: Altered Sensation (Fingers and Toes)

Feelings in the fingers, toes and limbs may become altered through a variety of conditions, many of them serious. It is sometimes quite difficult to define exactly what altered sensation is, but it may often be caused by nerve and neurological problems. Frost Bite or Raynaud's Phenomenon should be excluded if the individual has been exposed to cold conditions.

POSSIBLE CONDITIONS

• Alcohol or Narcotics

Cancer of the Spine

Carpal Tunnel Syndrome

Cauda Equine Syndrome

Cervical Rib

Cervical Spondylosis

• Diabetes

Frost Bite

Guillain-Barre Syndrome

Hyperventilation

Ischaemic Contracture

Leprosy

Median Nerve Damage

Multiple Sclerosis

• Nerve Injury including Peripheral Neuropathy

Peripheral Vascular Disease

Pernicious Anaemia

Prolapsed Cervical Disc

Raynaud's Phenomenon

Ross River Fever

Sciatica

Spinal Cord Injury

Spinal Cord Tumours

Ulnar Nerve Damage

Vitamin B12 (Cyanocobalamin) Deficiency

Finger: Clubbing

Fingers become clubbed, most usually as a result of a problem with respiration and breathing. This is normally a sign of serious illness, and medical help should be sought. While an important indicator, it is unlikely this is going to be the most significant or pressing of symptoms.

POSSIBLE CONDITIONS

Allergic Alveolitis

Bronchiectasis

Cancers of the Oesophagus, Stomach, Bowel, Kidney, Lung and Pancreas

• Cirrhosis of the Liver

• Crohn's Disease

Cystic Fibrosis

Endocarditis

Extrinsic Allergic Alveolitis

Fibrosing Alveolitis

Heart Disease (inherited)

• Lung Cancer

Pneumoconiosis

• Pulmonary Fibrosis

Tuberculosis

• Ulcerative Colitis

Finger: Itching (Fingers and Toes)

Fingers feel itchy have little sensation. There are two most likely causes: either Dermatitis or a fungal infection if itchy; Frost Bite or Chilblains if numb.

POSSIBLE CONDITIONS
Athlete's Foot
Dermatitis

Finger: Nails Unusual in Colour, Shape or Texture

State of health may be indicated by fingernails and finger beds. If the finger beds are bluish, this is an indication of cyanosis, too little oxygen reaching body tissues, and a sign of respiratory or heart problems. This is an important sign and medical help should be sought if cyanosis is suspected.

POSSIBLE CONDITIONS [those associated with cyanosis are identified by (c)]
Anaemia
Athlete's Foot
Bronchitis (c)
Choking
Dermatitis
Endocarditis
Extrinsic Allergic Alveolitis (c)
Fibrosing Alveolitis (c)
•Fungal Infections of the Skin and Nail (c)
Heart Failure
Heart Disease (c)
Hypothermia
Injury to the Nails
Kidney Disease or Failure
Laryngeal Oedema (c)
Lichen Planus
Peripheral Vascular Disease (c)
Pneumoconiosis (c)
Pneumonia (c)
•Psoriasis
Pulmonary Embolism (c)

Pulmonary Fibrosis (c)
Pulmonary Oedema
Shock

Finger: Numbness (Fingers and Toes)

Fingers go numb and have little sensation. There are two most likely causes: either Dermatitis or a fungal infection if itchy; Frost Bite or Chilblains if numb.

POSSIBLE CONDITIONS
Adverse Drug Reaction
Alcohol or Narcotics
Carpal Tunnel Syndrome
Cauda Equine Syndrome
Cervical Rib
Cervical Spondylosis
Chilblains
•Diabetes
Frost Bite
Guillain-Barre Syndrome
Leprosy
Multiple Sclerosis
Nerve Damage
Peripheral Vascular Disease

Finger: Swollen or Distorted

Finger or fingers become swollen or distorted in shape, either the fingers themselves or the joints. This may be an indication of damage to or infection of the structures of the fingers, as well as arthritis.

POSSIBLE CONDITIONS
•Dupuytren's Contracture
Flexor Sheath Infection
Gout
Injury to the Nails

Ischaemic Contracture
Mallet Finger and Thumb
•Osteoarthritis
Rheumatoid Arthritis
Trigger Finger

Fit or Convulsions

Often heralded by an aura or feeling something is about to happen, followed by unconsciousness and twitching movements of the limbs, and possibly urinary incontinence. Usually the individual will regain consciousness although there will be a period of drowsiness and confusion. It may be a sign of serious underlying disease, and medical help should be sought if there is not a history of Epilepsy.

POSSIBLE CONDITIONS
•Alcohol or Narcotics
Brain Abscess
•Epilepsy
Fever
Hepatitis
Huntington's Chorea
Hydrocephalus
Kidney Disease or Failure
Meningitis
Pregnancy
Rabies
Sleeping Sickness
Stroke
Subarachnoid Haemorrhage
Subdural Haemorrhage
Toxoplasmosis

Flashing Lights: Eye

The individual experiences flashing lights before their eyes. Common causes are rising too quickly from sitting, a blow or injury to the head or eye, or the aura which heralds a Migraine.

POSSIBLE CONDITIONS
Detached Retina
Flashing Lights
Head Injury
Injury to the Eye
•Migraine
Temporal Lobe Epilepsy

Floaters

Floaters in the eye are brown or black patches or lines in the field of vision. These move across the vision as the individual looks in different directions or focuses on different objects. They may have no serious cause, although poor eyesight and damage to the eye can both cause floaters. This sign may also be an indication of serious damage to the eye, such as a Detached Retina. If the individual experiences a spot affecting the vision which retains the same position, then this is probably a 'Blind Spot': see the relevant section.

POSSIBLE CONDITIONS
Detached Retina
•Floaters
Injury to the Eye
Poor Eyesight
Vitreous Haemorrhage

Foot: Infected or Ulcerated

Foot or feet become infected or ulcerated, which may be directly from infections but also from nerve damage or peripheral vascular disease. Some of the causes may be minor, such as Veruccas or Warts, but ulcerated feet will often be an indication of neglect and/or serious disease.

POSSIBLE CONDITIONS
Alcohol or Narcotics
• Athlete's Foot
Cellulitis
• Dermatitis
Diabetes
Frost Bite
Ingrown Toenail
Lymphoedema
Multiple Sclerosis
• Peripheral Neuropathy
• Peripheral Vascular Disease
Raynaud's Phenomenon
Syphilis
Varicose Veins
Warts

Foot: Pain

Pain is experienced in the foot. This may be caused by relatively minor conditions such as Veruccas (Warts) or an Ingrown Toenail, but may also have more serious causes.

POSSIBLE CONDITIONS
• Athlete's Foot
Gout
Hallux Rigidus
Hallux Valgus
• Ingrown Toenail
Morton's Metatarsalgia
• Osteoarthritis
Peripheral Neuropathy
Pes Cavus

Plantar Fasciitis
Polio
Spina Bifida
Warts

Giddiness: Vertigo

The ears are also involved with balance and the concept of position, and consequently infections and other problems with the ear will affect balance as well as hearing.

POSSIBLE CONDITIONS
Acoustic Neuroma
Cholesteamota
Cold, Common
Ear Wax
Inner Ear Infection
• Meniere's Disease
Otosclerosis
• Vertebrabasilar Insufficiency
Vestibulitis

Groin: Blisters

Blisters may develop around the groin, usually as the result of an infection.

POSSIBLE CONDITIONS
Adverse Drug Reaction
Herpes Simplex
Molluscum Contagiosum
Pemphigus Vulgaris
Shingles

Groin: Loss of Pubic Hair

Hair is lost from the groin and the pubic area. This may be as a result of Pregnancy or the Menopause, but can unusually be the sign of serious illness — although there will usually be more pressing symptoms than hair loss.

POSSIBLE CONDITIONS
Addison's Disease
• Adverse Drug Reaction
AIDS
Alcohol or Narcotics
Alopecia
• Alopecia Areata
Cirrhosis of the Liver
Dermatitis
Hypopituitarism
Hypothyroidism
Menopause
Pregnancy
Psoriasis

Groin: Lumps, Sores and Ulcers

Lumps (small or large), sores and ulcers may develop in or around the groin. Although lumps may be just ordinary Warts or Boils, it is probably worth seeking medical help to rule out more serious conditions.

POSSIBLE CONDITIONS
Adverse Drug Reaction
Bartholin's Cyst
Behcet's Syndrome
Boil
Cancer of the Skin
Carbuncle
Chancroid
Femoral Artery Aneurysm
• Hernia, Inguinal
Hodgkin's Disease

Lipoma
• Lymphadenopathy
Metastasis
Plague
Sarcoidosis
Scabies
Syphilis
Tuberculosis
Undescended Testicle
Varicose Veins
Warts

Groin: Pain Between Legs (Men)

Pain or aching between the legs, usually caused by an injury such as falling astride, although there may be a more serious condition.

POSSIBLE CONDITIONS
Cancer of the Prostate
Enlarged Prostate
• Injury to Groin
Prostatitis

Gums: Bleeding

Bleeding gums can be caused by brushing teeth too vigorously, but may be the sign of infection. If bleeding gums persist, consult a dentist.

POSSIBLE CONDITIONS
Disorders of Blood Clotting
Trauma to Gums
Vitamin C (Ascorbic Acid) Deficiency

Hair: Excessive Body Hair

The amount of body hair that an individual has is largely determined by their genes. It is not unusual for women to have more body hair than the fashionable norm, but it is unusual for excessive body hair to be caused by underlying disease.

POSSIBLE CONDITIONS
Acromegaly
Adrenal Tumour
Adverse Drug Reaction
Congenital Adrenal Hyperplasia
Cushing's Syndrome
Hirsutism (Idiopathic)
Menopause
Ovarian Tumour
• Polycystic Ovaries
Porphyria Cutanea Tarda

Hair: Hair Loss and Baldness

Hair loss and baldness is a natural occurrence in many men, characterised by male pattern baldness. Hair can also become thinner in women as they grow older. In both cases, this is determined by genes. Baldness or hair loss may also be an indication of underlying disease.

POSSIBLE CONDITIONS
Adverse Drug Reaction
AIDS
• Alopecia
• Alopecia Areata
Dermatitis
Hypopituitarism
Hypothyroidism
Kwashiorkor
Menopause
Morphoea
Pregnancy
Psoriasis

Ringworm

Hair: Loss of Pubic Hair

Hair is lost from the groin and the pubic area. This may be as a result of Pregnancy or the Menopause, but can unusually be the sign of serious illness – although there will usually be more pressing symptoms than hair loss.

POSSIBLE CONDITIONS
Addison's Disease
Adverse Drug Reaction
AIDS
Alcohol or Narcotics
• Alopecia
• Alopecia Areata
Cirrhosis of the Liver
Dermatitis
Hypopituitarism
Hypothyroidism
Menopause
Pregnancy
Psoriasis

Halitosis and Bad or Foul Breath

Bad or foul-smelling breath is usually caused either by the consumption of spiced foods or alcohol, indigestion, or by problems with teeth or gums. It may, however, be associated with more serious disease, although it is unlikely that Halitosis is going to be one of the most significant symptoms.

POSSIBLE CONDITIONS
Adverse Drug Reaction
Appendicitis
Bronchiectasis

Bronchitis
Cancer of the Larynx
Cancer of the Mouth
Cancer of the Nose
Cancer of the Oesophagus
Cancer of the Stomach
Cancer in the Chest
Chest Infection
Cirrhosis of the Liver
Cold, Common
Cystic Fibrosis
• Dental Infections
Dentures
Diabetes
Emphysema
• Food and Drink
Hay Fever
Hepatitis
Kidney Disease or Failure
Laryngitis
Ludwig's Angina
Lung Abscess
Lung Cancer
Mouth Breathing
Nasal Polyps
Pharyngitis
Poisoning
• Poor Oral Hygiene
Pyorrhoea Alveolaris
Rhinitis
Sinusitis
Sjogren's Syndrome
Smoking
• Tonsillitis
• Tooth Decay and Abscess
Tuberculosis

Halitosis: Combined with Cough

Bad or foul-smelling breath is usually caused either by the consumption of spiced foods or alcohol, indigestion or by problems with teeth or gums. When combined with a persistent cough, however, it may be a sign of Bronchitis, cancer or other lung problems.

POSSIBLE CONDITIONS
• Bronchiectasis
• Bronchitis
Cystic Fibrosis
Hay Fever
Lung Abscess
Lung Cancer
Rhinitis
Tracheitis
Tuberculosis

Hallucinations

Experiencing sensations, sounds or visions which are not real. Dreams can be regarded as hallucinations, but these only happen when asleep, while in this context hallucinations take place when the individual is fully conscious. If this is the case, and there is not illness which would cause fever, this is usually an indication of mental illness.

POSSIBLE CONDITIONS
• Adverse Drug Reaction
• Alcohol or Narcotics
Anxiety
• Dementia
Depression and Manic Depression
Fever
Schizophrenia

Temporal Lobe Epilepsy

Hand: Swollen

Hand becomes swollen, usually as a result of fluid retention. This may also be an indication of serious illness.

POSSIBLE CONDITIONS
• Arthritis
Axillary Vein Thrombosis
Carpal Tunnel Syndrome
Chilblains
Hypothyroidism
Lymphoedema
Menstruation – as normal variation throughout cycle
Osteoarthitis
Pregnancy
Rheumatoid Arthitis

Hand: Trembling

Hands noticeably tremble or shake. From time to time, many individuals' hands will do this, and unless it is prolonged and particularly pronounced it is not a matter for concern. In some cases it can be an indication of serious illness, although there will often be other symptoms if this is the case.

POSSIBLE CONDITIONS
• Alcohol Withdrawal
Anxiety
Brain Tumours
• Essential Tremor
Friedreich's Ataxia
Hepatolentricular Degeneration
Huntington's Chorea
Hyperthyroidism

Multiple Sclerosis
Parkinson's Disease
Stroke

Head: Bulging or Sunken Places (babies)

Bumps and lumps on the head can be caused by injury, boils or similar infections. In babies, the skull takes some time to fuse, and soft areas (fontanelles) can be felt between the bones of the skull. If these areas become particularly sunken or bulging, it is an indication of a serious underlying problem.

POSSIBLE CONDITIONS
Brain Tumours
• Dehydration
Hydrocephalus
Meningitis
Paget's Disease
• Raised Intracranial Pressure

Head: Headache and Pain

Headaches are very common, and are usually only an indication that the individual is suffering from tiredness, stress or tension, Migraine or toothache. Occasionally headache may be a sign of serious underlying disease, but this will usually be combined with other symptoms.

POSSIBLE CONDITIONS
Adverse Drug Reaction
Alcohol or Narcotics
• Anxiety
Brain Abscess
Brain Tumours
Carbon Monoxide Poisoning

Cluster Headache
Cold, Common
Dental Infections
Erythema Multiforme
• Fever
Flu
Gastroenteritis
Head Injury
Heat Exhaustion
Heat Stroke
High Blood Pressure
Laryngitis
Meningitis
Meninogococcal Septicaemia
Menstruation (premenstrual tension)
• Migraine
Mountain Sickness
Nasal Septal Necrosis
Pharyngitis
Pituitary Tumours
Poisoning
Polio
Polycythaemia
Post-Viral Syndrome
Pyorrhoea Alveolaris
Q Fever
Raised Intracranial Pressure
Sinusitis
Sleeping Sickness
• Stress
Stroke
Subarachnoid Haemorrhage
Subdural Haemorrhage
Teething Pain
Temporal Arteritis
Tension Headache

Tonsillitis
Tooth Decay and Abscess
Tracheitis
Typhoid Fever
Typhus Fever
Viral Infection
Yellow Fever

Head: Overly Large

The size of head in proportion to the body varies from individual to individual. Where it is particularly large and increasing in size, this is most usually a sign of some underlying condition.

POSSIBLE CONDITIONS
• Acromegaly
Hydrocephalus
• Paget's Disease

Head: Pain, Headache and Fever

Usually will be a sign of viral infection such as a Cold or Flu, but may be an indication of more serious illness.

POSSIBLE CONDITIONS
Brain Abscess
Brucellosis
• Cold, Common
• Flu
Glandular Fever
Malaria
Meningitis
Meninogococcal Septicaemia
Polio
Sinusitis
Temporal Arteritis

73

Typhus Fever

• Viral Infection

Weil's Disease

Head: Prominent Blood Vessels

Most usually an indication of Temporal Arteritis with typically tender, inflamed arteries.

POSSIBLE CONDITIONS

Temporal Arteritis

Head: Running Nose, Sore Eyes and Headache

Combination of symptoms which usually indicates the Common Cold, but there are other conditions, some mild, some serious, which can also fit these symptoms.

POSSIBLE CONDITIONS

Cancer of the Nose

• Cold, Common

• Flu

Foreign Body in Nose

• Hay Fever

Head Injury

Nasal Polyps

• Rhinitis

Sinusitis

Headache and Head Pain

Headaches are very common, and are usually only an indication that the individual is suffering from tiredness, stress or tension, Migraine or toothache. Occasionally headache may be a sign of serious underlying disease, but this will usually be combined with other symptoms.

POSSIBLE CONDITIONS

Adverse Drug Reaction

Alcohol or Narcotics

• Anxiety

Brain Abscess

Brain Tumours

Cancer of the Pituitary

Carbon Monoxide Poisoning

Cluster Headache

Cold, Common

Dental Infections

Erythema Multiforme

• Fever

Flu

Gastroenteritis

Head Injury

Heat Exhaustion

Heat Stroke

High Blood Pressure

Laryngitis

Meningitis

Meninogococcal Septicaemia

Menstruation (premenstrual tension)

• Migraine

Mountain Sickness

Nasal Septal Necrosis

Pharyngitis

Poisoning

Polio

Polycythaemia

Post-Viral Syndrome

Pyorrhoea Alveolaris

Q Fever

Raised Intracranial Pressure

Sinusitis

Sleeping Sickness

• Stress
Stroke
Subarachnoid Haemorrhage
Subdural Haemorrhage
Temporal Arteritis
• Tension Headache
Tonsillitis
Tooth Decay and Abscess
Tracheitis
Travel Sickness
Typhoid Fever
Typhus Fever
• Viral Infection
Yellow Fever

Headache: Fever

Usually will be a sign of viral infection such as a Cold or Flu, but may be an indication of more serious illness.

POSSIBLE CONDITIONS
Brain Abscess
Brucellosis
• Cold, Common
Encephalitis
• Flu
Glandular Fever
Malaria
Meningitis
Meninogococcal Septicaemia
Polio
Sinusitis
Temporal Arteritis
Typhus Fever
• Viral Infection
Weil's Disease

Hearing Problems and Deafness (Adults)

Deafness may be from birth or acquired during life, and it is normal for older individuals to have some degree of hearing impairment. Many conditions can make an individual temporarily deaf or deafer, even Ear Wax, but it may also be a sign of a serious condition.

POSSIBLE CONDITIONS
Acoustic Neuroma
Adverse Drug Reaction
Artery Disease
Brittle Bone Disease
Cholesteamota
• Ear Wax
Head Injury
Inner Ear Infection
• Loud Noises
Meniere's Disease
Meningitis
Mumps
• Otosclerosis
Paget's Disease
• Presbyacusis
Rubella
Syphilis
Turner's Syndrome

Hearing Problems and Deafness (Children)

Deafness may be from birth or acquired during early life. Many conditions can make an individual temporarily deaf or deafer, even Ear Wax, but it may also be a sign of a serious condition.

POSSIBLE CONDITIONS
Adverse Drug Reaction
Brittle Bone Disease
•Ear Wax
Hypothyroidism
•Inner Ear Infection
Meningitis
Mumps
Rubella
Turner's Syndrome

Heart: Extra Beats

Extra heart beats are a relatively common phenomenon, and are not usually the sign of serious illness. Causes include consuming too much caffeine or alcohol, smoking, Anxiety, indigestion, or there may be no obvious cause. It may also be the sign of a serious problem.

POSSIBLE CONDITIONS
Adverse Drug Reaction
Alcohol or Narcotics
•Anxiety
•Caffeine
Cigarettes
Dyspepsia, Non-Ulcer
•Extra Heart Beats (normal variant)
Fever
Heart Attack and Failure

Heart: Irregular Beating

The heart beats irregularly, or may appear to, although it is always difficult for an individual to gauge their own heart beat. This can be the sign of problems with the heart, although there will usually be other symptoms. Investigations will always be needed but sometimes there is no obvious disease or cause.

POSSIBLE CONDITIONS
•Atrial Fibrillation
•Extra Heart Beats
Polymyositis
Pulmonary Embolism
Rheumatic Fever
Sick Sinus Syndrome
•Sinus Arrhythmia

Heart: Rapid and Irregular Beat

The heart beats at a rapid, but irregular, beat, although it is always difficult for an individual to gauge their own heart beat. This may be the sign of serious underlying problems with the heart or respiratory system, although there will usually be other symptoms. Medical help should be sought as soon as possible and investigations undertaken.

POSSIBLE CONDITIONS
Alcohol or Narcotics
•Atrial Fibrillation
Constrictive Pericarditis
Endocarditis
Extra Heart Beats
Heart Attack and Failure
Hyperthyroidism
Ischaemic Heart Disease
Mitral Valve Disease
Rheumatic Fever

Heart: Rapid and Regular Beat

The heart beats at a regular, but much faster, rate than seems normal, although it is always difficult for an individual to gauge their own heart beat. This will usually have an innocent cause, such as vigorous exercise, nerves or anxiety. If, however, the rate does not return to normal when exercise or anxiety ceases, it may be a sign of serious underlying disease. There will usually be other symptoms.

POSSIBLE CONDITIONS
Adverse Drug Reaction
Alcohol or Narcotics
Allergic Reaction, Severe
Anaemia
• Anxiety
Bleeding
Caffeine
Cardiomyopathy
Cigarettes
Constrictive Pericarditis
Dehydration
Diphtheria
• Exercise
• Fever
Flu
Heart Failure
Heart Disease
Heat Exhaustion
Heat Stroke
Hyperthyroidism
Myocarditis
Paroxysmal Tachycardia
Pernicious Anaemia
Phaeochromocytoma
Polymyositis
Porphyria
Pregnancy
Rheumatic Fever
Shock

Vitamin B1 (Thiamine) Deficiency

Heart: Slow Beat

The heart beats at an unusually slow rate, although it is always difficult for an individual to gauge their own heart beat. This is relatively common in very fit individuals, but may be a sign of underlying problems with the heart.

POSSIBLE CONDITIONS
• Adverse Drug Reaction
Cardiomyopathy
Exercise
Hypothermia
• Hypothyroidism
Sick Sinus Syndrome

Heartburn, Indigestion or Dyspepsia

A range of symptoms associated with the upper part of the gastrointestinal tract, such as burning pain in the gullet, nausea, belching, flatulence and acid from the stomach being regurgitated into the mouth. If there are only occasional bouts which can be linked to eating certain foods or drinking too much alcohol, then this is nothing to worry about. If pain or discomfort are experienced often or persistently, it may be the sign of a serious underlying condition.

POSSIBLE CONDITIONS
Achalasia
Cancer of the Oesophagus
Cancer of the Stomach
Dyspepsia, Non-Ulcer
Gall Stones
Gastritis
Gastroenteritis

- Hernia, Hiatus
- Oesophagitis
Pancreatitis
- Peptic Ulcer
Pregnancy

Hip: Dislocation

Leg becomes dislocated from the hip joint in the pelvis. Medical help should be sought.

POSSIBLE CONDITIONS
Acquired Dislocation of the Hip
- Congenital Dislocation of the Hip (CDH)
Infective Dislocation of the Hip
Tuberculosis

Hip: Pain

Pain is experienced in or around the hip, often either from injury, fracture or dislocation, or from arthritis – or a combination.

POSSIBLE CONDITIONS
Acquired Dislocation of the Hip
Congenital Dislocation of the Hip (CDH)
Infective Dislocation of the Hip
Irritable Hip
- Osteoarthritis
Osteoporosis
Perthes' Disease
Rheumatoid Arthritis
Slipped Epiphysis
Subluxation of the Hip
Tuberculosis

Hot Flushes

Individual experiences hot flushes, most usually because of embarrassment or nerves. Hot flushes are associated with the Menopause and Fever, but may be an indication of other conditions.

POSSIBLE CONDITIONS
- Anxiety
Carcinoid Syndrome
Fever
Hyperthyroidism
- Menopause
Phaeochromocytoma

Hunger: Excessive or Abnormal

Appetite varies from individual to individual, and some people crave food more than others. Hunger can also be diminished when suffering from feverish illness or emotional upset, and with more serious conditions.

POSSIBLE CONDITIONS
Bulimia Nervosa
- Dyspepsia, Non-Ulcer
Hyperthyroidism
- Hypothalmic Disease
Low Blood Sugar
- Peptic Ulcer
Tapeworms

Hypothermia

The temperature of the internal body (normally maintained at 37 degrees Celsius) falls at least two degrees below this level. Those especially at risk at new-born babies and the elderly, both of whom have reduced ability to cope with low temperatures. Babies do not shiver. If an individual has hypothermia, they should be warmed slowly with blankets and warm drinks. Warming up the individual too quickly can be dangerous, and they should not be given alcohol.

POSSIBLE CONDITIONS
Adverse Drug Reaction
Alcohol or Narcotics
• Hypothermia
• Hypothyroidism
Myxoedema

Hysteria

The definition of this symptom is difficult to pin down: to most people, it is wild and uncontrolled behaviour, while in medicine is usually taken to mean symptoms, such as paralysis of a limb or blindness, for which there is no obvious underlying physical condition and no intention to deceive. Identified most in women between 30 and 50 years old. It will usually be necessary to exclude physical illness.

POSSIBLE CONDITIONS
• Anxiety
Brain Tumours
Dementia
• Hyperventilation
• Hysteria

Impotence or Difficulty Maintaining Erection

Many men suffer problems with impotence and maintaining an erection from time to time, especially if they are tired, drunk, stressed or suffering from any debilitating illness. As men get older, it also takes them longer to regain an erection after ejaculation. It is generally thought that problems with impotence are usually psychological in nature, especially if problems are only experienced with one partner. There are possible physical causes as well, such as blood flow problems, neurological disease, damage to nerves following surgery, and problems with hormones. Psychological causes such as depression or tension within a relationship may be helped by counselling.

POSSIBLE CONDITIONS
• Adverse Drug Reaction
Alcohol or Narcotics
• Anxiety
Artery Disease
Cushing's Syndrome
Damage to Testicles
Depression and Manic Depression
Diabetes
• Hypogonadism
Hypopituitarism
Multiple Sclerosis
Peripheral Neuropathy
Peripheral Vascular Disease

Incontinence: Urine or Dribbling Urine

Incontinence of urine is the unintentional or accidental passing or dribbling of urine. This can have a range of causes, many of them serious.

POSSIBLE CONDITIONS
Alcohol or Narcotics
Bladder Neck Obstruction
Cancer of the Prostate
Cancer of the Urethra
Cauda Equine Syndrome
Enlarged Bladder

Enlarged Prostate
Epilepsy
Hydrocephalus
• Irritable Bladder
Multiple Sclerosis
Prostatitis
Sciatica
Spina Bifida
Spinal Cord Injury
• Stress Incontinence
Stroke
Urethral Stricture
• Urinary Tract Infection
• Womb Prolapse

Indigestion, Dyspepsia or Heartburn

A range of symptoms associated with the upper part of the gastrointestinal tract, such as burning pain in the gullet, nausea, belching, flatulence and acid from the stomach being regurgitated into the mouth. If there are only occasional bouts which can be linked to eating certain foods or drinking too much alcohol, then this is nothing to worry about. If pain or discomfort are experienced often or persistently, it may be the sign of a serious underlying condition.

POSSIBLE CONDITIONS
Achalasia
Cancer of the Oesophagus
Cancer of the Stomach
Dyspepsia, Non-Ulcer
Gall Stones
• Gastritis
Gastroenteritis
• Hernia, Hiatus
• Oesophagitis

Pancreatitis
• Peptic Ulcer
Pregnancy

Infertility: Male

Ability to reproduce varies from individual to individual, but about one third of couples cannot conceive because of problems with male fertility. If sexual intercourse is occurring at the right time in the woman's cycle, it is usual for a sperm count to be done and to check that sperm in normal. Fertility can be reduced by and following serious illness.

POSSIBLE CONDITIONS
Adverse Drug Reaction
Alcohol or Narcotics
• Damage to Testicles
Ectopic Testicle
Mumps
Undescended Testicle
Varicocele

Insomnia and Difficulty Sleeping

The amount of sleep needed varies from individual to individual, and most people can survive on less then they believe. Difficulty getting a good night's rest can be caused by drinking too much coffee, alcohol, cat-napping during the day, tension, stress, anxiety and depression.

POSSIBLE CONDITIONS
Adverse Drug Reaction
• Anxiety
Depression and Manic Depression

Irritability and Emotional Instability

Varies greatly from individual to individual, and many people can be very highly strung without suffering from any underlying disease. More importantly are changes in an individual, such as more pronounced irritability and mood swings, which are out of character.

POSSIBLE CONDITIONS
Adverse Drug Reaction
Alcohol or Narcotics
• Anxiety
Brain Tumours
Dementia
Depression and Manic Depression
Head Injury
Meningitis
Menopause
Polio
• Premenstrual Syndrome
Rabies
Schizophrenia
Syphilis
Vitamin B12 (Cyanocobalamin) Deficiency

Itching With No Rash

Itching is usually just a normal response, but it can be caused by problems such as Scabies, Lice or Threadworms. In some cases it is also an indication of serious underlying disease.

POSSIBLE CONDITIONS
• Adverse Drug Reaction
Angioneurotic Oedema
Biliary Colic
Bite, Insect

Cancer of the Pancreas
Dandruff
• Dermatitis
Fibreglass
Hepatitis
Hodgkin's Disease
• Hyperthyroidism
Hypothyroidism
Leukaemia
Lice
Lymphoma
Pancreatitis
Polycythaemia
Pregnancy
Scabies
Sclerosing Cholangitis (Adult)
Threadworm
Uraemia

Jaundice: Abdominal Pain and Vomiting

Combination of symptoms which indicates serious illness. Medical help should be sought immediately.

POSSIBLE CONDITIONS
• Biliary Colic
Cancer of the Liver
Cancer of the Pancreas
Cancer of the Stomach
• Gall Stones
Hepatitis
Pancreatitis
Sickle Cell Anaemia

Jaundice: Weight Loss

Persistent weight loss combined with jaundice,

caused by problems with the liver or associated organs. It is a serious combination of symptoms, and often indicates cancer.

POSSIBLE CONDITIONS
Cancer of the Bile Ducts
Cancer of the Gall Bladder
•Cancer of the Liver
Cancer of the Pancreas
Cancer of the Stomach
Cirrhosis of the Liver

Joint: Pain or Inflammation

Joints become painful or inflamed, or both, affecting either a few or many joints of the body. This may be caused by a range of conditions, some relatively mild such as Colds and Flu, others much more serious. Any long-term problem should prompt a visit to a doctor. In many of the conditions, this will not be the only symptom: there will be other signs of illness from an infection. If there is no obvious infection, pain or inflammation, then medical help should be sought.

POSSIBLE CONDITIONS
Adverse Drug Reaction
Allergic Alveolitis
Ankylosing Spondylitis
•Arthritis
Behcet's Syndrome
Cat Scratch Fever
Chondritis
Cold, Common
Endocarditis
Flu
Gastroenteritis
Gonorrhoea

•Gout
Haemophilia
Henoch's Purpura
•Osteoarthritis
Psoriasis
Reiter's Disease
Rheumatic Fever
•Rheumatoid Arthritis
Ross River Fever
•Septicaemia
Sickle Cell Anaemia
Syphilis
Systemic Lupus Erythematosis (SLE)
Typhus Fever
•Viral Infection

Joint: Swollen with Nodules

Joints become inflamed with nodules, affecting either a few or many joints of the body. This is usually a problem with the joints themselves, and medical help should be sought.

POSSIBLE CONDITIONS
Alcohol or Narcotics
Bursitis
Charcot's Joints
•Gout
Hallux Rigidus
Hallux Valgus
•Osteoarthritis
Rheumatic Fever
•Rheumatoid Arthritis
Spina Bifida
Syphilis

Knee: Locked or Giving Way

Knee locks or gives way when any weight is put on it. This is usually caused by dislocation or injury, including damage to the ligaments or cartilage.

Possible Conditions
•Cartilage Tear (Knee)
Dislocation of the Knee Cap
Ligamentous Tear (Knee)
•Loose Body in the Knee
Osteoarthritis

Knee: Pain

Pain experienced in or around the knee. The most likely cause is going to be injury or damage to the structures of the knee, including ligaments and cartilage.

Possible Conditions
Bursitis
•Cartilage Tear (Knee)
Dislocation of the Knee
Dislocation of the Knee Cap
Fractures of the Knee Cap (Patella)
Fractures of the Lower Leg (femur, tibia and fibula)
•Injury
Ligamentous Tear (Knee)
•Osteoarthritis
Upper Tibial Epiphysis and Apophysis

Leg: Bowlegged

Legs are bowlegged and the knees are unusually far apart. The most common cause is Knock Knees, but it can be a sign of serious problems, such as Rickets (Vitamin D Deficiency).

Possible Conditions
Charcot's Joints
Knock Knees
Osteoarthritis
•Paget's Disease
Rickets
•Vitamin D (Calciferol) Deficiency

Leg: Swollen

Ankle and/or leg may become swollen, usually from injury, from a build of fluid, or because of Deep Vein Thrombosis (DVT). Swollen ankles may be the result of water retention during Menstruation Cycle, but it may also more unusually be an indication of heart or kidney problems. If one leg suddenly becomes swollen and pale then this may be an indication of DVT.

Possible Conditions
Anaemia
Cellulitis
•Deep Vein Thrombosis
Heart Failure
•Injury to the Ankle
Kidney Disease or Failure
Lymphoedema
•Menstruation (normal cyclical variation in fluid retention)
Mitral Valve Disease
Myocarditis
Myxoedema
Nephrotic Syndrome
Phlegmasia Alba Dolens
Pregnancy
•Varicose Veins
Vitamin B1 (Thiamine) Deficiency

Leg: Waddling Walk

Individual walks with an unusually waddling gait.

POSSIBLE CONDITIONS
Congenital Dislocation of the Hip (CDH)
Muscular Dystrophy

Leg: Weak

Leg becomes very weak and unable to bear weight. This may be a result of any long period of inaction, such as being bedridden, arthritis or nerve or neurological problems.

POSSIBLE CONDITIONS
Adverse Drug Reaction (including steroids)
• Alcohol or Narcotics
Bedridden
Brain Tumour
Guillain Barré Syndrome
Hyperthyroidism
Hypothyroidism
Motor Neurone Disease
Multiple Sclerosis
Muscular Dystrophy
Myopathy
Polio
Polymyositis
Rheumatoid Arthritis
Spinal Tumours or Compression
Steriod Use
• Stroke
Vitamin D Deficiency (Osteomalacia)

Lips: Bluish or Purplish

Often the sign of underlying problems with the heart or lungs resulting in too little oxygen getting to body tissues. This makes these areas go bluish or purpley (cyanosis), and is particularly apparent on the lips, beds of the fingernails and earlobes. It can, however, be a sign that the individual is cold or even has hypothermia. In any event, persistent bluish or purple tinge should be treated seriously and medical help should be sought.

POSSIBLE CONDITIONS
Asthma
Bronchiolitis
• Bronchitis
Carcinoid Syndrome
• Chest Infection
Choking
• Cold Temperature Exposure
Congenital Atresia of the Oesophagus
Diphtheria
Drowning
Emphysema
Epiglottitis
Extrinsic Allergic Alveolitis
• Fibrosing Alveolitis
Heart Failure
Heart Disease
Hypothermia
Laryngeal Oedema
Laryngitis
• Peripheral Vascular Disease
Pneumoconiosis
Pneumonia
Pneumothorax
Pulmonary Embolism
• Pulmonary Fibrosis
Pulmonary Oedema
Shock
Suffocation

Lips: Cracked, Chapped, Sores or Discoloured Areas

This covers a range of problems with the lips, from chapped or dry lips, to sores, ulcers, white patches or even lumps. The causes can range from the mild to the severe.

POSSIBLE CONDITIONS
• Anaemia
Aphthous Ulcer
Behcet's Syndrome
Cancer of the Mouth
• Candidiasis
Dermatitis
Erythema Multiforme
• Herpes Simplex
• Impetigo
Leukoplakia
Lichen Planus
Motor Neurone Disease
Mucocele
Multiple Sclerosis
Parkinson's Disease
Poisoning
Shingles
Stroke
Syphilis
Vitamin C (Ascorbic Acid) Deficiency

Lump: Breast

Lump develops in the breast. Although this may often may be a harmless lump, medical help should be sought immediately to exclude serious disease.

POSSIBLE CONDITIONS
Cancer of the Breast

Duct Papilloma
Fat Necrosis in Breast
• Fibroadenoma
• Fibrocystic Disease
Mastitis
Metastasis

Lumps: Abdomen

A lump, mass or swelling which can be felt in the stomach or abdomen (apart from Pregnancy) is usually a sign of serious underlying disease.

POSSIBLE CONDITIONS
Aortic Aneurysm
Appendicitis
Cancer of the Bile Ducts
Cancer of the Bladder
Cancer of the Cervix
Cancer of the Colon or Rectum (Bowel)
Cancer of the Gall Bladder
Cancer of the Kidney
Cancer of the Liver
Cancer of the Ovaries
Cancer of the Pancreas
Cancer of the Stomach
Cancer of the Womb
Cirrhosis of the Liver
Diverticulitis
Enlarged Bladder
Gall Bladder Infection
Hepatitis
• Hernia, Inguinal
• Hernia, Umbilical
Injury to the Lower Chest or Pelvis
Jejunal Diverticulitis
Kala-azar

Leukaemia
Malaria
Myelofibrosis
Ovarian Cyst
Pancreatitis
Pregnancy
Tapeworms
Wilms' Tumour

Lumps: Back

Range of lumps from the small and numerous to a hump can affect the back. Causes range from Boils, Warts and Acne to more serious illness.

Possible Conditions
• Acne Vulgaris
• Boil
Cancer of the Skin
Carbuncle
Cellulitis
Kyphosis
Lipoma
Metastasis
Scoliosis
• Sebaceous Cyst
Spina Bifida
Tuberculosis
Warts

Lumps: Eyelid

Various types of lumps can develop on the eyelid. The most common are Styes or Warts, but there may be more serious problems.

Possible Conditions
Dacryocystitis

Infected Meibomian Cyst
Rodent Ulcer
• Stye
Warts

Lumps: Face

Nodules or bumps develop on the face, which may be caused by Gout or very rarely Leprosy.

Possible Conditions
• Acne Vulgaris
Gout
Leprosy
Metastases
Rodent Ulcer
Sarcoma
• Sebaceous cysts
Tuberculosis
Tumours of salivary glands
Tumours of sinuses

Lumps: In Ear

Lump or boil develops in the ear.

Possible Conditions
• Boil
Ear Polyp
Herpes Simplex
Ramsay-Hunt Syndrome

Lumps: Joint

Joints become inflamed with nodules, affecting either a few or many joints of the body. This is usually a problem with the joints themselves, and medical help should be sought.

POSSIBLE CONDITIONS
Alcohol or Narcotics
Bursitis
Charcot's Joints
•Gout
Hallux Rigidus
Hallux Valgus
•Osteoarthritis
Rheumatic Fever
•Rheumatoid Arthritis
Spina Bifida
Syphilis

Lumps: Mouth

Mouth (Aphthous) Ulcer or Ulcers are relatively common and are the most likely cause, although ulcers may also be present as a result of the Herpes virus. Unusually, this may be an indication of serious underlying disease.

POSSIBLE CONDITIONS
•Aphthous Ulcer
Behcet's Syndrome
Cancer of the Mouth
Cancrumoris
Crohn's Disease
Erythema Multiforme
Leukaemia
Pemphigus Vulgaris
Syphilis
Tuberculosis
Vincent's Angina

Lumps: Neck

Lumps or other swellings can develop on the neck. Most usually these are simply harmless boils or cysts, but they may be an indication of serious underlying illness, particularly if the area is swollen from structures within the neck rather than there being a distinct lump on the skin.

POSSIBLE CONDITIONS
•Boil
Carbuncle
Cervical Rib
Diffuse Thyroid Gland Enlargement
•Isolated Thyroid Nodule
Lipoma
•Lymph Node Enlargement
Pharyngeal Pouch
Ramsay-Hunt Syndrome
Sarcoidosis
Sarcoma
•Sebaceous Cyst
Squamous Cell Carcinoma
Sternomastoid Tumour
Submandibular Duct Stone
Submandibular Tumour
Thyroglossal Cyst
Tuberculosis

Lumps: On Ear

Lump or boil develops on the outside structure of the ear. Most usually this will be caused by Warts or Boils, but occasionally it may be a sign of serious illness. A very misshapen ear will often have been caused by repeated trauma.

POSSIBLE CONDITIONS
•Auricular Appendage
•Boil
Cancer of the Skin
Cauliflower Ear

Gout

Warts

Lumps: Skin

Most usually lumps found on the skin are caused by harmless conditions such as spots, pimples or warts. Occasionally it may be a sign of serious underlying disease.

POSSIBLE CONDITIONS

• Acne Vulgaris

• Boil

Cancer of the Skin

Carbuncle

Cat Scratch Fever

Dermoid Cysts

Ganglion

• Lipoma

Lymphoma

Metastasis

Molluscum Contagiosum

Pyogenic Granuloma

Rheumatoid Arthritus

Rodent Ulcer

Sarcoma

• Sebaceous Cyst

Squamous Cell Carcinoma

• Warts

Lumps: Swollen Lymph Nodes

The lymphatic system is used by the body to fight off infection and disease. When this is the case, lymph nodes become swollen, and if this only lasts for a few days it is of little significance. If lymph nodes remain swollen for a week or more, it may be the indication of serious underlying disease such as cancer.

POSSIBLE CONDITIONS

Adverse Drug Reaction

AIDS

Cancer of the Breast

Cancer of the Colon or Rectum (Bowel)

Cancer of the Larynx

Cancer of the Mouth

Cancer of the Nose

Cancer of the Prostate

Cancer of the Stomach

Cancer of the Womb

Cancer in the Chest

Cancrumoris

Cat Scratch Fever

Chancroid

Dental Infections

Diphtheria

Epiglottitis

• Glandular Fever

Hodgkin's Disease

Kala-azar

Leukaemia

Lung Cancer

Lymphangitis

Lymphoma

Metastases

Mumps

Peritonsillar Abscess

Ross River Fever

Rubella

Sarcoidosis

Squamous Cell Carcinoma

Submandibular Tumour

Syphilis

Tonsillitis

Toxoplasmosis

Tuberculosis
Vincent's Angina
•Viral Infection
Yaws

Lumps: Testicle and Scrotum

Lumps can develop on or in the testicles and the scrotum (the bag which holds the testicles). These are usually harmless, being minor infections or cysts, but any lumps on the testicles should be investigated.

POSSIBLE CONDITIONS
Cancer of the Testicles
•Epididymal Cyst
•Inguinal Hernia
Syphilis
Tuberculosis
•Varicocele

Lumps: Wrist

Lumps or swelling can develop on the wrist, usually because of the formation of a Ganglion or arthritis.

POSSIBLE CONDITIONS
•Ganglion
Osteoarthritis
Rheumatoid Arthritis
Tuberculosis

Mania

Frenetic and frantic behaviour including inability to sleep, rapid speech and thought, jittery, restlessness, sudden changes in topics of conversation, and even hallucinations.

POSSIBLE CONDITIONS
Adverse Drug Reaction
Alcohol or Narcotics
•Anxiety
Dementia
Depression and •Manic Depression
Hyperthyroidism
Schizophrenia

Memory: Poor or Reduced

Memory varies from individual to individual: some people are good at remembering faces and places, others names and phone numbers. The effectiveness of memory is generally agreed to reduce as individual get older. Elderly individuals, however, may not have a good short-term memory, while recalling minute details of their childhood.

POSSIBLE CONDITIONS
Alcohol or Narcotics
•Anxiety
•Dementia
Depression
Head Injury
Hypothyroidism
Stroke

Menstruation: Bleeding After Menopause

Older women who have gone through the Menopause may still experience periods of bleeding. This may also be a sign of an underlying problem.

POSSIBLE CONDITIONS
Cancer of the Cervix
Cancer of the Ovaries

• Cancer of the Womb
Cervical Polyp
• Menopause
Urethral Caruncle

Menstruation: Bleeding Between Periods

Bleeding, beyond what would be expected from periods, is experienced between menstruation. This may be a normal variation, but it may also be an indication of a miscarriage (see Pregnancy), Menopause, use of the Contraceptive Pill, and several other conditions.

POSSIBLE CONDITIONS
Cancer of the Cervix
Cancer of the Ovaries
Cancer of the Womb
• Cervical Polyp
Contraceptive Pill
• Erosion of the Cervix
Inflammation of the Vagina
Menopause
• Menstruation (normal variation)
Pregnancy
Urethral Caruncle

Menstruation: Delay in Starting

There is a delay in the onset of menstruation, most usually simply a normal variant between individuals, although this may be a sign of an underlying problem.

POSSIBLE CONDITIONS
Anorexia Nervosa
• Anxiety/Stress

Congenital Adrenal Hyperplasia
Cushing's Syndrome
• Menstruation (normal variation – some are later)
Polycystic Ovaries
Turner's Syndrome

Menstruation: Heavy

Periods are very heavy and produce a lot of blood, even with clots. The heaviness of periods does vary from individual to individual, but this may be a sign of an underlying problem.

POSSIBLE CONDITIONS
Cancer of the Cervix
Cancer of the Ovaries
Cancer of the Womb
Disorders of Blood Clotting
Endometriosis
• Fibroids
Hyperthyroidism
• Hypothyroidism
• Menstruation (normal variation)
Pelvic Inflammatory Disease
Pregnancy

Menstruation: Irregular

Periods should occur around every 28 days, although there is some variation from individual to individual, and periods may be irregular in girls who have only recently started menstruating. Irregular menstruation in older women may herald the onset of the Menopause. This can also be a sign of an underlying conditions, particularly if found in younger women.

POSSIBLE CONDITIONS

Cancer of the Cervix
Cancer of the Ovaries
Fibroids
Menopause (normal variation)
Menstruation (normal variation)
• Polycyctic Ovarian Syndrome
Prolactin Excess

Menstruation: Period Pain

Pain is experienced during the menstrual cycle, sometime quite severe in intensity. This may be a normal variant between individuals, but may also be an indication of an underlying condition.

POSSIBLE CONDITIONS
• Endometriosis
Fibroids
• Menstruation (normal variation)
Pelvic Inflammatory Disease

Menstruation: PMT

Pre-Menstrual Tension affects many women, although symptoms, and their severity, vary from individual to individual.

POSSIBLE CONDITIONS
Menstruation (normal variation)

Menstruation: Rare or Absent

Menstruation occurs rarely or is not present at all (in women of child-bearing age). This may happen in women who are very fit, those suffering from Anorexia Nervosa, Anxiety or from use of the Contraceptive Pill. Two other obvious causes are Pregnancy and Menopause, although the latter is more unlikely the younger the woman. This sign may

also be a symptom of underlying disease.

POSSIBLE CONDITIONS
• Anorexia Nervosa
• Anxiety/Stress
Congenital Adrenal Hyperplasia
Contraceptive Pill
Cushing's Syndrome
Excess of Prolactin
• Exercise
Hyperthyroidism
HypothalamicDisease
Hypothyroidism
• Low Body Weight
• Menopause (normal)
Pituitary Tumours
Polycystic Ovaries
• Pregnancy

Mental Impairment

Lack of mental faculties to deal with everyday living. This can either be because of an inherited condition from birth or acquired.

POSSIBLE CONDITIONS
• Cerebral Palsy
• Dementia
Friedreich's Ataxia
Head Injury
Hepatitis
Hydrocephalus
Kidney Disease or Failure
Malnutrition
Myxoedema
Phenylketonuria (PKU)
Stroke
Syphilis

91

Mouth: Cleft Lip or Palate

Birth defect resulting in a cleft lip and palate when tissues have not formed properly.

POSSIBLE CONDITIONS
Cleft Lip and Palate

Mouth: Difficult to Open

Opening the mouth is difficult or even impossible, caused either by extreme pain or inflammation of structures within the mouth. Causes range from the mild, such as Mouth Ulcers, to serious underlying problems.

POSSIBLE CONDITIONS
Aphthous Ulcer
Cold, Common
• Dental Infections
Glandular Fever
Mumps
Osteoarthritis
• Peritonsillar Abscess
Poisoning
Scleroderma
Tetanus
Tonsillitis
Tooth Decay and Abscess
Wisdom Teeth

Mouth: Dry

Mouth feeling dry is most likely to be caused by being dehydrated, through fear or anxiety, or because the individual habitually breathes through the mouth. It can also be caused by some antidepressants and as a result of anaesthetics. Rarely it is a sign of serious underlying disease.

POSSIBLE CONDITIONS
• Adverse Drug Reaction
• Anxiety
• Dehydration
Mouth Breathing
Salivary Gland Calculus
Sjogren's Syndrome
Uraemia

Mouth: General Infection

The tissues within the mouth, such as the tongue, gums, palate and the inside of the mouth, can become generally and severely infected. This is unusual and is caused by very poor oral and dental hygiene. Medical help should be sought immediately.

POSSIBLE CONDITIONS
Cancrumoris
• Candidiasis (may be due to other disease)
Vincent's Angina
• Poor Oral Hygiene

Mouth: Skin Around Mouth is Pale

Most usually a sign of Scarlet Fever.

POSSIBLE CONDITIONS
Scarlet Fever

Mouth: Ulcers

Mouth (Aphthous) Ulcer or Ulcers are relatively common and are the most likely cause, although ulcers may also be present as a result of the Herpes virus. Unusually, this may be an indication of serious underlying disease.

POSSIBLE CONDITIONS
• Aphthous Ulcer
Behcet's Syndrome
Cancer of the Mouth
Cancrumoris
Crohn's Disease
Erythema Multiforme
Leukaemia
Lupus
Pemphigus Vulgaris
Syphilis
Tuberculosis
Vincent's Angina

Mouth: White Spots (Mouth and Throat)

This is usually a sign of potentially serious conditions such as Thrush (Candidiasis), Tonsillitis or Measles. If the spots do not resolve and persist in the mouth, and cannot be easily removed, medical help should be sought.

POSSIBLE CONDITIONS
• Aphthous Ulcer
• Candidiasis
Leukoplakia
Lichen Planus
Measles
Tonsillitis

Muscle: Loss of Strength and Wasting

There is a prolonged and relentless wastage and reduction of strength in muscles, either generally throughout the body or one part of the body. This may be caused by any period of long-term physical inaction, such as being bedridden or having a limb immobilised. If there is no obvious cause such as this, medical help should be sought as this is a serious sign.

POSSIBLE CONDITIONS
Adverse Drug Reaction (including steroids)
• Alcohol or Narcotics
Bedridden
Brain Tumour
Guillain Barré Syndrome
Hyperthyroidism
Hypothyroidism
Motor Neurone Disease
Multiple Sclerosis
Muscular Dystrophy
Myopathy
Polio
Polymyositis
Rheumatoid Arthritis
Spinal Tumours or Compression
Steriod Use
• Stroke
Vitamin D Deficiency (Osteomatacia)

Muscle: Pain, Aches and Cramp

Pain, aches or cramps are experienced in muscles. The most common cause will be contact sports, vigorous exercise or injury caused by accidents. This should resolve in a few days. Feverish illness will also cause aching and muscle pain. Prolonged pain or aches without any obvious cause may be a sign of serious illness, although it is unlikely this will be the more obvious or serious of symptoms.

POSSIBLE CONDITIONS
Adverse Drug Reaction
Cholera

Cold, Common

Dermatomyositis

•Exercise

•Flu

•Fever

Heat Exhaustion

Lung Cancer

Meningitis

Meninogococcal Septicaemia

Menstruation

•Muscle Cramp

Muscle Injury

Peripheral Vascular Disease

Polymyalgia Rheumatica

Polymyositis

Post-Viral Syndrome

Q Fever

Rabies

Tetanus

•Viral Infection

Vitamin B1 (Thiamine) Deficiency

Muscle: Weak but No Wasting

Muscle bulk remains the same but the individual is very weak. This may be a serious symptoms, and if there is no obvious cause, then medical help should be sought.

POSSIBLE CONDITIONS

Aldosteronism

Cushing's Syndrome

Hypercalcaemia

Myopathy

Potassium Deficiency

Sarcoidosis

•Viral Infection

Nausea, Vomiting and Regurgitation of Food

Vomiting and nausea may result from a relatively mild cause — such as minor food poisoning (Gastroenteritis), drinking too much, travel sickness, Pregnancy or Migraines — to severe illness. Vomit will usually and initially consist of undigested food and is yellow, frothy and smells unpleasant, but persistent sickness results in the vomit becoming thin, green, mucousy and slimy. If vomit is brown, black or appears to have coffee grains, this is an indication that there is blood. See the relevant section on Vomit: Blood. In any event medical help should be sought should this be the case or if vomiting persists for a long time.

POSSIBLE CONDITIONS

Achalasia

Addison's Disease

Adverse Drug Reaction

Alcohol or Narcotics

Appendicitis

Biliary Colic

Botulism

Brain Abscess

Brain Tumours

Bulimia Nervosa

Cancer of the Oesophagus

Cancer of the Stomach

Chagas' Disease

Cholera

Cirrhosis of the Liver

Congenital Atresia of the Oesophagus

Diabetes

Diuretics

Dyspepsia, Non-Ulcer

Epididymitis
Gall Bladder Infection
Gall Stones
•Gastritis
•Gastroenteritis
Heat Exhaustion
Heat Stroke
•Hernia, Hiatus
Hernia, Inguinal (obstructed)
Hernia, Umbilical (obstructed)
Hypercalcaemia
Intestinal Ischaemia
Intestinal Obstruction
Kidney Disease or Failure
Kidney Stones
Meniere's Disease
Meningitis
Meninogococcal Septicaemia
Mesenteric Adenitis
Mesenteric Vascular Occlusion
Migraine
Mountain Sickness
Oesophageal Varices
Oesophagitis
Pancreatitis
Peptic Ulcer
Peritonitis
Phaeochromocytoma
Poisoning
Polio
Porphyria
Porphyria Cutanea Tarda
Post-Gastrectomy Syndrome
Pregnancy
Pyloric Stenosis
Raised Intracranial Pressure

Salpingitis
Sarcoidosis
Shock
Subarachnoid Haemorrhage
Torsion
Travel Sickness
Uraemia
Urinary Tract Infection
Vestibulitis

Neck: Lumps or Swellings

Lumps or other swellings can develop on the neck. Most usually these are simply harmless boils or cysts, but they may be an indication of serious underlying illness, particularly if the area is swollen from structures within the neck rather than there being a distinct lump on the skin.

POSSIBLE CONDITIONS
•Boil
Carbuncle
Cervical Rib
•Diffuse Thyroid Gland Enlargement
Isolated Thyroid Nodule
Lipoma
Pharyngeal Pouch
Sarcoma
•Sebaceous Cyst
Squamous Cell Carcinoma
Sternomastoid Tumour
Submandibular Duct Stone
Submandibular Tumour
Thyroglossal Cyst

Neck: Pain or Stiffness

Stiffness or pain in the neck, particularly if there are

SYMPTOMS SIGNS AND CONDITIONS

no other symptoms, is usually an indication of trauma to the structures in the neck, either slight, from sleeping awkwardly, or a serious whiplash injury. When combined with other symptoms, such as sensory changes in the limbs or severe headache and rash, it is a sign of serious illness. Meningitis may be a cause, in which case medical help should be sought immediately, and any persistent pain and stiffness should be investigated.

POSSIBLE CONDITIONS
Bursitis
Cervical Rib
Cervical Spine Infection
•Cervical Spondylosis
Meningitis
Meninogococcal Septicaemia
Polio
Prolapsed Cervical Disc
Rheumatoid Arthritis
Spinal Cord Tumours
Subarachnoid Haemorrhage
Thyroiditis
•Viral Infection
Whiplash Injury
Wryneck

Neck: Prominent Blood Vessels

This is usually a sign of serious underlying disease, and medical help should be sought and investigations undertaken.

POSSIBLE CONDITIONS
Asthma
Cancer in the Chest
•Chronic Bronchitis
Constrictive Pericarditis

•Heart Failure
Pericarditis
Pulmonary Fibrosis
Suffocation

Neck: Swollen Lymph Nodes

The lymphatic system is concerned with fighting infection, and enlarged lymph nodes or glands are usually a sign the body is fighting off infection, either localised to one area of the body or a general infection such as a Cold. More unusually it can be an indication of serious underlying disease, especially if the nodes remain enlarged for long periods, such as more than a couple of weeks, and there are other prolonged symptoms. Also see other sections on lymph nodes or glands.

POSSIBLE CONDITIONS
AIDS
Cancer of the Larynx
Cancer of the Mouth
Cancer in the Chest
Cancrumoris
Cold, Common
Dental Infections
Diphtheria
Epiglottitis
•Glandular Fever
Hodgkin's Disease
Leukaemia
Lymphoma
Mumps
Peritonsillar Abscess
•Rubella
Sarcoidosis
Squamous Cell Carcinoma

Submandibular Tumour
• Tonsillitis
Toxoplasmosis
Tuberculosis
Vincent's Angina
• Viral Infection

Night Blindness

Most individuals see much better in bright daylight than at night. Night blindness or greatly impaired vision in darker conditions will be exacerbated if the individual has poor eyesight. It may also be an indication of a lack of Vitamin A.

POSSIBLE CONDITIONS
Malnutrition
• Poor Eyesight
Retinitis Pigmentosa
• Vitamin A Deficiency

Nipple: Discharge

Discharge from the nipple. This may be caused by several conditions, and medical help should be sought unless the woman is pregnant or has a young baby. A discharge of milk from the breast is possible before giving birth.

POSSIBLE CONDITIONS
Breast Abscess
Cancer of Ducts in the Breast
Cancer of the Breast
Duct Ectasia
Duct Papilloma
• Excess of Prolactin
• Fibrocystic Disease of the Breast
Paget's Disease of the Nipple

• Pregnancy

Nipple: Retraction

Nipple is retracted. This may be a normal variation if present from birth, and should cause no problems except possibly for breast feeding. If a nipple becomes retracted in later life, this may be a sign of Breast Cancer.

POSSIBLE CONDITIONS
Cancer of the Breast
• Retraction of the Nipple

Nose: Blocked

Nose is blocked and it is difficult or impossible to breath through the nose. Most common causes are infections and injury to the nose. Medical help should be sought if there has been severe trauma to the nose as it may be broken.

POSSIBLE CONDITIONS
Adenoids
• Cold, Common
Foreign Body in Nose
Injury to the Nose
• Nasal Polyps
Rhinitis
Septal Deviation
Sinusitis

Nose: Misshapen

Most common cause for nose which is misshapen is a direct injury or a blow. Medical help should be sought if there has been severe trauma to the nose as it may be broken. Rarely this may be a sign of cancer, or even Leprosy.

POSSIBLE CONDITIONS
Cancer of the Nose
•Injury to the Nose
Leprosy
Nasal Septal Necrosis
Rhinophyma

Nose: No Sense of Smell

Individual has no or a very reduced sense of smell. The most likely cause is infection or allergy, such as Cold or Rhinitis. Occasionally, and if other signs of these conditions are not present, it may be an indication of injury, nerve or neurological problems.

POSSIBLE CONDITIONS
Adenoids
Brain Tumours
•Cold, Common
Foreign Body in Nose
Head Injury
Injury to the Nose
Nasal Polyps
•Rhinitis
Sinusitis
Smoking

Nose: Nosebleed

Nose bleeds are relatively common, and are rarely a sign of any serious problem. Medical help should be sought if there has been severe trauma to the nose as it may be broken. Prolonged bleeding from the nose for no apparent reason may be a cause for concern.

POSSIBLE CONDITIONS
Adverse Drug Reaction

Cancer of the Nose
Cold, Common
Disorders of Blood Clotting
Foreign Body in Nose
High Blood Pressure
•Injury to the Nose
Nasal Polyps
•Picking Nose
Sinusitis

Nose: Running

Nose runs with phlegm, either clear, yellow or green, watery or viscous. By far the most common causes are Cold, flu, Rhinitis and Hay Fever.

POSSIBLE CONDITIONS
Alcohol or Narcotics
Cancer of the Nose
•Cold, Common
Flu
Foreign Body in Nose
•Hay Fever
Nasal Polyps
•Rhinitis
Sinusitis

Nose: Very Red

Nose looks especially red, even when compared to the rest of the face.

POSSIBLE CONDITIONS
•Acne Rosacea
Erysipelas
Rhinophyma
Staphylococcal Infection of the Nose

PMT

Pre-Menstrual Tension affects many women, although symptoms, and their severity, vary from individual to individual.

POSSIBLE CONDITIONS
• Menstruation

Pain: Abdomen (Severe and Persistent)

Severe and persistent pain in the abdomen is usually a sign of serious disease, and medical help should be sought immediately.

POSSIBLE CONDITIONS
Abcess (abdominal, bowel, kidney, pancreas, liver)
Aortic Aneurysm
Bladder Neck Obstruction
Cholangitis
Crohn's Disease
Diverticulitis
• Gastritis
Injury to the Lower Chest or Pelvis
Intestinal Ischaemia
Mesenteric Vascular Occlusion
Pancreatitis
Peptic Ulcer
Perforated Viscus
Peritonitis
Pyelonephritis
Salpingitis
Ulcerative Colitis
Urinary Tract Infection
Vertebral Collapse/Fracture

Pain: Abdomen (Severe and Intermittent)

Severe pain in the abdomen which appears to resolve but then recurs. If this goes on for any length of time, particularly if not associated with food poisoning or similar condition, medical help should be sought immediately.

POSSIBLE CONDITIONS
• Biliary Colic
• Constipation
Crohn's Disease
Diverticulitis
Fibroids
Injury to the Lower Chest or Pelvis
Intestinal Obstruction
Irritable Bladder
Jejunal Diverticulitis
• Kidney Stones
Peptic Ulcer
Ulcerative Colitis
Urinary Tract Infection
Vertebral Collapse/Fracture

Pain: Abdomen and Collapse

Collapse in any individual is a serious condition, and combined with abdominal pain can indicate a variety of conditions. Also see the sections on Collapse, Fever and Abdominal Pain. Some of the conditions which can cause collapse are listed below.

POSSIBLE CONDITIONS
Cholangitis
Crohn's Disease
Diverticular Abcess
Gall Bladder Infection

Gastroenteritis
Intestinal Ischaemia
Intestinal Obstruction
Pancreatitis
Perforated Peptic Ulcer
• Perforated Viscus
Septicaemia
Ulcerative Colitis

Pain: Abdomen and Constipation

A sign of inflammatory bowel disease or Irritable Bowel Syndrome. Also consult the sections on Constipation and on Abdominal Pain.

POSSIBLE CONDITIONS
Adverse Drug Reaction
Bowel Cancer
Crohn's Disease
Hypercalcaemia
Intestinal Obstruction
• Irritable Bowel Syndrome
Peritonitis

Pain: Abdomen and Diarrhoea

Usually an indication of minor food poisoning or Gastroenteritis, but may be a sign of serious disease.

POSSIBLE CONDITIONS
Adverse Drug Reaction
Cancer of the Colon or Rectum (Bowel)
Carcinoid Syndrome
Cholera
Crohn's Disease
Dysentery
• Gastroenteritis

Henoch's Purpura
Intestinal Ischaemia
• Irritable Bowel Syndrome
Jejunal Diverticulitis
Pancreatitis
Phaeochromocytoma
Post-Gastrectomy Syndrome
Typhoid Fever
Ulcerative Colitis

Pain: Abdominal and Persistent Weight Loss

Pain in the abdomen and long-term weight loss may be a sign of serious disease, and medical help should be sought.

POSSIBLE CONDITIONS
Cancer of the Colon or Rectum (Bowel)
Cancer of the Kidney
Cancer of the Liver
Cancer of the Pancreas
Cancer of the Stomach
• Coeliac Disease
• Crohn's Disease
Diabetes
Metastases
Pancreatitis
• Peptic Ulcer
Ulcerative Colitis

Pain: Abdominal and Vomiting

An indication of minor food poisoning or Gastroenteritis, but may be a sign of serious disease.

POSSIBLE CONDITIONS
Adverse Drug Reaction
Appendicitis
Biliary Colic
Cancer of the Stomach
Cholecystitis
Diabetes
• Gastroenteritis
Hernia, Inguinal (obstructed)
Hernia, Umbilical (obstructed)
Intestinal Ischaemia
Intestinal Obstruction
Kidney Disease or Failure
Kidney Stones
Meckel's Diverticulum
Mesenteric Adenitis
Ovarian Cyst
Pancreatitis
• Peptic Ulcer
Peritonitis
Porphyria
Salpingitis

Pain: Abdominal and Vomiting Blood

A sign of serious underlying disease, and medical help should be sought.

POSSIBLE CONDITIONS
Adverse Drug Reaction
Blood Clotting Disorders
Cancer of the Oesophagus
Cancer of the Stomach
Cirrhosis of the Liver
• Gastritis
Hernia, Hiatus
Mallory-Weiss Tear

Oesophageal Varices
Oesophagitis
• Peptic Ulcer
• Yellow Fever

Pain: Abdominal and Vomiting and Fever

An indication of food poisoning, Gastroenteritis or Urinary Tract Infection, but may be a sign of serious disease.

POSSIBLE CONDITIONS
Abcess
Appendicitis
Cholecystitis
Gall Stones
• Gastroenteritis
Intestinal Obstruction
Meckel's Diverticulum
Pancreatitis
Pelvic Inflammatory Disease
Porphyria
Septicaemia
• Urinary Tract Infection
• Viral Infection

Pain: Abdominal and Vomiting and Jaundice

Combination of symptoms which indicates serious illness. Medical help should be sought immediately.

POSSIBLE CONDITIONS
• Biliary Colic
Cancer of the Liver
Cancer of the Pancreas
Cancer of the Stomach

- Cholecystitis
- Gall Stones
Hepatitis
Pancreatitis
Sickle Cell Anaemia

Pain: Ankle

Pain is experienced in or around the ankle, and the joint is weak or cannot bear weight. This is most likely an indication of injury or fracture of the ankle.

POSSIBLE CONDITIONS
Broken Ankle
Cellulitis
- Injury to the Ankle

Pain: Back

Back pain is very common, but can be very severe in intensity. It may be caused by a huge range of conditions, from simple strain, Slipped Disc or Period Pain to cancer and Tuberculosis. Pain is not always related to severity.

POSSIBLE CONDITIONS
Ankylosing Spondylitis
- Back Strain
Cancer of the Cervix
Cancer of the Ovaries
Cancer of the Spine
Cancer of the Womb
Cauda Equine Syndrome
- Cervical Spondylosis
Coccydynia
Crohn's Disease
Kyphosis
- Menstruation

- Osteoarthritis
Osteoporosis
Pancreatitis
Pelvic Inflammatory Disease
Peptic Ulcer
Sciatica
Scoliosis
Shingles
- Slipped Disc
Spinal Cord Injury
Tuberculosis
Ulcerative Colitis
Urinary Tract Infection
Vertebral Fracture
Vitamin D (Calciferol) Deficiency

Pain: Bone

Pain is experienced in bones. The most obvious cause is injury or fracture , although this may be a sign of serious illness such as cancer or Tuberculosis.

POSSIBLE CONDITIONS
Ankylosing Spondylitis
- Broken Bone
Broken Collarbone
Broken Lower Arm Bones (Radius, Ulna and wrist)
Broken Upper Arm Bone (Humerus)
Cancer of the Bones
Cushing's Syndrome
Dengue
Hypercalcaemia
Hyperparathyroidism
- Injury
Metastases
Osteoarthritis

Osteomyelitis
Osteoporosis (with fracture)
Rheumatoid Arthritis
Tuberculosis (of bone)
Vitamin D (Calciferol) Deficiency

Pain: Breast

Pain is experienced in or around the breast. This will usually be because of changes during a woman's menstrual cycle or Pregnancy, but may be a sign of an underlying condition.

POSSIBLE CONDITIONS
Breast Abscess
• Fibrocystic Disease
Injury
Mastitis
• Menstruation
Pregnancy

Pain: Chest (Persistent or Recurrent)

Persistent or recurrent pain, which may be severe, but varies in intensity over a prolonged period. This may be mild, but it can also be the indication of serious underlying problems.

POSSIBLE CONDITIONS
Angina
Aortic Aneurysm
Chest Infection
Chest Injury
Chondritis
Fibromyalgia
Gall Bladder Infection
Gall Stones
Heart Attack

Heart Disease
Hernia, Hiatus
Lung Abscess
Lung Cancer
Mesothelioma
Oesophagitis
Pancreatitis
Peptic Ulcer
Pericarditis
Pleurisy
Pneumonia

Pain: Chest (Sudden Onset)

The sudden onset of severe pain, particularly if concentrated in the centre of the chest but radiates into the left arm or jaw, may be the sign of a Heart Attack. Other problems, some milder, some as severe, can also cause sudden chest pain.

POSSIBLE CONDITIONS
• Angina
Aortic Aneurysm
• Chest Injury
Heart Attack
Nerve Irritation in Chest
Oesophaged Spasm
Oesophagitis
Pancreatitis
Peptic Ulcer
Pericarditis
• Pleurisy
Pneumothorax
Pulmonary Embolism
Viral Infection

Pain: Chest and Breathlessness

A combination of symptoms which may indicate a serious or even life-threatening condition, such as a Heart Attack, Pleurisy or Lung Cancer.

POSSIBLE CONDITIONS
Aortic Aneurysm
• Chest Infection
• Heart Attack and Failure
Heart Disease
Lung Abscess
Lung Cancer
Pericarditis
Pleurisy
• Pneumonia
Pneumothorax
Pulmonary Embolism

Pain: Chest, Bloody Phlegm and Chest Pain

Chest pain combined with a cough, which also produces phlegm, which may be yellow or green in colour, but is also streaked or contains blood. This is most usually the result of a serious problem such as severe and prolonged Chest Infections, Pneumonia or Lung Cancer. Medical help should be sought as soon as possible.

POSSIBLE CONDITIONS
• Chest Infection
Chest Injury
Lung Cancer
• Pneumonia
Pulmonary Embolism
Q Fever

Pain: Chest, No Appetite and Weight Loss

Combination of symptoms which often indicates a serious underlying disease.

POSSIBLE CONDITIONS
Bone Cancer
Cancer of the Stomach
• Chest Infection
Gall Bladder Infection
Metastases
Lung Cancer
Mesothelioma
Oesophagitis
• Pneumonia
Peptic Ulcer
Tuberculosis

Pain: Ear

Earache and pain, experienced in or around the ear. This may be caused by conditions ranging from relatively mild to very severe, and pain may be referred from the teeth or mouth. Severe and prolonged pain should prompt a visit to the doctor or dentist.

POSSIBLE CONDITIONS
• Boil
Cancer of the Ear
Cancer of the Mouth
• Cold, Common
Dental Infections
• Ear Infection
Ear Wax
Eustachian Catarrh
Inner Ear Infection

Mastoiditis
Perichondritis
Ramsay-Hunt Syndrome
Rodent Ulcer
Tonsillitis
Tooth Decay and Abscess
Trigeminal Neuralgia
•Viral Infection

Pain: Elbow

Pain is experienced in or around the elbow. This will usually be caused either by an injury, arthritis or fracture, or damage to nerves.

POSSIBLE CONDITIONS
Broken Lower Arm Bones (Radius, Ulna and wrist)
Broken Upper Arm Bone (Humerus)
Bursitis
Gout
•Injury
Osteoarthritis
Rheumatoid Arthritis
•Tennis Elbow
Ulnar Nerve

Pain: Eye (Acute)

Severe pain in the eye or eyes should not be ignored as it may be the sign of a serious problem. A foreign body in or injury to the eye can cause pain, and there are also several conditions causing the same sign, including Glaucoma and Iritis.

POSSIBLE CONDITIONS
•Conjunctivitis
Corneal Ulcer
•Foreign Body in Eye

Glaucoma
Injury to the Eye
Iritis
Multiple Sclerosis
Retrobulbar Neuritis
Shingles

Pain: Eye (Mild)

Mild pain in the eye is not uncommon, and may have innocent causes, such as rubbing the eye too much or being in a very dry atmosphere. Flu, Colds, infections or feverish illness will also make the eyes sore. This may also be the sign of serious illness.

POSSIBLE CONDITIONS
Cancer of the Eye
Cold, Common
•Conjunctivitis
Dacryocystitis
•Eye Strain
Fever
Flu
Glaucoma
Optic Neuritis
Sinusitis

Pain: Face

Facial pain may be an indication of many conditions, including dental problems, pain referred to the face from other parts of the body, nerve problems or even cancer.

POSSIBLE CONDITIONS
Bell's Palsy
Cancer of the Mouth
Cancer of the Nose

Dental Infections
Migraine
Paget's Disease
Post-Herpetic Neuralgia
•Sinusitis
Temporal Arteritis
Tooth Decay and Abscess
Trigeminal Neuralgia

Pain: Foot

Pain is experienced in the foot. This may be caused by relatively minor conditions such as Veruccas (Warts) or an Ingrown Toenail, but may also have more serious causes.

POSSIBLE CONDITIONS
Abcess
Athlete's Foot
Cellulitis
Gout
Hallux Rigidus
Hallux Valgus
Ingrown Toenail
Injury
Morton's Metatarsalgia
•Osteoarthritis
Peripheral Neuropathy
Pes Cavus
Plantar Fasciitis
Warts

Pain: General and Recurrent

Pain in different parts of the body or general aches or pains. This pain is constant or recurs and remits. Pain thresholds vary from individual to individual, and some people may constantly complain of general aches and pains without there being any identifiable underlying disease.

POSSIBLE CONDITIONS
Arthitis
Depression and Manic Depression
Diabetes
Fractures
Gout
Hyperparathyroidism
•Osteoarthritis
Polymyalgia Rheumatica
Rheumatoid Arthritis
Sickle Cell Anaemia
Syphilis
Viral Infection
Vitamin D Deficiency

Pain: Head and Fever

Usually will be a sign of viral infection such as a Cold or Flu, but may be an indication of more serious illness.

POSSIBLE CONDITIONS
Brain Abscess
Brucellosis
•Cold, Common
•Flu
Glandular Fever
Malaria
Meningitis
Meninogococcal Septicaemia
•Sinusitis
Temporal Arteritis
Typhus Fever
•Viral Infection
Weil's Disease

Pain: Head and Headache

Headaches are very common, and are usually only an indication that the individual is suffering from tiredness, stress or tension, Migraine or toothache. Occasionally headache may be a sign of serious underlying disease, but this will usually be combined with other symptoms.

POSSIBLE CONDITIONS
Adverse Drug Reaction
Alcohol or Narcotics
Anxiety
Brain Abscess
Brain Tumours
Carbon Monoxide Poisoning
Cluster Headache
Cold, Common
Dental Infections
Erythema Multiforme
Fever
Flu
Gastroenteritis
• Head Injury
Heat Exhaustion
Heat Stroke
High Blood Pressure
Laryngitis
Meningitis
Meninogococcal Septicaemia
Menopause
Menstruation
• Migraine
Mountain Sickness
Nasal Septal Necrosis
Pharyngitis
Pituitary Tumour

Poisoning
Polycythaemia
Pyorrhoea Alveolaris
Q Fever
Raised Intracranial Pressure
Sinusitis
Sleeping Sickness
Stroke
Subarachnoid Haemorrhage
Subdural Haemorrhage
Teething Pain
Temporal Arteritis
• Tension Headache
Tonsillitis
Tooth Decay and Abscess
Typhoid Fever
Typhus Fever
• Viral Infection
Yellow Fever

Pain: Headache and Tiredness

Combination of symptoms which indicate a headache caused by tiredness, tension or stress, and there is rarely any more sinister cause. It may also be the onset of a feverish illness. This is a sign of a serious underlying illness, although it will rarely be the most pressing of symptoms.

POSSIBLE CONDITIONS
Adverse Drug Reaction
Anxiety
Brain Abcess
Brain Tumours
Carbon Monoxide Poisoning
Cluster Headache
Cold, Common

Dental Infection
Fever
High Blood Pressure
Meningitis
Menigococcal Septicaemia
Menstruation
Migraine
Mountain Sickness
Pituitary Tumour
Poisoning
Polycythaemia
Sinusitis
Subarachnoid Haemorrhage
Temporal Arteritis
Viral Infection

Pain: Headache, Chills and Fever

Most usually the symptoms of a viral illness, normally mild but occasionally there may be a serious underlying condition. If there are further symptoms affecting other parts of the body, also consult those sections, as well as tropical fevers and fever.

POSSIBLE CONDITIONS
Chest Infection
•Cold, Common
•Flu
Lung Abscess
Malaria
Meningitis
Mumps
Osteomyelitis
Septicaemia
Temporal Arteritis
Typhus Fever
•Viral Infection

Pain: Headache, Running Nose and Sore Eyes

Combination of symptoms which usually indicates the Common Cold, but there are other conditions, some mild, some serious, which can also fit these symptoms.

POSSIBLE CONDITIONS
Cancer of the Nose
•Cold, Common
Foreign Body in Nose
•Hay Fever
Head Injury
Nasal Polyps
Rhinitis
Sinusitis

Pain: Hip

Pain is experienced in or around the hip, often either from injury, fracture or dislocation, or from arthritis – or a combination.

POSSIBLE CONDITIONS
Acquired Dislocation of the Hip
Congenital Dislocation of the Hip (CDH)
Fracture of the Hip
Infective Dislocation of the Hip
Irritable Hip
•Osteoarthritis
Osteoporosis (hip fracture)
Perthes' Disease
Rheumatoid Arthritis
Slipped Epiphysis
Subluxation of the Hip
Tuberculosis

Pain: Joint

Joints become painful or inflamed, or both, affecting either a few or many joints of the body. This may be caused by a range of conditions, some relatively mild such as Colds and Flu, others much more serious. Any long-term problem should prompt a visit to a doctor. In many of the conditions, this will not be the only symptom: there will be other signs of illness from an infection. If there is no obvious infection, pain or inflammation, then medical help should be sought.

POSSIBLE CONDITIONS
Allergic Alveolitis
Ankylosing Spondylitis
Behcet's Syndrome
Cat Scratch Fever
Chondritis
Cold, Common
Endocarditis
Flu
Gastroenteritis
Gonorrhoea
Gout
Haemophilia
Henoch's Purpura
•Injury
Osteoarthritis
Psoriasis
Reiter's Disease
Rheumatic Fever
Rheumatoid Arthritis
Ross River Fever
Sickle Cell Anaemia
Syphilis
Systemic Lupus Erythematosis (SLE)

Torn Cartilage
Typhus Fever
•Viral Infection

Pain: Knee

Pain experienced in or around the knee. The most likely cause is going to be injury or damage to the structures of the knee, including ligaments and cartilage.

POSSIBLE CONDITIONS
Arthritis
Bursitis
Cartilage Tear (Knee)
Dislocation of the Knee
Dislocation of the Knee Cap
Fractures of the Knee Cap (Patella)
Fractures of the Lower Leg (femur, tibia and fibula)
•Gout
Injury
•Ligamentous Tear (Knee)
Trauma
Osteoarthritis
Upper Tibial Epiphysis and Apophysis

Pain: Menstruation

Pain is experienced during the menstrual cycle, sometime quite severe in intensity. This may be a normal variant between individuals, but may also be an indication of an underlying condition.

POSSIBLE CONDITIONS
Endometriosis
Fibroids
•Menstruation
Pelvic Inflammatory Disease

Pain: Muscle

Pain, aches or cramps are experienced in muscles. The most common cause will be contact sports, vigorous exercise or injury caused by accidents. This should resolve in a few days. Feverish illness will also cause aching and muscle pain. Prolonged pain or aches without any obvious cause may be a sign of serious illness, although it is unlikely this will be the more obvious or serious of symptoms.

POSSIBLE CONDITIONS
Adverse Drug Reaction
Cholera
•Cold, Common
Dermatomyositis
Exercise
•Fever
Flu
Heat Exhaustion
Lung Cancer
Meningitis
Meninogococcal Septicaemia
•Menstruation
Muscle Cramp
•Muscle Injury
Peripheral Vascular Disease
Polymyalgia Rheumatica
Polymyositis
•Post-Viral Syndrome
Q Fever
Rabies
Tetanus
•Viral Infection
Vitamin B1 (Thiamine) Deficiency

Pain: Neck Pain or Stiffness

Stiffness or pain in the neck, particularly if there are no other symptoms, is usually an indication of trauma to the structures in the neck, either slight, from sleeping awkwardly, or a serious whiplash injury. When combined with other symptoms, such as sensory changes in the limbs or severe headache and rash, it is a sign of serious illness. Meningitis may be a cause, in which case medical help should be sought immediately, and any persistent pain and stiffness should be investigated.

POSSIBLE CONDITIONS
Cervical Rib
Cervical Spine Infection
•Cervical Spondylosis
Meningitis
Meninogococcal Septicaemia
Osteoarthritis
Prolapsed Cervical Disc
Rheumatoid Arthritis
Spinal Cord Tumours
Subarachnoid Haemorrhage
Thyroiditis
•Viral Infection
Whiplash Injury
•Wryneck

Pain: Penis

Penis becomes painful, usually caused by an infection or direct injury to the organ. Less commonly this may be a sign of serious illness.

POSSIBLE CONDITIONS
•Balanitis
Cancer of the Penis

Chlamydia
Gonorrhoea
• Injury to the Penis
Kidney Stones
Non-Specific Urethritis
Paraphimosis
Peyronie's Disease
Phimosis
Urinary Tract Infection

Pain: Period

Pain is experienced during the menstrual cycle, sometime quite severe in intensity. This may be a normal variant between individuals, but may also be an indication of an underlying condition.

POSSIBLE CONDITIONS
Endometriosis
Fibroids
• Menstruation
Pelvic Inflammatory Disease

Pain: Rectum or Anus

Pain around the rectum or anus can be caused by passing hard faeces or anal intercourse: either of these can damage the wall of the bowel. Piles (haemorrhoids) may also be extremely painful. This may also be a sign of a more serious underlying condition.

POSSIBLE CONDITIONS
Anal Abscess
Anal Fissure
Crohn's Disease
Diabetes
• Fistula-In-Ano

Injury
• Piles

Pain: Sex

Pain is experienced during sexual intercourse. This is most commonly because of tension in the woman, but less usually is a sign of some underlying condition.

POSSIBLE CONDITIONS
Cancer of the Vagina
Candidiasis
Endometriosis
Failure to Orgasm
Herpes Simplex
Menopause (dryness of vagina)
Salpingitis
• Vaginismus

Pain: Shoulder

Pain is experienced in or around the shoulder. This may be caused most obviously by injury or fracture, but may be a sign of serious illness.

POSSIBLE CONDITIONS
Broken Collarbone
Broken Upper Arm Bone (Humerus)
• Cervical Spondylitis
Frozen Shoulder
Gout
Injury
• Osteoarthritis
Painful Arc Syndrome (Shoulder)
Polymyalgia Rheumatica
Prolapsed Cervical Disc
Rheumatoid Arthritis

Rotator Cuff Tear (Shoulder)
Shoulder Dislocation
Tuberculosis

Pain: Swallowing Problems

Pain in the throat combined with swallowing problems is most usually an indication of an infection, such as Tonsillitis or Laryngitis. Rarely it is a sign of serious underlying disease, such as cancer, particularly if there is also prolonged weight loss and poor appetite, and long-term hoarseness.

POSSIBLE CONDITIONS
Cancer of the Larynx
Cancer of the Lung
Cancer of the Oesophagus
Candidiasis
Diphtheria
Epiglottitis
Herpes Simplex
Laryngitis
Ludwig's Angina
Oesophageal Pouch
Oesophageal Spasm
•Oesophageal Stricture
Oesophagitis
Peritonsillar Abscess
Pharyngitis
Scleroderma
Shingles
•Tonsillitis
•Viral Infection

Pain: Testicle

Several conditions can cause pain in the testicles, not least a kick or blow in the groin. This can be exquisitely painful to begin with, and ache for some little time afterwards. As long as there is normal urine with no blood, this will resolve.

POSSIBLE CONDITIONS
Cancer of the Testicle
Epididymitis
•Hernia, Inguinal
Hydrocele
Kidney Stones
Mumps
•Orchitis
Pancreatitis
•Torsion
Varicocele

Pain: Throat and Fever

Usually an indication of common infections, such as Colds, Tonsillitis or Laryngitis, although occasionally this combination may be associated with more serious conditions.

POSSIBLE CONDITIONS
Adverse Drug Reaction
Cancrumoris
•Cold, Common
Dental Infections
•Flu
Glandular Fever
Laryngitis
Ludwig's Angina
Pharyngitis
Rabies
Rheumatic Fever
Tonsillitis
Tracheitis
Vincent's Angina

• Viral Infection

Pain: Urinating

Sign of Cystitis or Urinary Tract Infections, although it may be an indication of more serious illness.

POSSIBLE CONDITIONS
Bilharzia
Cystitis
Gonorrhoea
Kidney Disease or Failure
Non-Specific Urethritis
Prostatitis
• Urinary Tract Infection

Pain: Urinating and Blood in Urine

Most likely cause is Cystitis or Urinary Tract Infections, but it may be an indication of more serious illness.

POSSIBLE CONDITIONS
Bilharzia
Cystitis
Kidney Disease or Failure
Kidney Stones
Prostatitis
• Urinary Tract Infection

Pain: Vagina

Pain is experienced in or around the vagina. If this is persistent, then it is likely to be an indication of a potentially serious problem. Medical help should be sought, even if only to exclude any disease.

POSSIBLE CONDITIONS
Cancer of the Vagina

Candidiasis
Chlamydia
Endometriosis
Gardnerella
Gonorrhoea
Herpes Simplex
Menopause (dryness of vagina)
Pelvic Inflammatory Disease
Trichomonas
• Vaginitis
• Vaginismus

Pain: Wrist

Pain is experienced in or around the wrist. This will usually be caused either by an injury, arthritis or fracture, or damage to nerves.

POSSIBLE CONDITIONS
Broken Lower Arm Bones (Radius, Ulna and wrist)
Menstruation
• Osteoarthritis
Rheumatoid Arthritis
Synovitis
Tuberculosis
• Wrist Sprain

Palpitations

The heart beats at a regular, but much faster, rate than seems normal, although it is always difficult for an individual to gauge their own heart beat. This will usually have an innocent cause, such as vigorous exercise, nerves or anxiety. If, however, the rate does not return to normal when exercise or anxiety ceases, it may be a sign of serious underlying disease. There will usually be other symptoms.

POSSIBLE CONDITIONS
Adverse Drug Reaction
Alcohol or Narcotics
Allergic Reaction, Severe
Anaemia
• Anxiety
• Atrial Fibrillation
Bleeding
• Caffeine
Cardiomyopathy
• Cigarettes
Constrictive Pericarditis
Diphtheria
Exercise
Fever
Flu
Heart Attack and Failure
Heart Disease
Heat Exhaustion
Heat Stroke
Hyperthyroidism
Myocarditis
Paroxysmal Tachycardia
Pernicious Anaemia
Phaeochromocytoma
Polymyositis
Porphyria
Pregnancy
Rheumatic Fever
Shock
Vitamin B1 (Thiamine) Deficiency

Paralysis: Rapid Onset

Part of the body becomes paralysed and cannot be moved. The arm or leg is most likely affected, but it may be the eye, swallowing or even breathing. This is rarely a minor problem, and medical help should always be sought.

POSSIBLE CONDITIONS
Brain Abscess
Brain Tumours
Encephalitis
Guillain-Barre Syndrome
Head Injury
Hysteria
Multiple Sclerosis
Intracranial Haemorrhage
Periodic Paralysis
Peripheral Vascular Disease
Polio
Rabies
Spinal Cord Injury
Spinal Cord Tumours
• Stroke
Subarachnoid Haemorrhage

Paralysis: Slow Onset

Paralysis in part of the body, although it takes some time to develop. This will not normally be the only sign that something is wrong, and medical help should be sought.

POSSIBLE CONDITIONS
Brain Tumours
• Guillain-Barre Syndrome
Huntington's Chorea
Intracranial Haemorrhage
Motor Neurone Disease
Multiple Sclerosis
Nerve Injury
Polio
Spinal Cord Tumours

Vitamin B12 (Cyanocobalamin) Deficiency

Passing Out

The individual passes out for a short time, caused by flow of blood to the brain being interrupted. This usually has a simple and harmless cause, such as standing for too long, too little food, or not having enough sleep. It may also be a sign of serious underlying disease.

POSSIBLE CONDITIONS
• Anxiety
Aortic Stenosis
Atrial Fibrillation
Bleeding
Cardiomyopathy
Constrictive Pericarditis
Epilepsy
• Faint
Heart Attack
Heart Block
Heart Disease
Heat Exhaustion
• Low Blood Pressure
Mountain Sickness
Paroxysmal Tachycardia
Pregnancy
Sick Sinus Syndrome
Stroke

Penis: Curved

It is not unusual for the penis to be slightly curved, and this will not normally cause any problems. In rare cases, it can be so curved that sexual intercourse is difficult or impossible. This can be rectified by surgery.

POSSIBLE CONDITIONS
Peyronie's Disease

Penis: Discharge

It is not normal for the penis to have a discharge other than sperm, seminal fluid or urine. Residual fluid can occur some time after sex or ejaculation, and it is possible for a man to have some seminal fluid without ejaculating. Any persistent clear or coloured discharge, however, not occurring because of sexual activity is probably from a sexually transmitted disease.

POSSIBLE CONDITIONS
Balanitis
Cancer of the Penis
• Chlamydia
Epididymitis
Gonorrhoea
• Non-Specific Urethritis
Trichomonas
Urinary Tract Infection

Penis: Foreskin Problems

Foreskin of the penis can become infected, causing cracking and scar tissue. This may make urinating or sexual intercourse difficult and painful.

POSSIBLE CONDITIONS
Balanitis
Cancer of the Penis
• Paraphimosis
• Phimosis

Penis: Impotence or Difficulty Maintaining Erection

Many men suffer problems with impotence and maintaining an erection from time to time, especially if they are tired, drunk, stressed or suffering from any debilitating illness. As men get older, it also takes them longer to regain an erection after ejaculation. It is generally thought that problems with impotence are usually psychological in nature, especially if problems are only experienced with one partner. There are possible physical causes as well, such as blood flow problems, neurological disease, damage to nerves following surgery, and problems with hormones. Psychological causes such as depression or tension within a relationship may be helped by counselling.

POSSIBLE CONDITIONS
• Adverse Drug Reaction
• Alcohol or Narcotics
• Artery Disease
Cushing's Syndrome
Damage to Testicles
Depression and Manic Depression
• Diabetes
• Hypogonadism
Hypopituitarism
Multiple Sclerosis
Prolactin Excess

Penis: Pain

Penis becomes painful, usually caused by an infection or direct injury to the organ. Less commonly this may be a sign of serious illness.

POSSIBLE CONDITIONS
• Balanitis
Cancer of the Penis
Chlamydia
Gonorrhoea
• Injury to the Penis
Kidney Stones
Non-Specific Urethritis
• Paraphimosis
Peyronie's Disease
• Phimosis
Urinary Tract Infection

Penis: Premature Ejaculation

Premature ejaculation is ejaculation sooner than intended or is desirable. It is actually difficult to define exactly when this is, and the level of excitement may be a factor. Generally, premature ejaculation does not give the partner time to achieve satisfaction.

POSSIBLE CONDITIONS
Premature Ejaculation
• Psychological

Penis: Prolonged Erection

Most men will get an erection when they are sexually aroused. It is possible that an erection can occur with no sexual desire, and is maintained despite the circumstances. In most cases this is not anything sinister, and may be a result of heavy sexual activity. If an erection does not subside, tests may be needed to exclude any underlying disease.

POSSIBLE CONDITIONS
• Adverse Drug Reaction

• Clotting Problems
Leukaemia
Sickle Cell Anaemia

Period: Bleeding Between Periods

Bleeding, beyond what would be expected from periods, is experienced between menstruation. This may be a normal variation, but it may also be an indication of a miscarriage (see Pregnancy), Menopause, use of the Contraceptive Pill, and several other conditions.

POSSIBLE CONDITIONS
Cancer of the Cervix
Cancer of the Ovaries
Cancer of the Womb
• Cervical Polyp
Contraceptive Pill
Erosion of the Cervix
Inflammation of the Vagina
• Menopause
• Menstruation (normal)
Pregnancy
Urethral Caruncle

Period: Heavy

Periods are very heavy and produce a lot of blood, even with clots. The heaviness of periods does vary from individual to individual, but this may be a sign of an underlying problem.

POSSIBLE CONDITIONS
Cancer of the Cervix
Cancer of the Ovaries
Cancer of the Womb
Disorders of Blood Clotting

Endometriosis
• Fibroids
Hypothyroidism
Menopause
• Menstruation (normal)
Pelvic Inflammatory Disease
Pregnancy

Period: Irregular

Periods should occur around every 28 days, although there is some variation from individual to individual, and periods may be irregular in girls who have only recently started menstruating. Irregular menstruation in older women may herald the onset of the Menopause. This can also be a sign of an underlying conditions, particularly if found in younger women.

POSSIBLE CONDITIONS
Cancer of the Cervix
Cancer of the Womb
Fibroids
• Menopause
• Menstruation (normal)
• Polycystic Ovary Syndrome

Period: Rare or Absent

Menstruation occurs rarely or is not present at all (in women of child-bearing age). This may happen in women who are very fit, those suffering from Anorexia Nervosa, Anxiety or from use of the Contraceptive Pill. Two other obvious causes are Pregnancy and Menopause, although the latter is more unlikely the younger the woman. This sign may also be a symptom of underlying disease.

POSSIBLE CONDITIONS
- Anorexia Nervosa
- Anxiety

Congenital Adrenal Hyperplasia

Contraceptive Pill

Cushing's Syndrome

Excess of Prolactin
- Exercise

Hyperthyroidism

Hypothyroidism
- Menopause

Polycystic Ovaries
- Pregnancy

Personality Change

Change in the normal personality of an individual, over and above what would be thought of as normal. This will most usually be because of stress or anxiety, but can be the sign of serious underlying disease.

POSSIBLE CONDITIONS

Adverse Drug Reaction
- Alcohol or Narcotics
- Anxiety

Brain Tumours
- Dementia
- Depression and Manic Depression

Head Injury

Rabies

Schizophrenia

Stroke

Phlegm

Phlegm collects in the throat, causing coughing or often persistent attempts to clear the throat. This is usually an indication of Rhinitis – such as that induced by change in temperature or humidity, or Hay Fever – or infection, the latter   likely if the phlegm is yellow or green. It is rarely an indication of serious underlying disease.

POSSIBLE CONDITIONS

Bronchiectasis
- Bronchitis

Cancer of the Nose
- Chest Infection

Croup

Hay Fever

Lung Abcess

Nasal Polyps

Rhinitis

Sinusitis

Tuberculosis

Phlegm: Bloody and Cough

A cough with the production of phlegm, which may be yellow or green in colour, but is also streaked or contains blood. This is most usually the result of a serious problem such as severe Chest Infections, Pneumonia or Lung Cancer. Medical help should be sought as soon as possible.

POSSIBLE CONDITIONS

Bleeding

Bronchiectasis
- Chest Infection

Heart Disease

Lung Cancer

Mitral Valve Disease
- Pneumonia

Pulmonary Embolism

Q Fever

Tuberculosis

Phlegm: Bloody, Cough and Chest Pain

Chest pain combined with a cough, which also produces phlegm, which may be yellow or green in colour, but is also streaked or contains blood. This is most usually the result of a serious problem such as severe and prolonged Chest Infections, Pneumonia or Lung Cancer. Medical help should be sought as soon as possible.

POSSIBLE CONDITIONS
• Chest Infection
Chest Injury
Lung Cancer
• Pneumonia
Pulmonary Embolism
Tuberculosis
Q Fever

Phlegm: Cough

A cough with the production of phlegm, which may be yellow or green in colour. This is most usually the result of infections such as Colds or Chest Infections, although it may be a sign of more serious illness, particularly if it lasts for a long time and is very productive.

POSSIBLE CONDITIONS
Adverse Drug Reaction
AIDS
Bronchiectasis
• Bronchitis
• Chest Infection
Choking
• Cold, Common
Cystic Fibrosis
Emphysema

Flu
Lung Abscess
Pneumonia
Q Fever
Tuberculosis
Whooping Cough

Phlegm: Headache, Running Nose and Sore Eyes

Combination of symptoms which usually indicates the Common Cold, but there are other conditions, some mild, some serious, which can also fit these symptoms.

POSSIBLE CONDITIONS
Cancer of the Nose
• Cold, Common
Foreign Body in Nose
Hay Fever
Head Injury
Nasal Polyps
Rhinitis
Sinusitis
• Viral Infection

Phlegm: Nose

Nose runs with phlegm, either clear, yellow or green, watery or viscous. By far the most common causes are Cold, flu, Rhinitis and Hay Fever.

POSSIBLE CONDITIONS
Alcohol or Narcotics
Cancer of the Nose
• Cold, Common
Flu
Foreign Body in Nose

• Hay Fever
Nasal Polyps
• Rhinitis
Sinusitis

Posture: Hunched or Stooped

Posture of the individual is hunched and they may move in a stiff or restricted way. The most common cause is the changes associated with ageing, although this will vary from individual to individual.

POSSIBLE CONDITIONS
Ankylosing Spondylitis
Kyphosis or Kyphoscoliosis
Osteomyelitis of spine
Osteoporosis (vertebral fracture)
Paget's Disease
Parkinson's Disease
Tuberculosis
Vertebral Fracture
Vitamin D (Calciferol) Deficiency

Prominent Blood Vessels: Abdomen

Prominent blood vessels become apparent on the stomach or abdomen. This may be a sign of serious underlying disease, and medical help should be sought and investigations undertaken.

POSSIBLE CONDITIONS
• Cirrhosis of the Liver
Malignant Ascites

Prominent Blood Vessels: Head

Most usually an indication of Temporal Arteritis.

POSSIBLE CONDITIONS
Temporal Arteritis

Prominent Blood Vessels: Neck

This is usually a sign of serious underlying disease, and medical help should be sought and investigations undertaken.

POSSIBLE CONDITIONS
• Asthma Bronchitis
Cancer in the Chest
Constrictive Pericarditis
• Emphysema
• Heart Failure
Pericarditis
Suffocation

Pupil: Irregular in Shape

Pupils of the eyes are irregularly shaped. This is an unusual sign, and is an indication of a serious underlying condition.

POSSIBLE CONDITIONS
• Adverse Drug Reaction
Brain Tumours
• Injury or Previous Surgery
Iritis
Multiple Sclerosis
Syphilis

Pupil: Very Large

Size of the pupil of the eye varies with the intensity of light, so that in bright light it is very small, in dark conditions it is much larger to let in as much light as possible. Large pupils may also be the sign of several conditions.

POSSIBLE CONDITIONS
- •Adie's Pupil
- •Adverse Drug Reaction
- •Anxiety
- Blindness
- Botulism
- Coma
- Injury to the Eye
- Multiple Sclerosis
- Nerve Palsies of the Eye
- Stroke
- Third Nerve Palsy

Pupil: Very Small

Size of the pupil of the eye varies with the intensity of light, so that in bright light it is very small, in dark conditions it is much larger to let in as much light as possible. Small pupils may also be the sign of several conditions.

POSSIBLE CONDITIONS
- •Adverse Drug Reaction
- Brain Tumours
- •Horner's Syndrome
- Iritis
- Longsightedness
- Lung Cancer
- Multiple Sclerosis

Rash: Blisters or Peeling

Rashes which have or develop blisters or peeling are often caused by infections or skin inflammation.

POSSIBLE CONDITIONS
- •Adverse Drug Reaction
- •Athlete's Foot

Chickenpox
Dermatitis
Erythema Multiforme
- •Fungal Infection
Herpes Simplex
Impetigo
Pemphigoid
Pemphigus
Psoriasis
Shingles
- •Sunburn
Yaws

Rash: Itchy

This will usually be caused by Dermatitis, infestations, bites, reaction to plants (such as nettles) or infections.

POSSIBLE CONDITIONS
- •Adverse Drug Reaction
- •Bite, Insect
- •Dermatitis
- •Fungal Infections of the Skin
- •Lice
- Lichen Simplex
- Nodular Prurigo
- Pityriasis Rosea
- •Scabies
- •Urticaria

Rash: Localised

Rash which is localised to one specific area, most usually caused by conditions such as Acne or Sunburn.

POSSIBLE CONDITIONS
- Acne Rosacea
- Acne Vulgaris
- Allergic Reaction, Severe
- Fungal Infection
- Ringworm
- Sunburn

Syphilis

Toxoplasmosis

Typhoid Fever

Vasculitis

Rash: Rash of Dark Spots or Areas

Rashes which have dark spots, such as red, purple or black in colour may be caused by Measles, Rubella or even Meningitis.

POSSIBLE CONDITIONS
- Adverse Drug Reaction

Henoch's Purpura

Measles

Meninogococcal Septicaemia

Polio

Rubella
- Senile Purpura

Tinea Versicolor

Vitamin C (Ascorbic Acid) Deficiency

Rash: Widespread

Widespread rash which covers most of the body and is not localised to one specific area will often be caused by infections or skin irritation. Sometimes it is an indication of a serious underlying condition.

POSSIBLE CONDITIONS
- Adverse Drug Reaction

Bleeding Disorders

Chickenpox

Dengue
- Dermatitis

Endocarditis

Erythema Multiforme

Measles

Porphyria Cutanea Tarda

Psoriasis
- Purpura

Rheumatic Fever

Roseola

Ross River Fever

Rubella

Scalded Skin Syndrome

Scarlet Fever

Sunburn

Tinea Versicolor

Typhus Fever
- Urticaria
- Viral Infection

Vitamin A Deficiency

Rectum: Blood from

It is not unusual to get blood coming from the anus if the individual has Piles (haemorrhoids). If this is the case, the blood will be fresh and bright red. It may be an indication of serious underlying disease, however, particularly if the blood is black, dark or tar-like.

POSSIBLE CONDITIONS

Adverse Drug Reaction

Anal Fissure

Bleeding

Cancer of the Colon or Rectum (Bowel)

Cirrhosis of the Liver
Disorders of Blood Clotting
Diverticulitis
Dysentery
Henoch's Purpura
Intestinal Polyps
Intussusception
Jejunal Diverticulitis
Mallory-Weiss Tear
Meckel's Diverticulum
Mesenteric Vascular Occlusion
Oesophageal Varices
Peptic Ulcer
•Piles
Pregnancy

Rectum: Itching (Rectum and Anus)

It is not unusual for the anus to become itchy, particularly if the individual spends a long time sitting in a sweaty environment, has Piles, Threadworms or an infection. Occasionally it is a sign of more serious illness.

POSSIBLE CONDITIONS
Anal Fissure
•Candidiasis
Diabetes
Fistula-In-Ano
•Piles
Pilonidal Sinus
•Threadworm

Rectum: Pain (Rectum or Anus)

Pain around the rectum or anus can be caused by passing hard faeces or anal intercourse: either of these can damage the wall of the bowel. Piles

(haemorrhoids) may also be extremely painful. This may also be a sign of a more serious underlying condition.

POSSIBLE CONDITIONS
Anal Abscess
Anal Fissure
Crohn's Disease
Diabetes
•Fistula-In-Ano
•Piles

Regurgitation of Food, Vomiting and Nausea

Vomiting and nausea may result from a relatively mild cause – such as minor food poisoning (Gastroenteritis), drinking too much, travel sickness, Pregnancy or Migraines – to severe illness. Vomit will usually and initially consist of undigested food and is yellow, frothy and smells unpleasant, but persistent sickness results in the vomit becoming thin, green, mucousy and slimy. If vomit is brown, black or appears to have coffee grains, this is an indication that there is blood. See the relevant section on Vomit: Blood. In any event medical help should be sought should this be the case or if vomiting persists for a long time.

POSSIBLE CONDITIONS
Achalasia
Addison's Disease
Alcohol or Narcotics
Anorexia Nervosa
Appendicitis
Biliary Colic
Botulism
Brain Abscess

Brain Tumours
Cancer of the Oesophagus
Cancer of the Stomach
Chagas' Disease
Cholera
Cirrhosis of the Liver
Coeliac Disease
Congenital Atresia of the Oesophagus
Diabetes
Dyspepsia, Non-Ulcer
Epididymitis
Gall Bladder Infection
Gall Stones
• Gastritis
• Gastroenteritis
Heat Exhaustion
Heat Stroke
Hernia, Hiatus
Hernia, Inguinal
Hernia, Umbilical
Hypercalcaemia
Intestinal Ischaemia
Intestinal Obstruction
Kidney Disease or Failure
Kidney Stones
Meniere's Disease
Meningitis
Meninogococcal Septicaemia
Mesenteric Adenitis
Mesenteric Vascular Occlusion
Migraine
Mountain Sickness
Oesophageal Varices
• Oesophagitis
Pancreatitis
• Peptic Ulcer

Peritonitis
Phaeochromocytoma
Poisoning
Polio
Porphyria
Porphyria Cutanea Tarda
Post-Gastrectomy Syndrome
Pregnancy
Pyloric Stenosis
Raised Intracranial Pressure
Salpingitis
Sarcoidosis
Shock
Subarachnoid Haemorrhage
Torsion
Travel Sickness
Uraemia
Urinary Tract Infection
Vestibulitis

Regurgitation: Swallowing Problems

Combination of symptoms which are usually caused by acid from the stomach coming into the gullet, and may be an indication of serious disease. Any long-standing problems with swallowing should be investigated.

POSSIBLE CONDITIONS
Achalasia
Cancer of the Lung
Cancer of the Oesophagus
Cancer of the Stomach
Congenital Atresia of the Oesophagus
Hernia, Hiatus
• Oesophagitis
• Peptic or Oesophageal Stricture

Pharyngeal Pouch

Saliva: Excessive Amounts

Saliva is usually present in the mouth, although from time to time individuals may notice an excessive amount (or a completely dry mouth). A lot of saliva can be caused by smoking, infections such as Tonsillitis, and the mouth will feel full of salty saliva before vomiting. Rarely, this sign may be caused by more serious illness.

POSSIBLE CONDITIONS
Bell's Palsy
Cancer of the Oesophagus
Cancrumoris
Congenital Atresia of the Oesophagus
Glandular Fever
Motor Neurone Disease
Multiple Sclerosis
Parkinson's Disease
Peritonsillar Abscess
Pharyngitis
Rabies
Smoking
Teething Pain
Tonsillitis
Vincent's Angina
• Vomiting and Nausea

Scrotum: Lumps (Testicles and Scrotum)

Lumps can develop on or in the testicles and the scrotum (the bag which holds the testicles). These are usually harmless, being minor infections or cysts, but any lumps on the testicles should be investigated.

POSSIBLE CONDITIONS
Cancer of the Testicles
• Epididymal Cyst
Syphilis
Tuberculosis
• Varicocele

Scrotum: Swollen (Testicles and Scrotum)

The testicles and/or the scrotum (the bag which holds them) becomes swollen. This is an indication of a serious condition and medical help should be sought.

POSSIBLE CONDITIONS
Cancer of the Testicles
Epididymitis
Filariasis
• Hernia, Inguinal
• Hydrocele
Mumps
Orchitis
Torsion
• Varicocoele

Sex: Disinterest and Frigidity

Disinterest in sex or low sex drive. Interest in sex varies from individual to individual, and there is no right or wrong, only what suits a person or couple. It may be a sign of Depression, boredom or tensions within a relationship.

POSSIBLE CONDITIONS
• Depression and Manic Depression
• Low or Absent Sexual Drive

Sex: Early Puberty in Males

Most males do not proceed to become adolescents until ten or older, with the development of body hair, the breaking of the voice, and changes in the penis. Although not common, if boys develop these characteristics early may be a sign of serious underlying disease.

POSSIBLE CONDITIONS
• Hypothalmic Disease

Sex: Failure to Orgasm

Woman fails to orgasm or reach a climax. This is rarely caused by an underlying disease, and most commonly because of poor technique by a partner, or tension or anxiety experienced by the woman.

POSSIBLE CONDITIONS
• Anxiety
• Failure to Orgasm

Sex: Infertility

Infertility may be caused by a range of factors, but it should be remembered that some couples can just not conceive: there is nothing physically wrong. Infertility may also be caused by a range of conditions in both men and women.

POSSIBLE CONDITIONS
Adverse Drug Reaction
Endometriosis
Gonorrhoea
Hypogonadism
Hypopituitarism
Infertility
Klinefelter's Syndrome

Non-Specific Urethritis
Orchitis
Ovarian Failure
Pelvic Inflammatory Disease
Prolactin Excess
Salpingitis
Turner's Syndrome

Sex: Male Changes in Females

The amount of body hair that an individual has is largely determined by their genes. It is not unusual for women to have more body hair than the fashionable norm, but it is unusual for excessive body hair to be caused by underlying disease.
Woman may experience other physical, and possibly mental, changes normally associated with males, such as hair loss and a lower voice. This should be investigated, and medical help should be sought, especially if it occurs in the younger woman.

POSSIBLE CONDITIONS
Acromegaly
Adverse Drug Reaction
Congenital Adrenal Hyperplasia
Cushing's Syndrome
• Hirsutism
Menopause
• Polycystic Ovaries
Porphyria Cutanea Tarda
Turner's Syndrome

Sex: Male Infertility

Ability to reproduce varies from individual to individual, but about one third of couples cannot conceive because of problems with male fertility. If sexual intercourse is occurring at the right time in the woman's cycle, it is usual for a sperm count to be done and to check that sperm in normal. Fertility can be reduced by and following serious illness.

POSSIBLE CONDITIONS
Adverse Drug Reaction
Alcohol or Narcotics
Damage to Testicles
Ectopic Testicle
Hypogonadism
Hypopituitarism
Klinefelter's Syndrome
Mumps
Orchitis
Undescended Testicle
Varicocele

Sex: Pain

Pain is experienced during sexual intercourse. This is most commonly because of tension in the woman, but less usually is a sign of some underlying condition.

POSSIBLE CONDITIONS
• Anxiety
Cancer of the Vagina
Candidiasis
Endometriosis
Herpes Simplex
• Menopause
Salpingitis
Vaginismus

Shock

Condition characterised by pale skin, sweating, confusion, weak pulse and even collapse, caused by a dramatic fall in blood pressure from trauma, blood loss or serious infection. This is a potentially life-threatening condition and medical help should be sought as soon as possible. This is opposed to the normal meaning of the shock experienced by an individual who has had an emotional or panic reaction.

POSSIBLE CONDITIONS
• Allergic Reaction, Severe
• Bleeding
Chest Injury
Dehydration
Diabetes
• Heart Attack and Failure
Low Blood Pressure
Mesenteric Vascular Occlusion
Perforated Viscus
Pericarditis
• Peritonitis
• Septicaemia
Shock

Shock: Collapse or Coma

Serious combination of symptoms and should be treated as a medical emergency. The individual is pale, has clammy skin, weak pulse and a blue tinge because of a lack of oxygen getting to tissues. This then progresses to shock, unconsciousness or coma. See other sections on Collapse and on Coma. Causes of collapse progressing to unconsciousness include severe pain or infection, while others are listed below.

POSSIBLE CONDITIONS
Alcohol or Narcotics
• Allergic Reaction, Severe

Aortic Aneurysm (leaking)
•Bleeding
Burns
Coma
Dehydration
Diabetes
Heart Attack and Failure
Heart Disease
Low Blood Pressure
Pericarditis
Septicaemia
Stroke

Shoulder: Pain

Pain is experienced in or around the shoulder. This may be caused most obviously by injury or fracture, but may be a sign of serious illness.

POSSIBLE CONDITIONS
Broken Collarbone
Broken Upper Arm Bone (Humerus)
Cervical Spondylitis
•Frozen Shoulder
Gout
•Osteoarthritis
•Painful Arc Syndrome (Shoulder)
Pelvic Inflammatory Disease
Polymyalgia Rheumatica
Prolapsed Cervical Disc
Rheumatoid Arthritis
Rotator Cuff Tear (Shoulder)
Shoulder Dislocation
Tuberculosis

Skin: Around Mouth Pale

Most usually a sign of Scarlet Fever.

POSSIBLE CONDITIONS
Appendicitis
Scarlet Fever

Skin: Black Spots or Patches

Areas of the skin are black or dark in colour. These are caused most commonly by bruising or Moles, but may be an indication of more serious conditions such as Skin Cancer or rarely gangrene.

POSSIBLE CONDITIONS
Acanthosis Nigricans
Black Eye
•Bruise
Burns
Cancer of the Skin
Gangrene
Injury to the Eye
Leprosy
•Mole
Mongolian Blue Spot

Skin: Bleeding Under the Skin and Bruising

The most common cause of bruising or bleeding under the skin is non-penetrating injury which results in bruising. It may be the sign of a serious condition.

POSSIBLE CONDITIONS
Adverse Drug Reaction
Bite, Animal
•Bruise
Cushing's Syndrome
•Disorders of Blood Clotting
Haemophilia

Henoch's Purpura

Leukaemia

Meninogococcal Septicaemia

Purpura

•Senile Purpura

Vitamin C (Ascorbic Acid) Deficiency

Skin: Blue Areas or Patterns

A few conditions can cause blue areas or patterns on the skin, most commonly Raynaud's Phenomenon. Bluish lips or finger nail beds or generalised bluey tone to the skin may be a sign of serious disease. Consult these sections.

POSSIBLE CONDITIONS

•Livido Reticularis

Mongolian Blue Spot

Raynaud's Phenomenon

Skin: Blue Tinge (Generalised)

Skin looks blue or has a bluish tinge, particularly noticeable on the lips and the fingernail beds. This may be a serious symptom, and may be caused by too little oxygen being sent around the body. It can also be caused in fingers and toes by low temperature: if this is the case, it should resolve after they are warmed.

POSSIBLE CONDITIONS

Adverse Drug Reaction

Alcohol or Narcotics

•Bronchitis

Cancer of the Lung

Carcinoid Syndrome

Choking

Cystic Fibrosis

Diphtheria

Drowning

Emphysema

Epiglottitis

Extrinsic Allergic Alveolitis

Fibrosing Alveolitis

Heart Failure

Heart Disease

Hypothermia

Laryngeal Oedema

Ochronosis

Pneumoconiosis

•Pneumonia

Pneumothorax

Pulmonary Embolism

Pulmonary Oedema

•Raynaud's Phenomenon

Shock

Suffocation

•Vascular Disease

Skin: Bronze Coloured

A sign of Haemochromatosis (bronze diabetes).

POSSIBLE CONDITIONS

Haemochromatosis

Skin: Brown Areas or Patches

Brown areas or patches on the skin are usually caused by Freckles.

POSSIBLE CONDITIONS

Addison's Disease

•Bruise

•Fungal Infection of Skin

Mole

• Pregnancy
Varicose Veins
Venous Ulceration

Skin: Dry

The skin is dry and often flaky, usually an indication of conditions such as Sunburn, infection or Dermatitis. The dryness of skin also varies from individual to individual.

POSSIBLE CONDITIONS
• Dandruff
• Dermatitis
Dermatomyositis
Erythrasma
• Fungal Infections of the Skin
Heat Stroke
• Hypothyroidism
• Ichthyosis
Myxoedema
Uraemia
Vitamin A Deficiency

Skin: Hard or Thickened

Hard or thickened skin is most usually an indication that the area sees a lot of use or rubbing, and develops thicker skin as a protective measure.

POSSIBLE CONDITIONS
• Callus
Hallux Rigidus
Hallux Valgus
Ichthyosis
Keloid Scarring
Lymphoedema
Metastasis

Morphoea
Myxoedema
Scleroderma
Vitamin A Deficiency

Skin: Linear Marks

Linear marks on the skin, which are discreet and can be traced. There can be caused by problems with the lymphatic system, Scabies or Acanthosis Nigricans.

POSSIBLE CONDITIONS
Acanthosis Nigricans
• Injury
Lymphangitis
• Scabies

Skin: Lumps

Most usually lumps found on the skin are caused by harmless conditions such as spots, pimples or warts. Occasionally it may be a sign of serious underlying disease.

POSSIBLE CONDITIONS
• Acne Vulgaris
• Boil
Cancer of the Skin
Carbuncle
Cat Scratch Fever
Dermoid Cysts
Ganglion
Lipoma
Lymphoma
Metastasis
Molluscum Contagiosum
Pyogenic Granuloma
Rheumatoid Arthritis

Rodent Ulcer

Sarcoma

• Sebaceous Cyst

Squamous Cell Carcinoma

• Warts

Skin: Miniature Red Spots

Most commonly an indication of Campbell de Morgan Spots or Spider Naevi.

POSSIBLE CONDITIONS

• Campbell de Morgan Spots

• Spider Naevi

Skin: Orange

Most usually a sign of too large a consumption of foods or products containing the orange pigment Carotene.

POSSIBLE CONDITIONS

• Carotenaemia

Skin: Pale (Quick Onset)

Pallor of the skin beyond normal variation between individuals which develops over some minutes, hours or even days.

POSSIBLE CONDITIONS

• Adverse Drug Reaction

• Anaemia

• Anxiety

Bleeding

Diabetes

• Exercise

• Faint

Gastroenteritis

Heart Attack and Failure

Heart Disease

Leukaemia

• Low Blood Pressure

Low Blood Sugar

Menstruation

Perforated Viscus

Pneumonia

Phaeochromocytoma

Pulmonary Embolism

Shock

• Viral Infection

Skin: Pale (Slow Onset)

Pallor of the skin beyond normal variation between individuals which develops over some weeks and months. It should be remembered that some individuals are naturally pale skinned.

POSSIBLE CONDITIONS

• Anaemia

Anorexia Nervosa

Heat Exhaustion

Hookworms (human)

Hypopituitarism

Hypothermia

Hypothyroidism

Pregnancy

Sickle Cell Anaemia

Travel Sickness

Vitamin B12 (Cyanocobalamin) Deficiency

Vitiligo

Skin: Pale and Skin Problems

Pallid look to the skin combined with sores, rashes or other skin problems or changes.

POSSIBLE CONDITIONS
- •Adverse Drug Reaction
- Alcohol or Drug Addiction
- •Anaemia
- Hypopituitarism
- Malnutrition
- Rheumatoid Arthritis
- Systemic Lupus Erythematosis (SLE)
- Vasculitis
- •Viral Infection
- Vitamin B12 (Cyanocobalamin) Deficiency

Skin: Pale or Anaemia and Weight Loss

This is usually an indication of serious underlying disease, including cancer, or other problems such as alcoholism or drug addiction. Medical help should be sought.

POSSIBLE CONDITIONS
Anorexia Nervosa
Cancer of the Bile Ducts
Cancer of the Bladder
Cancer of the Cervix
Cancer of the Colon or Rectum (Bowel)
Cancer of the Kidney
Cancer of the Larynx
Cancer of the Mouth
Cancer of the Oesophagus
Cancer of the Ovaries
Cancer of the Stomach
Cancer in the Chest
Cirrhosis of the Liver
•Coeliac Disease
Crohn's Disease
Leukaemia
Lymphoma

Malnutrition
Oesophagitis
•Peptic Ulcer
Sprue
Tuberculosis
Ulcerative Colitis

Skin: Pale or Anaemic

Pallor of the skin beyond normal variation between individuals. There are many conditions which can cause pallor, including vomiting, chronic conditions, such as cancer, kidney failure or bleeding, but it is rare for looking pale to be the most significant symptom of these conditions.

POSSIBLE CONDITIONS
Adverse Drug Reaction
•Anaemia
•Bleeding
Bone Cancer
Cancer of the Bladder
Cancer of the Colon or Rectum (Bowel)
Cancer of the Kidney
Cancer of the Lung
Cancer of the Stomach
Crohn's Disease
Endocarditis
Hodgkin's Disease
Hookworms (human)
Intestinal Polyps
Kala-azar
Kidney Disease or Failure
Leukaemia
Lymphoma
Malaria
Malnutrition

Menstruation

Myelofibrosis

Oesophagitis

• Peptic Ulcer

Pernicious Anaemia

Pregnancy

Rheumatoid Arthritis

Systemic Lupus Erythematosis

Tuberculosis

Ulcerative Colitis

Vitamin B12 (Cyanocobalamin) Deficiency

Wilms' Tumour

Skin: Peeling, Flaking or Cracking

The surface of the skin peels, flakes or cracks, usually caused by conditions such as Dandruff, Sunburn, fungal infections or skin inflammation.

POSSIBLE CONDITIONS

Blepharitis

• Dandruff

• Dermatitis

Dermatomyositis

• Fungal Infections of the Skin

Otitis Externa

Sunburn

Skin: Pitted or Scarred

Pitting of the skin is an indication of previous inflammation or infection.

POSSIBLE CONDITIONS

Acne Vulgaris

Chicken Pox

Self Harm

Skin: Red

The skin can be red from many causes including local Sunburn, infections, or even exercise.

POSSIBLE CONDITIONS

Adverse Drug Reaction

• Burns

• Cellulitis

• Dermatitis

Erysipelas

Skin: Red (Generalised)

The skin can be red from many causes including Sunburn, viral infections, or even exercise.

POSSIBLE CONDITIONS

Adverse Drug Reaction

Burns

Cellulitis

Dermatitis

Psoriasis

Viral Infection

Skin: Red or Purple Patches

Red or purple patches on the skin are often birthmarks, although they may be a sign of a serious condition.

POSSIBLE CONDITIONS

Acne Rosacea

AIDS

• Burns

• Cellulitis

Chilblains

• Dermatitis

Erythrasma

Frost Bite
• Fungal Infections of the Skin
Henoch's Purpura
Kaposi's Sarcoma
Paget's Disease of the Nipple
Psoriasis
Salmon Patch Naevus
• Senile Purpura
• Sunburn
Tuberculosis

Skin: Scabs

Scabs on the skin are formed from damage, bursting blisters, and the leaking of blood and pus from the surface.

POSSIBLE CONDITIONS
Blisters
Chickenpox
• Dermatitis
• Herpes Simplex
Impetigo
Pemphigus Vulgaris
• Self Harm
• Shingles

Skin: Scaly

Usually an indication of skin inflammation or infection, but may be a sign of a serious condition.

POSSIBLE CONDITIONS
• Dermatitis
Dermatomyositis
Erythrasma
• Fungal Infections of the Skin
Ichthyosis

Paget's Disease of the Nipple
• Psoriasis
• Ringworm
Vitamin B3 (Niacin) deficiency

Skin: White or Pale (Generalised)

The skin looks pale all over, often a sign of Anaemia, but it can also be caused by Albinism, Leukaemia or Shock. It should also be remembered that many individuals have very pale skin, and that people can go white from fear or anger (as an adrenaline response).

POSSIBLE CONDITIONS
Albinism
• Anaemia
Biliary Colic
• Bleeding
Bronchiolitis
Heat Exhaustion
Hookworms (human)
Hypopituitarism
Hypothermia
Intestinal Polyps
Leukaemia
Menstruation
Pernicious Anaemia
Phaeochromocytoma
Phenylketonuria (PKU)
Shock
Sickle Cell Anaemia
Travel Sickness
• Viral Infection
Vitamin B12 (Cyanocobalamin) Deficiency

Skin: White or Pale Patches or Areas

Areas or patches of the skin are white or pale, caused by pigment problems, Raynaud's Phenomenon or (very rarely in developed countries) Leprosy.

POSSIBLE CONDITIONS

Addison's Disease
• Artery Disease
Blisters
Frost Bite
Halo Naevus
Herpes Simplex
Leprosy
Morphoea
Peripheral Vascular Disease
Phlegmasia Alba Dolens
• Raynaud's Phenomenon
• Tinea Versicolor
• Vitiligo

Skin: Yellow

The skin looks yellow or has a yellow tinge, usually caused by conditions which have jaundice as a symptom. Medical help should be sought.

POSSIBLE CONDITIONS

• Adverse Drug Reaction
Biliary Colic
Bruise
Cancer of the Bile Ducts
Cancer of the Liver
Cancer of the Pancreas
Cancer of the Stomach
Cirrhosis of the Liver
• Gall Stones

Gout
• Hepatitis
Hepatolentricular Degeneration
Malaria
Pancreatitis
Pernicious Anaemia
Sclerosing Cholangitis (Adult)
Sickle Cell Anaemia
Uraemia
Vitamin B12 (Cyanocobalamin) Deficiency
Weil's Disease
Yellow Fever

Sleeping: Problems

The amount of sleep needed varies from individual to individual, and most people can survive on less then they believe. Difficulty getting a good night's rest can be caused by drinking too much coffee, alcohol, cat-napping during the day, tension, stress, anxiety and depression.

POSSIBLE CONDITIONS

• Anxiety
• Depression and Manic Depression

Smell: No Sense of

Individual has no or a very reduced sense of smell. The most likely cause is infection or allergy, such as Cold or Rhinitis. Occasionally, and if other signs of these conditions are not present, it may be an indication of injury, nerve or neurological problems.

POSSIBLE CONDITIONS

Adenoids
Brain Tumours
• Cold, Common

Foreign Body in Nose
• Hay Fever
Head Injury
• Injury to the Nose
Nasal Polyps
• Rhinitis
Sinusitis
Smoking

Snoring: Rasping Breathing

Snoring may be extremely tiresome, particularly for a snorer's partner, but it is not usually a sign of underlying disease. Sometimes it may be a cause for concern.

POSSIBLE CONDITIONS
• Adenoids
Alcohol or Narcotics
Coma
• Obesity
Sleep Apnoea Syndrome
• Snoring
Stroke

Speech: Nasal Sounding

Voice sounds unusually nasal, although many individuals speak this way naturally. Other than this, most common causes are infections and injury to the nose. Medical help should be sought if there has been severe trauma to the nose as it may be broken.

POSSIBLE CONDITIONS
Adenoids
Cleft Lip and Palate
• Cold, Common
Foreign Body in Nose

• Injury to the Nose
• Nasal Polyps
Rhinitis
Septal Deviation
Sinusitis

Speech: Slurred, Muffled or Altered

Slurred or muffled speech can be caused by many conditions, most of them not a cause for concern, such as Colds, problems with adenoids, habit or infections. It may also be an indication that the individual has been using alcohol or drugs, or that the nose or other structures have been damaged. Rarely it can be an indication of serious underlying neurological disease or even cancer. Some of the causes are listed below, and also see the sections on Voice: Hoarse and Swallowing Problems, and Voice: Hoarse or Loss of.

POSSIBLE CONDITIONS
Adenoids
Adverse Drug Reaction
Alcohol or Narcotics
Cancer of the Larynx
Cancer of the Mouth
Cancer of the Nose
Cleft Lip and Palate
• Cold, Common
Hepatolentricular Degeneration
Motor Neurone Disease
Multiple Sclerosis
Nasal Polyps
Parkinson's Disease
Septal Deviation
Sinusitis
Stroke

Tonsilar Abscess

Squint

Eyes appear to look in different directions. Most usually this will be found in children due to natural variation between individuals. It should be corrected, if possible, because it can lead to problems with sight if left untreated. It may also be a sign of serious underlying disease.

POSSIBLE CONDITIONS
Blindness
Grave's Disease
Nerve Palsies of the Eye
Pituitory Tumour
Stroke
• Squint
Tumours of the Eye or of structures behind the Eye

Stomach: Feeling Full on Eating Little

How much food it takes to make an individual feel full varies from person to person, and their emotional state. Nerves or anxiety can reduce appetite. Surgery to remove part of the stomach will obviously reduce the amount of food that can be consumed. In some cases it may be a sign of serious disease. Also see the other sections on Appetite.

POSSIBLE CONDITIONS
Adverse Drug Reaction
• Anxiety
Ascites
Cancer of the Stomach
Cirrhosis of Liver
Pancreatitis
• Peptic Ulcer

Post-Gastrectomy Syndrome
Pyloric Stenosis

Stomach: Indigestion, Dyspepsia or Heartburn

A range of symptoms associated with the upper part of the gastrointestinal tract, such as burning pain in the gullet, nausea, belching, flatulence and acid from the stomach being regurgitated into the mouth. If there are only occasional bouts which can be linked to eating certain foods or drinking too much alcohol, then this is nothing to worry about. If pain or discomfort are experienced often or persistently, it may be the sign of a serious underlying condition.

POSSIBLE CONDITIONS
Achalasia
Adverse Drug Reaction
Cancer of the Oesophagus
Cancer of the Stomach
• Dyspepsia, Non-Ulcer
Gall Stones
• Gastritis
Gastroenteritis
• Hernia, Hiatus
• Oesophagitis
Pancreatitis
• Peptic Ulcer
Pregnancy

Suffocation

Feelings of suffocation are usually caused by blockage of the airways, either caused by a physical problem such as piece of food, allergic reactions or Epiglottitis. It is also possible that a Heart Attack might have similar symptoms. This is a serious symptom and medical help should be sought immediately. The Heimlich manoeuvre may be needed to dislodge a piece of food or other item from the windpipe.

POSSIBLE CONDITIONS
Allergic Reaction, Severe
• Angioneurotic Oedema
Bite, Insect
Bronchitis
Chest Injury
• Choking
Croup
Diphtheria
Drowning
Emphysema
Epiglottitis
Haert Failure
Laryngeal Oedema
Laryngitis
Pneumoconiosis
Pneumothorax
Poisoning
Pulmonary Embolism
Suffocation
Tracheitis

Swallowing: Problems and Fever

This combination of symptoms is usually an indication of infections, such as Tonsillitis and Laryngitis, and rarely will be an indication of serious underlying illness.

POSSIBLE CONDITIONS
Cancer of th Lung
Cancer of the Oesophagus
Epiglottitis

Erythema Multiforme (Steven Johnson's Syndrome)
Laryngitis
Ludwig's Angina
• Pharyngitis
• Tonsillitis

Swallowing: Problems and Hoarse Voice

Swallowing problems combined with hoarseness are usually simply an indication of an infection involving the throat, such as Laryngitis. If the problems persist, and there is no obvious infection, it may be an indication of cancer, particularly if combined with weight loss and poor appetite. In any event, if this combination of symptoms becomes long term, medical help should be sought and investigations undertaken.

POSSIBLE CONDITIONS
Cancer of the Larynx
Cancer of the Oesophagus
Choking
• Laryngitis
Motor Neurone Disease
Multiple Sclerosis
Myasthenia Gravis
• Pharyngitis

Swallowing: Problems and Pain

Pain in the throat combined with swallowing problems is most usually an indication of an infection, such as Tonsillitis or Laryngitis. Rarely it is a sign of serious underlying disease, such as cancer, particularly if there is also prolonged weight loss and poor appetite, and long-term hoarseness.

POSSIBLE CONDITIONS
Achalasia
Cancer of the Larynx
Cancer of the Oesophagus
Candidiasis
Diphtheria
Epiglottitis
Herpes Simplex
Hiatus Hernia
Laryngitis
Ludwig's Angina
Oesophageal Spasm
• Oesophagitis or Ulceration
Peptic or Oesophaged Structure
Peritonsillar Abscess
• Pharyngitis
Scleroderma
Shingles
Tonsillitis

Swallowing: Problems and Regurgitation or Vomiting

Combination of symptoms which are usually caused by acid from the stomach coming into the gullet, and may be an indication of serious disease. Any long-standing problems with swallowing should be investigated.

POSSIBLE CONDITIONS
Achalasia
Cancer of the Oesophagus
Cancer of the Stomach
Congenital Atresia of the Oesophagus
Hernia, Hiatus
Oesophagitis
Peptic or Oesophageal Stricture

Pharyngeal Pouch

Swallowing: Problems and Weight Loss

This combination of symptoms is usually an indication of serious underlying disease. If weight loss is unexplained and persistent, medical help should be sought and investigations made.

POSSIBLE CONDITIONS
Cancer of the Lung
Cancer of the Oesophagus
Cancer of the Stomach
Chagas' Disease
Guillain-Barre Syndrome
Hepatolentricular Degeneration
Motor Neurone Disease
Multiple Sclerosis
Myasthenia Gravis
Parkinson's Disease
• Peptic or Oesophageal Stricture
Scleroderma
Systemic Lupus Erythematosis (SLE)

Sweating: Heavy

Sweating is the body's way of reducing temperature. Some individuals, particularly if they are unfit or obese, may sweat a lot more during exercise. Heavy sweating can also be a sign of underlying disease, such as fever caused by infection (see separate sections).

POSSIBLE CONDITIONS
Abscess – Ling, Abdomen, Bowel, Kidney
Acromegaly
• Anxiety

Cancer of Lung, Bowel, Kidney, Ovary
Carcinoid Syndrome
• Exercise
Fever
Heat Exhaustion
Hyperthyroidism
Kala-azar
Kidney Stones
Low Blood Sugar
Lung Abscess
Malaria
• Menopause
Perforated Viscus
Phaeochromocytoma
Rabies
Septicaemia
Tuberculosis
Shock
Urinary Tract Infection
• Viral Infection

Sweating: Heavy at Night

Many viral illnesses can cause a variety of symptoms including profuse sweating at night. This should normally only last a couple of days. Should heavy sweating at night persist for weeks it may be a sign of serious underlying disease such as infections or abscesses. Also see the other sections on fever.

POSSIBLE CONDITIONS
Adverse Drug Reaction
AIDS
Brucellosis
Cencer of Lung, Bowel, Kidney, Ovary
Endocarditis

Fever
Flu
Hodgkin's Disease
Hyperthyroidism
Leukaemia
Lymphoma
Menopause
Tuberculosis
Urinary Tract Infection
Viral Infection

Sweating: Normal

Individuals sweat as a way of lowering body temperature by the evaporation of the sweat from the skin. The amount of sweating varies from individual to individual, as people's reaction to stress, nerves or anxiety can also result in sweating. The most obvious causes are exercise and hot ambient surroundings, although it is also an indication of fever. Any condition which has severe pain as symptom will also cause sweating.

POSSIBLE CONDITIONS
Adverse Drug Reaction
AIDS
Alcohol or Narcotics
• Anxiety
• Exercise
Fever
Low Blood Sugar
Tuberculosis

Swollen Abdomen: Adults

A swollen-looking abdomen can be caused by being overweight, wind or constipation, pregnancy or menstruation. It may also be the sign of a more serious condition.

POSSIBLE CONDITIONS
Adverse Drug Reaction
• Ascites
Cancer of the Colon or Rectum (Bowel)
Cancer of Liver, Kidneys, Ovaries or Womb
Cirrhosis of the Liver
• Constipation
Constrictive Pericarditis
Crohn's Disease
Diverticulitis
Fibroids
• Flatulence
Heart Attack and Failure
Hypothyroidism
Intestinal Obstruction
Irritable Bowel Syndrome
Jejunal Diverticulitis
Malignant Ascites
Meckel's Diverticulum
Mesenteric Vascular Occlusion
• Obesity
Ovarian Cyst
Pancreatitis
Perforated Viscus
• Pregnancy
Relapsing Fever
Typhoid Fever
Ulcerative Colitis

Swollen Abdomen: Children

Children can have a swollen stomach or abdomen for various reasons, not least they are constipated. It may be the indication of serious underlying illness, although this will usually be combined with other signs.

POSSIBLE CONDITIONS
Ascites
Cancer of Adrenal Glands or Kidneys
Coeliac Disease
• Constipation
Cystic Fibrosis
• Flatulence
Hirschsprung's Disease
Hypothyroidism
Intussusception
Kwashiorkor
• Obesity
Typhoid Fever

Swollen Abdomen: Constipation

Many individuals will suffer from bouts of constipation from time to time, and anyway frequency and consistency of motions varies from person to person. A change in bowel habit may be significant, although this combination of signs may simply be the result of too much refined food, too little fluid or too little roughage. If it persists for a long time, and cannot be related to lifestyle changes, it is possible that this may be an indication of a serious condition.

POSSIBLE CONDITIONS
Adverse Drug Reaction
Cancer of the Colon or Rectum (Bowel)
• Constipation
Diverticulitis
• Flatulence
Hypercalcaemia
Hypothyroidism
• Irritable Bowel Syndrome

141

Swollen Abdomen: Diarrhoea

Most individuals will suffer from bouts of diarrhoea from time to time, and the frequency and consistency of motions varies from person to person. A change in bowel habit may be significant, although often this is simply the result of too much rich food, alcohol, fruit or roughage, nerves, or minor food poisoning. If it persists for a long time, and cannot be related to lifestyle changes, it is possible that this may be an indication of serious conditions.

POSSIBLE CONDITIONS
Cancer of the Colon or Rectum (Bowel)
• Constipation
Crohn's Disease
Diverticulitis
Flatulence
Gastroenteritis
• Irritable Bowel Syndrome
• Laxatives
Ulcerative Colitis

Swollen Lymph Nodes

The lymphatic system is used by the body to fight off infection and disease. When this is the case, lymph nodes become swollen, and if this only lasts for a few days it is of little significance. If lymph nodes remain swollen for a week or more, it may be the indication of serious underlying disease such as cancer.

POSSIBLE CONDITIONS
Adverse Drug Reaction
AIDS
Cancer of the Breast
Cancer of the Colon or Rectum (Bowel)
Cancer of the Larynx

Cancer of the Mouth
Cancer of the Nose
Cancer of the Prostate
Cancer of the Stomach
Cancer of the Thyroid
Cancer of the Womb
Cancer in the Chest
Cancrumoris
Cat Scratch Fever
Chancroid
Cold, Common
Dental Infections
Diphtheria
Epiglottitis
• Glandular Fever
Hodgkin's Disease
Kala-azar
Leukaemia
Lung Cancer
Lymphangitis
Lymphoma
Metastases
Mumps
Peritonsillar Abscess
Ross River Fever
Rubella
Sarcoidosis
Squamous Cell Carcinoma
Submandibular Tumour
Syphilis
Tonsillitis
Toxoplasmosis
Tuberculosis
Vincent's Angina
• Viral Infection
Yaws

Swollen Lymph Nodes: Neck

The lymphatic system is concerned with fighting infection, and enlarged lymph nodes or glands are usually a sign the body is fighting off infection, either localised to one area of the body or a general infection such as a Cold. More unusually it can be an indication of serious underlying disease, especially if the nodes remain enlarged for long periods, such as more than a couple of weeks, and there are other prolonged symptoms. Also see other sections on lymph nodes or glands.

POSSIBLE CONDITIONS
Adverse Drug Reaction
AIDS
Cancer of the Larynx
Cancer of the Mouth
Cancer of the Thyroid
Cancer in the Chest
Cancrumoris
Cold, Common
Dental Infections
Diphtheria
Epiglottitis
•Glandular Fever
Hodgkin's Disease
Leukaemia
Lymphoma
Mumps
Peritonsillar Abscess
Rubella
Sarcoidosis
Squamous Cell Carcinoma
Submandibular Tumour
Tonsillitis
Toxoplasmosis
Tuberculosis
Vincent's Angina
•Viral Infection

Teeth: Loose

Most usually a sign of gum or dental problems, prompting a visit to the dentist.

POSSIBLE CONDITIONS
•Dental Infections
Pyorrhoea Alveolaris
•Tooth Decay and Abscess

Teeth: Sensitive

Most usually a sign of over vigorous brushing of teeth, but it may be caused by gum or dental problems. If the sensitivity persists, and particularly if combined with toothache or bleeding gums, a dentist should be visited.

POSSIBLE CONDITIONS
•Dental Infections
Pyorrhoea Alveolaris
•Tooth Decay and Abscess

Teeth: Toothache and Teething Pain

In adults, most usually a sign of dental or gum problems, prompting a visit to the dentist.

POSSIBLE CONDITIONS
•Dental Infections
Pyorrhoea Alveolaris
Teething Pain
•Tooth Decay and Abscess
Wisdom Teeth

Teething Pain and Toothache

In adults, most usually a sign of dental or gum problems, prompting a visit to the dentist.

POSSIBLE CONDITIONS
• Dental Infections
Pyorrhoea Alveolaris
Teething Pain
• Tooth Decay and Abscess
Wisdom Teeth

Temperature: Low and Hypothermia

The temperature of the internal body (normally maintained at 37 degrees Celsius) falls at least two degrees below this level. Those especially at risk at new-born babies and the elderly, both of whom have reduced ability to cope with low temperatures. Babies do not shiver. If an individual has hypothermia, they should be warmed slowly with blankets and warm drinks. Warming up the individual too quickly can be dangerous, and they should not be given alcohol.

POSSIBLE CONDITIONS
Adverse Drug Reaction
Alcohol or Narcotics
• Hypothermia
• Hypothyroidism
Myxoedema

Testicle: Absent

Testicles can moved in the scrotum and even up into the abdomen, particularly during sexual activity or when the individual is very cold or frightened. In a small number of boys, however, the testicles do not descend into the scrotum as normal, and it is also possible that the testicle may get stuck in the abdomen.

POSSIBLE CONDITIONS
Ectopic Testicle
• Retractile Testicle
• Undescended Testicle

Testicle: Lumps (Testicles and Scrotum)

Lumps can develop on or in the testicles and the scrotum (the bag which holds the testicles). These are usually harmless, being minor infections or cysts, but any lumps on the testicles should be investigated.

POSSIBLE CONDITIONS
Cancer of the Testicles
• Epididymal Cyst
Hydrocoele
Inguinal Hernia
Syphilis
Tuberculosis
Varicocele

Testicle: Pain

Several conditions can cause pain in the testicles, not least a kick or blow in the groin. This can be exquisitely painful to begin with, and ache for some little time afterwards. As long as there is normal urine with no blood, this will resolve.

POSSIBLE CONDITIONS
Epididymitis
Hernia, Inguinal
Hydrocele
• Injury

Kidney Stones
Mumps
• Orchitis
Pancreatitis
Torsion
Varicocele

Testicle: Swollen (Testicles and Scrotum)

The testicles and/or the scrotum (the bag which holds them) becomes swollen. This is an indication of a serious condition and medical help should be sought.

POSSIBLE CONDITIONS
Cancer of the Testicles
Epididymitis
Filariasis
Hernia, Inguinal
• Hydrocele
Mumps
Orchitis
Torsion
• Varicocoele

Thirst: Excessive

Excessive thirst can have many causes, some of them quite innocent such as simply not drinking enough fluid or vigorous exercise, while others may be more serious, such as periods of vomiting, diarrhoea or bleeding. Babies and elderly people can become dehydrated very quickly, and extra care should be taken if suspected in these groups.

POSSIBLE CONDITIONS
Adverse Drug Reaction

Aldosteronism
Asthma
Bleeding
Cholera
• Dehydration
• Diabetes Mellitus
Diabetes Insipidus
Diuretics
Exercise
Fever
Hypercalcaemia
Hypothalamic Problems
Pituitary Tumours
Rabies

Thirst: Excessive and Dehydration

This combination of symptoms tends to suggest any condition which more fluid is lost from the body than replaced, such as vomiting, diarrhoea, sweating including fevers, blood loss and haemorrhaging, and even from breathing from asthma. Symptoms of dehydration include thirst, urine being dark and smelly, dry skin, and even confusion and collapse. Babies and elderly people can become dehydrated very quickly, and extra care should be taken if suspected in these groups.

POSSIBLE CONDITIONS
Adverse Drug Reaction
Alcohol or Narcotics
Asthma
Bleeding
Cholera
Diabetes Mellitus
Diabetes Insipidus
Diuretics

Exercise
Gastroenteritis
Heat Exhaustion
Heat Stroke
Hypercalcaemia
Hypothalamic Problems
Kidney Disease or Failure
Pituitary Tumours
Rabies
Sarcoidosis
Viral Infection

Thirst: Excessive and Excessive Urination

This combination of symptoms can simply be caused by drinking a lot of fluids but may be a result of Diabetes.

POSSIBLE CONDITIONS
Adverse Drug Reaction
Aldosteronism
Diabetes Mellitus
Diabetes Insipidus
Diuretics
Hypercalcaemia
Hypothalamic Problems
Kidney Disease or Failure
Pituitary Tumours
Potassium Deficiency

Throat: Hoarse or Loss of Voice

The voice becomes hoarse, making it difficult to talk, or it may even become impossible to talk. This usually has an obvious cause such as shouting or talking for long periods or infections. If hoarseness persists for more than a couple of weeks, it may be an indication of serious underlying illness and medical help should be sought and tests undertaken.

POSSIBLE CONDITIONS
Cancer of the Larynx
Cancer of the Oesophagus
Cancer of the Thyroid
Cancer in the Chest
Choking
• Cold, Common
Croup
Epiglottitis
Isolated Thyroid Nodule
• Laryngitis
Lung Cancer
Myasthenia Gravis
Myxoedema
Sarcoidosis
Sjogren's Syndrome
• Viral Infection
Vocal Nodules

Throat: Pain and Fever

Usually an indication of common infections, such as Colds, Tonsillitis or Laryngitis, although occasionally this combination may be associated with more serious conditions.

POSSIBLE CONDITIONS
Adverse Drug Reaction
Cancrumoris
• Cold, Common
Dental Infections
Flu
Glandular Fever
• Laryngitis
Ludwig's Angina

Pharyngitis
Rabies
Rheumatic Fever
Tonsillitis
Tracheitis
Vincent's Angina

Throat: Phlegm

Phlegm collects in the throat, causing coughing or often persistent attempts to clear the throat. This is usually an indication of Rhinitis – such as that induced by change in temperature or humidity, or Hay Fever – or infection, the latter likely if the phlegm is yellow or green. It is rarely an indication of serious underlying disease.

POSSIBLE CONDITIONS
Bronchiectasis
•Bronchitis
Cancer of the Nose
•Chest Infection
Croup
Hay Fever
Nasal Polyps
•Pharyngitis
Rhinitis
Sinusitis
Tuberculosis
•Viral Infection

Throat: Slurred, Muffled or Altered Speech

Slurred or muffled speech can be caused by many conditions, most of them not a cause for concern, such as Colds, problems with adenoids, habit or infections. It may also be an indication that the individual has been using alcohol or drugs, or that the nose or other structures have been damaged. Rarely it can be an indication of serious underlying neurological disease or even cancer. Some of the causes are listed below, and also see the sections on Voice: Hoarse and Swallowing Problems, and Voice: Hoarse or Loss of.

POSSIBLE CONDITIONS
Adenoids
Adverse Drug Reaction
•Alcohol or Narcotics
Cancer of the Larynx
Cancer of the Lung
Cancer of the Mouth
Cancer of the Nose
Cleft Lip and Palate
•Cold, Common
Hepatolentricular Degeneration
Motor Neurone Disease
Multiple Sclerosis
Nasal Polyps
Parkinson's Disease
Septal Deviation
Sinusitis
Stroke
•Viral Infection

Throat: Swallowing Problems and Fever

This combination of symptoms is usually an indication of infections, such as Tonsillitis and Laryngitis, and rarely will be an indication of serious underlying illness.

POSSIBLE CONDITIONS
Cancer of the Oesophagus

Candidiasis
Epiglottitis
Erythema Multiforme – Stevens Johnson Syndrome
• Laryngitis
Ludwig's Angina
• Tonsillitis
• Viral Infection

Throat: Swallowing Problems and Hoarse Voice

Swallowing problems combined with hoarseness are usually simply an indication of an infection involving the throat, such as Laryngitis. If the problems persist, and there is no obvious infection, it may be an indication of cancer, particularly if combined with weight loss and poor appetite. In any event, if this combination of symptoms becomes long term, medical help should be sought and investigations undertaken.

POSSIBLE CONDITIONS
Cancer of the Larynx
Cancer of the Lung
Cancer of the Oesophagus
Cancer of the Thyroid
Choking
• Laryngitis
Myasthenia Gravis
Oesophageal Pouch
• Viral Infection

Throat: Swallowing Problems and Pain

Pain in the throat combined with swallowing problems is most usually an indication of an infection, such as Tonsillitis or Laryngitis. Rarely it is a sign of serious underlying disease, such as cancer,

particularly if there is also prolonged weight loss and poor appetite, and long-term hoarseness.

POSSIBLE CONDITIONS
Cancer of the Larynx
Cancer of the Lung
Cancer of the Oesophagus
Cancer of the Stomach
Candidiasis
Diphtheria
Epiglottitis
Herpes Simplex
• Laryngitis
Ludwig's Angina
Oesophageal Spasm
Oesophagitis
Peptic Stricture
Peritonsillar Abscess
Pharyngitis
Scleroderma
Shingles
• Tonsillitis
• Viral Infection

Throat: Swallowing Problems and Regurgitation or Vomiting

Combination of symptoms which are usually caused by acid from the stomach coming into the gullet, and may be an indication of serious disease. Any long-standing problems with swallowing should be investigated.

POSSIBLE CONDITIONS
Achalasia
Cancer of the Lung
Cancer of the Oesophagus
Cancer of the Stomach

Congenital Atresia of the Oesophagus
• Hernia, Hiatus
• Oesophagitis
• Peptic or Oesophageal Stricture
Pharyngeal Pouch

Throat: Swallowing Problems and Weight Loss

This combination of symptoms is usually an indication of serious underlying disease. If weight loss is unexplained and persistent, medical help should be sought and investigations made.

POSSIBLE CONDITIONS
Cancer of the Lung
Cancer of the Oesophagus
Cancer of the Stomach
Chagas' Disease
Guillain-Barre Syndrome
Hepatolentricular Degeneration
Motor Neurone Disease
Multiple Sclerosis
Myasthenia Gravis
Parkinson's Disease
Peptic or Oesophageal Stricture
Scleroderma
Systemic Lupus Erythematosis (SLE)

Throat: White Spots (Mouth and Throat)

This is usually a sign of potentially serious conditions such as Thrush (Candidiasis), Tonsillitis or Measles. If the spots do not resolve and persist in the mouth, and cannot be easily removed, medical help should be sought.

POSSIBLE CONDITIONS
• Aphthous Ulcer
• Candidiasis
Leukoplakia
Lichen Planus
Measles
Tonsillitis

Tinnitus

Noises are heard in the ear, such as ringing, singing or crackling. If the individual has been exposed to very loud noises, the ears may ring afterwards for a few days, but this will usually resolve. Long-term exposure to loud noises may cause hearing damage. This sign can also be caused by infections and more serious conditions.

POSSIBLE CONDITIONS
Acoustic Neuroma
Adverse Drug Reaction
Anaemia
Artery Disease
• Eustachian Catarrh
Heart Disease
Inner Ear Infection
• Meniere's Disease
Mitral Valve Disease
Otosclerosis
Paget's Disease
Presbyacusis

Tiredness: Fever

Illnesses which have fever as a symptom will also cause tiredness and fatigue. Any chronic inf
will cause fatigue. Also see sectic

POSSIBLE CONDITIONS
Abscess
Adverse Drug Reaction
AIDS
Cancer of the Bowel, Stomach, Kidney, Lung, Oesaphagus
Cellulitis
•Cold, Common
Endocarditis
•Flu
Glandular Fever
Rheumatic Fever
Rheumatoid Arthritis
Septicaemia
Systemic Lupus Syndrome
Tuberculosis
•Viral Infection

Tiredness: General

Many factors can make an individual feel tired, fatigued and sap their energy. Sometimes the most obvious is the most ignored: overexertion, either physically, mentally or emotionally. It is also often overlooked that being bored or inactive can actually be extremely tiring. Lack of sleep or disturbed sleep can sometimes by overemphasised. Most periods of tiredness will resolve with rest and relaxation. There are some serious conditions which have tiredness as a symptom, not least cancer, while some of the other causes are listed below. Also see the other sections on Tiredness.

POSSIBLE CONDITIONS
Adverse Drug Reaction
AIDS
Addison's Disease

Alcohol or Narcotics
•Anaemia
Anxiety
Coeliac Disease
Cancer of the Bowel, Stomach, Kidney, Lung, Oesophagus
Cellulitis
Constrictive Pericarditis
Depression and Manic Depression
Diabetes
Exercise
Fever
Heart Disease
Hyperthyroidism
Hypothyroidism
Hypopituitarism
Kidney Disease or Failure
Low Blood Pressure
Malnutrition
Myasthenia Gravis
Pernicious Anaemia
•Post-Viral Syndrome
Potassium Deficiency
Rheumatoid Arthritis
Sick Sinus Syndrome
Systemic Lupus Erythematosis (SLE)
Vitamin C (Ascorbic Acid) Deficiency
•Viral Infection

Tiredness: Headache

Combination of symptoms which indicate a headache caused by tiredness, tension or stress, and there is rarely any more sinister cause. It may also be the onset of a feverish illness. This is a sign of a serious underlying illness, although it will rarely be the most pressing of symptoms.

POSSIBLE CONDITIONS
Adverse Drug Reaction
• Anxiety
Brain Tumours
Carbon Monoxide Poisoning
Flu
High Blood Pressure
Menstruation
• Migraine
Mountain Sickness
Stroke
Subarachnoid Haemorrhage
• Viral Infection

Toe: Altered Sensation (Fingers and Toes)

Feelings in the fingers, toes and limbs may become altered through a variety of conditions, many of them serious. It is sometimes quite difficult to define exactly what altered sensation is, but it may often be caused by nerve and neurological problems. Frost Bite or Raynaud's Phenomenon should be excluded if the individual has been exposed to cold conditions.

POSSIBLE CONDITIONS
Acromagely
Adverse Drug Reaction
• Alcohol or Narcotics
Cancer of the Bowel
Cancer of the Kidney
Cancer of the Ovaries
Cancer of the Testicles
Cancer of the Spine
Cancer of the Stomach
Cancer of the Womb
Carpal Tunnel Syndrome

Cauda Equine Syndrome
Cervical Rib
Cervical Spondylosis
• Diabetes
Frost Bite
Guillain-Barre Syndrome
Hyperventilation
Hypothyroidism
Leprosy
Multiple Sclerosis
• Nerve Injury
Peripheral Vascular Disease
Pernicious Anaemia
Prolapsed Cervical Disc
Raynaud's Phenomenon
Rheumatoid Arthritis
Ross River Fever
Sciatica
Spinal Cord Injury
Spinal Cord Tumours
Ulnar Nerve
Vitamin B12 (Cyanocobalamin) Deficiency

Toe: Itching or Numbness (Fingers and Toes)

Fingers feel itchy or go numb and have little sensation. There are two most likely causes: either Dermatitis or a fungal infection if itchy; Frost Bite or Chilblains if numb.

POSSIBLE CONDITIONS
Acromagely
Adverse Drug Reaction
• Alcohol or Narcotics
Cancer of the Bowel
Cancer of the Kidney

Cancer of the Ovaries
Cancer of the Testicles
Cancer of the Spine
Cancer of the Stomach
Cancer of the Womb
Carpal Tunnel Syndrome
Cauda Equine Syndrome
Cervical Rib
Cervical Spondylosis
• Diabetes
Frost Bite
Guillain-Barre Syndrome
Hyperventilation
Hypothyroidism
Leprosy
Multiple Sclerosis
• Nerve Injury
Peripheral Vascular Disease
Pernicious Anaemia
Prolapsed Cervical Disc
Raynaud's Phenomenon
Rheumatoid Arthritis
Ross River Fever
Sciatica
Spinal Cord Injury
Spinal Cord Tumours
Ulnar Nerve
Vitamin B12 (Cyanocobalamin) Deficiency

Toothache and Teething Pain

In adults, most usually a sign of dental or gum problems, prompting a visit to the dentist.

POSSIBLE CONDITIONS
• Dental Infections
Pyorrhoea Alveolaris

Teething Pain
• Tooth Decay and Abscess
Wisdom Teeth

Trembling or Shaking

Most individuals can shake or have trembling hands at different times, which can be exacerbated by nerves, excitement, anxiety, alcohol, coffee and other stimulants and drugs. There may be a hereditary component, and can get worse with age. While most shaking or trembling is quite normal, it can be a sign of disease.

POSSIBLE CONDITIONS
• Adverse Drug Reaction
Alcohol or Narcotics
• Anxiety
Brain Tumours
Caffeine
Head Injury
• Hyperthyroidism
Multiple Sclerosis
Parkinson's Disease
Shock
Stroke
Syphilis

Twitching

Spasmodic movements in limbs or elsewhere, usually not a sign of any underlying problem. It is possible to get twitching in one particular muscle, such as the thigh. This may twitch for several days before resolving by itself. Twitching can be a sign of underlying disease, although this is not common and other symptoms are likely to be more prevalent or noticeable.

Possible Conditions
Adverse Drug Reaction
• Anxiety
Epilepsy
Huntington's Chorea
Hypertension
Kidney Disease or Failure
Motor Neurone Disease
Multiple Sclerosis
Rabies
Rheumatic Fever
Spasmodic Torticollis
Tetanus
Tourette's Syndrome

Urine: Blood in

Blood passed in urine can look bright red or pink, or it may make urine look cloudy. Blood may also only be passed at the beginning or end of the act of urination. Blood in urine can be caused by relatively mild conditions, such as Cystitis (although it may feel anything but mild), but persistent blood in urine can be a sign of serious underlying illness.

Possible Conditions
Adverse Drug Reaction
Bilharzia
• Bleeding
Cancer of the Bladder
Cancer of the Kidney
Cancer of the Prostate
Cystitis
Disorders of Blood Clotting
Endocarditis
Enlarged Prostate
Exercise

Henoch's Purpura
Injury to the Lower Chest or Pelvis
Kidney Disease or Failure
Kidney Stones
Non Specific Urethritis
Prostatitis
Pyelonephritis
• Urinary Tract Infection
Wilms' Tumour
Yellow Fever

Urine: Blood in Urine and Pain Urinating

Most likely cause is Cystitis or Urinary Tract Infections, but it may be an indication of more serious illness.

Possible Conditions
Bilharzia
• Cystitis
Kidney Disease or Failure
Kidney Stones
Prostatitis
Pyelonephritis
• Urinary Tract Infection

Urine: Breath Smells of Urine

Most usually a sign of Kidney Failure, and medical help should be sought immediately. This is not likely to be the most significant symptom, but it can aid in diagnosis.

Possible Conditions
Kidney Disease or Failure
Uraemia

Urine: Cloudy

The most likely cause for cloudy urine is Cystitis or Urinary Tract Infections. It is not always the sign of disease, however, and concentrated urine, from dehydration or vigorous exercise, may look cloudy.

POSSIBLE CONDITIONS
Bilharzia
• Cystitis
Dehydration
Enlarged Prostate
Gonorrhoea
Kidney Stones
Prostatitis
Pyelonephritis
• Urinary Tract Infection

Urine: Dark, Discoloured or Concentrated

Urine is very dark in colour, and often smells much more strongly than usual. The cause may simply be that the individual have been vigorously exercising or sweating, and has not been taking enough fluids to replace that lost. If this is the cause, it should resolve within a day or so by drinking more water. Dark urine may be the sign of a serious underlying conditions.

POSSIBLE CONDITIONS
• Adverse Drug Reaction
Alkaptonuria
Cirrhosis
Cystitis
• Dehydration
• Food and Drugs
Gall Stones

Haemaglobinuria
Heat Exhaustion
Heat Stroke
Hepatitis
Jaundice
Kidney Disease or Failure
Kidney Stones
Malaria
Urinary Tract Infection

Urine: Excessive Urination and Thirst

This combination of symptoms can simply be caused by drinking a lot of fluids but may be a result of Diabetes.

POSSIBLE CONDITIONS
Aldosteronism
• Diabetes
• Diuretics
• Hypercalcaemia
Kidney Disease or Failure
Potassium Deficiency

Urine: Frequent or Excessive Urination

The need to urinate often and to produce excessive amounts of urine. The cause may be obvious, such as drinking alcohol or large quantities of fluid, or taking diuretics, but may be the sign of serious underlying conditions, such as Diabetes.

POSSIBLE CONDITIONS
Alcohol or Narcotics
Aldosteronism
Bilharzia
Bladder Neck Obstruction
Caffeine

Cancer of the Prostate

Cushing's Syndrome

Diabetes

Diuretics

Enlarged Prostate

Hypercalcaemia

Hypothalmic Disease

Irritable Bladder

Kidney Disease or Failure

Sarcoidosis

Urinary Tract Infection

Urine: Inability to Urinate

An indication of serious underlying disease, and medical help should be sought immediately. It may have suddenly become impossible to urinate, or it may have taken some time while the stream of urine gradually diminishes.

POSSIBLE CONDITIONS

•Adverse Drug Reaction

Cancer of the Bladder

Cancer of the Cervix

Cancer of the Colon or Rectum (Bowel)

Cancer of the Kidney

Cancer of the Ovaries

Cancer of the Prostate

Cancer of the Womb

•Constipation

•Enlarged Prostate

Injury to the Lower Chest or Pelvis

•Kidney Disease or Failure

Kidney Stones

Poisoning

Septicaemia

Shock

Spinal Cord Injury

Urethral Stricture

Urine: Incontinence or Dribbling Urine

Incontinence of urine is the unintentional or accidental passing or dribbling of urine. This can have a range of causes, many of them serious.

POSSIBLE CONDITIONS

Alcohol or Narcotics

Bladder Neck Obstruction

Cancer of the Prostate

Cancer of the Urethra

Cauda Equine Syndrome

Enlarged Bladder

•Enlarged Prostate

Epilepsy

Hydrocephalus

Irritable Bladder

Multiple Sclerosis

Prostatitis

Sciatica

Spina Bifida

Spinal Cord Injury

•Stress Incontinence

Stroke

Urethral Stricture

•Urinary Tract Infection

•Womb Prolapse

Urine: Pain When Urinating

Sign of Cystitis or Urinary Tract Infections, although it may be an indication of more serious illness.

POSSIBLE CONDITIONS

Bilharzia

• Cystitis
Gonorrhoea
Kidney Disease or Failure
Non-Specific Urethritis
Prostatitis
• Urinary Tract Infection

Urine: Urinating Problems

Problems with urinating include not being able to start, although the bladder feels full, the stream of urine is poor, and finding it difficult to stop or dribbling urine.

POSSIBLE CONDITIONS
Adverse Drug Reaction
Bladder Neck Obstruction
Cancer of the Urethra
Cancer of the Womb
Cauda Equine Syndrome
• Cystitis
Enlarged Bladder
• Enlarged Prostate
Gonorrhoea
Irritable Bladder
Kidney Stones
Multiple Sclerosis
Non-Specific Urethritis
Poisoning
Prostatitis
Reiter's Disease
Septicaemia
Shock
Slipped Disc
Spinal Cord Injury
Spinal Cord Tumours
• Stress Incontinence

Stroke
Urethral Stricture
• Urinary Tract Infection
Womb Prolapse

Vagina: Bleeding

Blood comes from the vagina, beyond that which would be expected during Menstruation. This may have many causes, many of them serious, such as miscarriage (see Pregnancy). If unexpected bleeding from the vagina persists and is heavy medical help should be sought.

POSSIBLE CONDITIONS
• Bleeding
Cancer of the Cervix
Cancer of the Ovaries
Cancer of the Womb
• Cervical Polyp
Contraceptive Pill
Disorders of Blood Clotting
Endometriosis
Erosion of the Cervix
Fibroids
Hypothyroidism
Inflammation of the Vagina
• Menopause
• Menstruation
Pelvic Inflammatory Disease
Pregnancy
Urethral Caruncle

Vagina: Discharge

Discharge from the vagina, beyond that which would be expected from a normal menstrual cycle. The consistency and odour of discharge does vary. If discharge is particularly profuse, coloured or smells unpleasant, medical help should be sought.

POSSIBLE CONDITIONS
Cancer of the Cervix
Cancer of the Colon or Rectum (Bowel)
Cancer of the Ovaries
Cancer of the Vagina
Cancer of the Womb
• Candidiasis
Cervical Polyp
Chlamydia
Erosion of the Cervix
Foreign Body in Vagina
Gardnerella
Gonorrhoea
Inflammation of the Vagina
• Menopause
• Menstruation
Non-Specific Urethritis
Pelvic Inflammatory Disease
Salpingitis
Sexual Abuse
Trichomonas
Womb Prolapse

Vagina: Pain

Pain is experienced in or around the vagina. If this is persistent, then it is likely to be an indication of a potentially serious problem. Medical help should be sought, even if only to exclude any disease.

POSSIBLE CONDITIONS
Cancer of the Vagina
Candidiasis
Chlamydia
Endometriosis

Gardnerella
Gonorrhoea
Herpes Simplex
• Menopause
• Pelvic Inflammatory Disease
Trichomonas

Vagina: Protrusion

Protrusion or swelling can be felt within the vagina. This is most usually an indication of a serious problem, and medical help should be sought.

POSSIBLE CONDITIONS
Cancer of the Vagina
Cancer of the Womb
Prolapse of the Bladder
Prolapse of the Rectum
• Womb Prolapse

Vagina: Unpleasant Smell

Unpleasant smell comes from the vagina, although this is extremely difficult to define, except in cases of infection (when there will be little doubt). Some women worry unnecessarily about their own odours. Odours also change during a woman's menstrual cycle.

POSSIBLE CONDITIONS
• Candidiasis
Cervical Polyp
Chlamydia
Foreign Body in Vagina
Gardnerella
Gonorrhoea
• Menstruation
Pelvic Inflammatory Disease
Trichomonas

Vagina: Vulval Itch

Area in and around the vagina becomes persistently itchy. This may be caused by a variety of conditions, from the mild to the severe.

POSSIBLE CONDITIONS
Cancer of the Skin
• Candidiasis
Chlamydia
Dermatitis
Foreign Body in Vagina
• Fungal Infections of the Skin
Gardnerella
Gonorrhoea
Inflammation of the Vagina
Leukoplakia
Lice
Non-Specific Urethritis
Pelvic Inflammatory Disease
Pregnancy
Psoriasis
Scabies
Threadworm
Trichomonas

Vertigo

Feeling of dizziness and giddiness with a spinning or falling sensation when the head is turned. Most usually a problem with the ear.

POSSIBLE CONDITIONS
Acoustic Neuroma
Adverse Drug Reaction
Botulism
Cervical Spondylosis
Inner Ear Infection
• Labyrinthitis
• Meniere's Disease
Stroke
Travel Sickness
Vestibulitis
• Viral Infection

Vertigo: Giddiness

The ears are also involved with balance and the concept of position, and consequently infections and other problems with the ear will affect balance as well as hearing.

POSSIBLE CONDITIONS
Acoustic Neuroma
Adverse Drug Reaction
• Cervical Spondylosis
Cholesteamota
Cold, Common
Ear Wax
Inner Ear Infection
• Labyrinthitis
• Low Blood Pressure
Meniere's Disease
Otosclerosis
Stroke
Travel Sickness
Vestibulitis
Viral Infection

Vision: Blurred

Vision becomes blurred, meaning that it is difficult or impossible to focus. The most common causes are poor eyesight (a visit to an optician is advisable), focusing for long periods on objects such as a computer screen, and excess alcohol consumption or drugs. Individuals who have problems with eyesight may find these are worse at night or when they are tired. This sign may also more unusually be an indication of a serious problem.

POSSIBLE CONDITIONS
Adverse Drug Reaction
Alcohol or Narcotics
Cataract
Detached Retina
Diabetes
Iritis
• Macular Degeneration
• Poor Eyesight

Vision: Distorted

Vision is distorted and fractured. This will usually be because of problems with the retina of the eye, but certain drugs can also cause this sign.

POSSIBLE CONDITIONS
Alcohol or Narcotics
Detached Retina
• Macular Degeneration
• Cataract

Vision: Double

Double vision is usually a serious sign, and should not be ignored. The most common cause will be a blow or injury to the head, but it may also be an indication of nerve or neurological problems or infection.

POSSIBLE CONDITIONS
Botulism
Head Injury
• Hyperthyroidism

Introcranial Haemorrhage
Meningitis
Multiple Sclerosis
Myasthenia Gravis
Nerve Pulses
• Stroke
Subcranial Haemorrhage
Systemic Lupus Erythematosis
Tumour of the Eye or behind the Eye

Vision: Sensitive to Light

Normal reaction of the pupil of the eye is to constrict in bright light. Going from a dark environment to a very bright one may hurt the eyes until they adjust, but this should be short term. Many infections make the eye especially sensitive to light, including Meningitis, as can injury to and infections of the eye.

POSSIBLE CONDITIONS
Abscess of the Brain
Adverse Drug Reaction
Albinism
Conjunctivitis
Corneal Ulcer
Dermatitis
Injury to the Eye
Iritis
Keratitis
Measles
Meningitis
• Migraine
Polio
Reddened Eyes
Subarachnoid Haemorrhage
• Viral Infection

Vision: Tunnel

Field of vision becomes narrower, and seems as if the individual is looking down a tunnel. If the field of vision becomes reduced, this is an indication of a serious problem with the eye or the structures in the brain concerned with vision. Medical help should be sought immediately.

POSSIBLE CONDITIONS
Brain Tumours
Cancer of the Eye
Carotid Aneurysm
Glaucoma
Hypothalmic Disease
Retinitis Pigmentosa
Syphilis

Voice: Hoarse and Swallowing Problems

Swallowing problems combined with hoarseness are usually simply an indication of an infection involving the throat, such as Laryngitis. If the problems persist, and there is no obvious infection, it may be an indication of cancer, particularly if combined with weight loss and poor appetite. In any event, if this combination of symptoms becomes long term, medical help should be sought and investigations undertaken.

POSSIBLE CONDITIONS
Cancer of the Larynx
Cancer of the Lung
Cancer of the Oesophagus
Choking
Laryngitis
Myasthenia Gravis

Pharyngitis
Pharyngeal Pouch
• Viral Infection

Voice: Hoarse or Loss of

The voice becomes hoarse, making it difficult to talk, or it may even become impossible to talk. This usually has an obvious cause such as shouting or talking for long periods or infections. If hoarseness persists for more than a couple of weeks, it may be an indication of serious underlying illness and medical help should be sought and tests undertaken.

POSSIBLE CONDITIONS
Cancer of the Larynx
Cancer of the Oesophagus
Cancer in the Chest
Choking
• Cold, Common
Croup
Epiglottitis
Isolated Thyroid Nodule
• Laryngitis
Lung Cancer
Myasthenia Gravis
Myxoedema
• Pharyngitis
Sarcoidosis
Sjogren's Syndrome
Vocal Nodules

Voice: Nasal Sounding

Voice sounds unusually nasal, although many individuals speak this way naturally. Other than this, most common causes are infections and injury to the nose. Medical help should be sought if there has been severe trauma to the nose as it may be broken.

POSSIBLE CONDITIONS
• Adenoids
Cleft Lip and Palate
Cold, Common
Foreign Body in Nose
Injury to the Nose
• Nasal Polyps
Septal Deviation
Sinusitis

Voice: Slurred, Muffled or Altered

Slurred or muffled speech can be caused by many conditions, most of them not a cause for concern, such as Colds, problems with adenoids, habit or infections. It may also be an indication that the individual has been using alcohol or drugs, or that the nose or other structures have been damaged. Rarely it can be an indication of serious underlying neurological disease or even cancer. Some of the causes are listed below, and also see the sections on Voice: Hoarse and Swallowing Problems, and Voice: Hoarse or Loss of.

POSSIBLE CONDITIONS
Adenoids
Adverse Drug Reaction
• Alcohol or Narcotics
Cancer of the Larynx
Cancer of the Mouth
Cancer of the Nose
Cleft Lip and Palate
• Cold, Common
Hepatolentricular Degeneration
Motor Neurone Disease
Multiple Sclerosis

Nasal Polyps
Parkinson's Disease
Septal Deviation
Sinusitis
Stroke
Viral Infection

Vomit: Blood in

Blood can be present in vomit. It may be bright red and fresh, or it may be black and like coffee grounds. Either way, this is usually a sign of a serious underlying problem, and medical help should be sought.

POSSIBLE CONDITIONS
Adverse Drug Reaction
Aortic Aneurysm
• Bleeding
Disorders of Blood Clotting
Gastritis
• Hernia, Hiatus
Intussusception
Mallory-Weiss Tear
• Oesophagitis
• Oesophageal Varices
• Peptic Ulcer
Yellow Fever

Vomiting, Nausea and Regurgitation of Food

Vomiting and nausea may result from a relatively mild cause — such as minor food poisoning (Gastroenteritis), drinking too much, travel sickness, Pregnancy or Migraines — to severe illness. Vomit will usually and initially consist of undigested food and is yellow, frothy and smells unpleasant, but persistent sickness results in the vomit becoming thin, green, mucousy and slimy. If vomit is brown, black or appears to have coffee grains, this is an indication that there is blood. See the relevant section on Vomit: Blood. In any event medical help should be sought should this be the case or if vomiting persists for a long time.

POSSIBLE CONDITIONS
Achalasia
Addison's Disease
Alcohol or Narcotics
Anorexia Nervosa
Appendicitis
Biliary Colic
Botulism
Brain Abscess
Brain Tumours
Cancer of the Oesophagus
Cancer of the Stomach
Chagas' Disease
Cholera
Cirrhosis of the Liver
Coeliac Disease
Congenital Atresia of the Oesophagus
Constipation
Diabetes
Diuretics
Dyspepsia, Non-Ulcer
Epididymitis
Gall Bladder Infection
Gall Stones
• Gastritis
• Gastroenteritis
Heat Exhaustion
Heat Stroke
• Hernia, Hiatus
Hernia, Inguinal (if obstruction)

Hernia, Umbilical (if obstruction)
Hypercalcaemia
Intestinal Ischaemia
Intestinal Obstruction
Kidney Disease or Failure
Kidney Stones
Meniere's Disease
Meningitis
Meninogococcal Septicaemia
Mesenteric Adenitis
Mesenteric Vascular Occlusion
Migraine
Mountain Sickness
Oesophageal Varices
• Oesophagitis
Pancreatitis
Peptic Ulcer
Peritonitis
Phaeochromocytoma
Poisoning
Polio
Porphyria
Porphyria Cutanea Tarda
Post-Gastrectomy Syndrome
Pregnancy
Pyloric Stenosis
Raised Intracranial Pressure
Salpingitis
Sarcoidosis
Shock
Subarachnoid Haemorrhage
Torsion
Travel Sickness
Uraemia
Urinary Tract Infection
Vestibulitis

Vomiting: Abdominal Pain

An indication of minor food poisoning or Gastroenteritis, but may be a sign of serious disease.

POSSIBLE CONDITIONS
Appendicitis
Biliary Colic
Cancer of the Bowel
Cancer of the Stomach
Diabetes
•Gastritis
•Gastroenteritis
Hernia, Umbilical
Hernia, Inguinal (if obstructed)
Intestinal Ischaemia
Intestinal Obstruction
Kidney Disease or Failure
Kidney Stones
Meckel's Diverticulum
Mesenteric Adenitis
Ovarian Cyst
Pancreatitis
Peptic Ulcer
Peritonitis
Porphyria
Salpingitis

Vomiting: Abdominal Pain and Fever

An indication of food poisoning, Gastroenteritis or Urinary Tract Infection, but may be a sign of serious disease.

POSSIBLE CONDITIONS
Appendicitis
Cancer of the Bowel

Cancer of the Kidney
Cancer of the Oesophagus
Cancer of the Stomach
Gall Stones
•Gastritis
•Gastroenteritis
Intestinal Obstruction
Meckel's Diverticulum
Pancreatitis
Pelvic Inflammatory Disease
Porphyria
•Urinary Tract Infection
Viral Infection

Vomiting: Abdominal Pain and Jaundice

Combination of symptoms which indicates serious illness. Medical help should be sought immediately.

POSSIBLE CONDITIONS
•Biliary Colic
Cancer of the Liver
Cancer of the Pancreas
Cancer of the Stomach
•Cholecystitis
•Gall Stones
Hepatitis
Pancreatitis
Sickle Cell Anaemia

Vomiting: Blood and Abdominal Pain

A sign of serious underlying disease, and medical help should be sought.

POSSIBLE CONDITIONS
Adverse Drug Reaction

Cancer of the Stomach
• Gastritis
Hernia, Hiatus
Mallory-Weiss Tear
• Oesophagitis
Oesophageal Varices
• Peptic Ulcer
Yellow Fever

Vomiting: Swallowing Problems

Combination of symptoms which are usually caused by acid from the stomach coming into the gullet, and may be an indication of serious disease. Any long-standing problems with swallowing should be investigated.

POSSIBLE CONDITIONS
Achalasia
Cancer of the Lung
Cancer of the Oesophagus
Cancer of the Stomach
Congenital Atresia of the Oesophagus
Hernia, Hiatus
• Oesophagitis
• Peptic or Oesophageal Stricture
Pharyngeal Pouch

Wasting

There is a prolonged and relentless wastage and reduction of strength in muscles, either generally throughout the body or one part of the body. This may be caused by any period of long-term physical inaction, such as being bedridden or having a limb immobilised. If there is no obvious cause such as this, medical help should be sought as this is a serious sign.

POSSIBLE CONDITIONS
Addison's Disease
Alcohol or Narcotics
Anorexia Nervosa
Bedridden
Brain Tumour
Cancer of Bone
Cancer of the Bowel
Cancer of the Breast
Cancer of the Kidney
• Cancer of the Lung
Cancer of the Ovary
Cancer of the Stomach
Carpal Tunnel Syndrome
• Coeliac Disease
Depression
Diabetes
• Hyperthyroidism
Hypopituitarism
Ischaemic Contracture
Kala-azar
Malabsorption
Metastases
Motor Neurone Disease
Multiple Sclerosis
Muscle Injury
Muscular Dystrophy
Myasthenia Gravis
Nerve Injury
Pituitary Tumour
Rheumatoid Arthritis
Spinal Cord Injury
Spinal Cord Tumours
Sprue

Weakness: Long-Term

Most individuals will experience weakness from time to time, but if this persists for a prolonged period there may be a serious underlying problem, especially if overwork or anxiety have been excluded as causes. Cancer, nerve and muscle disease can all produce prolonged fatigue and weakness.

POSSIBLE CONDITIONS
Addison's Disease
Adverse Drug Reaction
Alcohol or Narcotics
Anorexia Nervosa
Bedridden
Brain Tumour
Cancer of Bone
Cancer of the Bowel
Cancer of the Breast
Cancer of the Kidney
• Cancer of the Lung
Cancer of the Ovary
Cancer of the Stomach
Carpal Tunnel Syndrome
• Coeliac Disease
Depression
Diabetes
• Hyperthyroidism
Hypopituitarism
Ischaemic Contracture
Kala-azar
Malabsorption
Metastases
Motor Neurone Disease
Multiple Sclerosis
Muscle Injury
Muscular Dystrophy

Myasthenia Gravis
Nerve Injury
Pituitary Tumour
Rheumatoid Arthritis
Spinal Cord Injury
Spinal Cord Tumours
Sprue

Weakness: Quick Onset

Most individuals will suffer from bouts of weakness and sudden tiredness from time to time. This can herald the beginning of a viral infection (see other sections, including on fever), or may just be that the person has been running on adrenaline. Many individuals work too hard or for too long periods without rest and relaxation, then seem baffled when they are tired or even exhausted. Most causes of weakness will resolve with rest, although it can be an indication of several conditions.

POSSIBLE CONDITIONS
Addison's Disease
• Anxiety
Bleeding
• Cold, Common
Depression
• Flu
Guillain-Barre Syndrome
Heart Attack and Failure
Heart Disease
Hepatitis
Hyperthyroidism
Hypothyroidism
Low Blood Sugar
Mountain Sickness
Post-Viral Syndrome

Pregnancy
• Viral Infection

Weight Gain

The most common cause of weight gain is simple overeating combined with taking too little exercise. It is rarely caused by having a slow metabolism or having large bones. Obesity is an increasing problem in the developed world, and has health risks such as Heart Disease, Diabetes and arthritis. Weight loss can be achieved by sensible dieting, although some individuals find this difficult because of a lack of willpower, while in others there may actually be a difference in they way they are 'wired up' in that they do not 'feel full'. In rare cases hormonal disorders may be responsible for weight gain.

POSSIBLE CONDITIONS
Adverse Drug Reaction
Ascites
Cirrhosis
Contraceptive Pill
Cushing's Syndrome
Hypopituitarism
Hypothyroidism
• Menopause
• Obesity
Polycystic Ovaries

POSSIBLE CONDITIONS
Addison's Disease
Anorexia Nervosa
Cancer of the Bile Ducts
Cancer of the Bladder
Cancer of the Cervix
Cancer of the Colon or Rectum (Bowel)
Cancer of the Larynx
Cancer of the Mouth
Cancer of the Oesophagus
Cancer of the Ovaries
Cancer of the Stomach
Cancer in the Chest
• Coeliac Disease
Diabetes
Endocarditis
Heart Disease
Hypopituitarism
Hypothalamic Disease
Leukaemia
Lymphoma
Malnutrition
• Oesophagitis
• Peptic Ulcer
Pituitary Tumour
Sprue
Tuberculosis
Ulcerative Colitis

Weight Loss: Combined with Pallor or Anaemia

This is usually an indication of serious underlying disease, including cancer, or other problems such as alcoholism or drug addiction. Medical help should be sought.

Weight Loss: Jaundice

Persistent weight loss combined with jaundice, caused by problems with the liver or associated organs. It is a serious combination of symptoms, and often indicates cancer.

POSSIBLE CONDITIONS
Alcohol or Narcotic Abuse
Cancer of the Bile Ducts
Cancer of the Gall Bladder
• Cancer of the Liver
Cancer of the Pancreas
Cancer of the Stomach
Cirrhosis of the Liver
Hepatitis
Metastases
Vitamin B12 (Cyanocobalamin) Deficiency

Weight Loss: No Appetite

Unexplained weight loss combined with a lack of appetite is often a cause for concern, particularly in older individuals. Long-term disease and feverish illness can produce this combination, as can cancer in many parts of the body. Although rare, cancer should be investigated if there are also signs such as tiredness, unexplained pain, lumps or swellings, or blood coming from the mouth, vagina or in phlegm, vomit, faeces or urine.

POSSIBLE CONDITIONS
Adverse Drug Reaction
Alcohol or Narcotics
Anorexia Nervosa
Anxiety
Brucellosis
Cancer of the Bowel
Cancer of the Cervix
Cancer of the Kidney
Cancer of the Ovaries
Cancer of the Pancreas
Cancer of the Spine
Cancer of the Stomach

• Depression and Manic Depression
Fever
Hyperthyroidism
Hypopituitarism
Hypothalamic Problems
Lung Cancer
Metateses
• Peptic Ulcer
Rheumatic Fever
Septicaemia

Weight Loss: No Appetite and Chest Pain

Combination of symptoms which often indicates a serious underlying disease.

POSSIBLE CONDITIONS
Cancer of the Oesophagus
Cancer of the Stomach
Gall Bladder Infection
Heart Attack and Failure
Hernia, Hiatus
Lung Abcess
• Lung Cancer
Oesophagitis
• Peptic Ulcer
Tuberculosis

Weight Loss: Persistent

Weight loss which is persistent, progressive and unplanned. There can be many causes, many of which are listed below, including long-term Anxiety, Diabetes, cancer, infection and eating disorders.

POSSIBLE CONDITIONS
Achalasia

AIDS
• Anorexia Nervosa
• Anxiety
Brain Tumour
Bronchiectasis
Brucellosis
Cancer of the Kidney
Cancer of the Liver
Cancer of the Oesophagus
Cancer of the Pancreas
Cancer of the Spine
Cancer of the Stomach
Carcinoid Syndrome
Chagas' Disease
Coeliac Disease
Crohn's Disease
Cystic Fibrosis
• Depression
Diabetes
Gall Bladder Infection
Hernia, Hiatus
• Hyperthyroidism
Hypopituitarism
Kidney Disease or Failure
Lung Cancer
Multiple Sclerosis
Myasthenia Gravis
Pancreatitis
Parkinson's Disease
Peptic or Oesophageal Stricture
Pyloric Stenosis
Rheumatic Fever
Tuberculosis
Ulcerative Colitis

Weight Loss: Persistent and Abdominal Pain

Pain in the abdomen and long-term weight loss may be a sign of serious disease, and medical help should be sought.

POSSIBLE CONDITIONS
Cancer of the Bone
Cancer of the Colon or Rectum (Bowel)
Cancer of the Kidney
Cancer of the Liver
Cancer of the Pancreas
Cancer of the Stomach
Crohn's Disease
Diabetes
Gastritis
Oesophagitis
• Pancreatitis
• Peptic Ulcer
Ulcerative Colitis

Weight Loss: Swallowing Problems

This combination of symptoms is usually an indication of serious underlying disease. If weight loss is unexplained and persistent, medical help should be sought and investigations made.

POSSIBLE CONDITIONS
Cancer of the Oesophagus
Cancer of the Stomach
Chagas' Disease
Guillain-Barre Syndrome
Lung Cancer
Motor Neurone Disease
Multiple Sclerosis
Parkinson's Disease

• Peptic or Oesophageal Stricture
Myasthenia Gravis
Scleroderma
Systemic Lupus Erythematosis (SLE)

Wheezing

Wheezing is most likely to be caused by Asthma, a Foreign Body being in the gullet and blocking or partially blocking the windpipe, or a Chest Infection.

Possible Conditions
Adverse Drug Reaction
• Asthma
• Chest Infection
Choking
Hay Fever
Heart Failure
Laryngeal Oedema
Poisoning

Wheezing: Breathlessness

This combination of symptoms is not uncommon, and is caused by conditions which result in a narrowing of airways, either from infection or allergy.

Possible Conditions
Adverse Drug Reaction
Allergic Alveolitis
Allergic Reaction, Severe
Aspergillosis
• Asthma
Bronchiolitis
• Bronchitis
Carcinoid Syndrome
Chest Infection
Emphysema

Extrinsic Allergic Alveolitis
Hay Fever
Heart Disease
• Heart Failure
Hyperventilation
Myocarditis
Poisoning

Worms

Worms can infest the human body. The most common type found are threadworms, although others can also affect individuals. This will be very unusual except in those who have been travelling abroad.

Possible Conditions
Bilharzia
Hookworms (human)
Roundworms
Tapeworms
Threadworm

Wrist: Lump or Swelling

Lumps or swelling can develop on the wrist, usually because of the formation of a Ganglion or arthritis.

Possible Conditions
• Ganglion
Osteoarthritis
Rheumatoid Arthritis
Tuberculosis

Wrist: Pain

Pain is experienced in or around the wrist. This will usually be caused either by an injury, arthritis or fracture, or damage to nerves.

Symptoms Signs and Conditions

Possible Conditions
Broken Lower Arm Bones (Radius, Ulna and wrist)
Carpal Tunnel Syndrome
Ganglion
• Injury
• Osteoarthritis
Rheumatoid Arthritis
Tuberculosis
Ulnar Nerve
Wrist Sprain

Section Two: Conditions

These are extensively cross-referenced, but if there is difficulty finding a particular condition, try it under any possible combination (ie Breast Cancer or Cancer of the Breast).

A–Z

Abdominal Injury

see INJURY TO THE LOWER CHEST OR PELVIS

Acanthosis Nigricans

Appearance of black lines of pigmentation about the armpit, face and neck, and the groin. It is usually associated with malignant cancer, but can be associated with conditions where there is resistance to the actions of the hormone, insulin.

SIGNS
- Black lines of pigmentation on the skin

> NOTE
> This is an extremely rare condition.

Achalasia

Difficulty with swallowing food and the passage of food into the stomach. Although there is no obvious mechanical obstruction, achalasia is caused by poor relaxation of the muscles in the gullet.

SYMPTOMS
- Difficulty when swallowing especially with solids
- Vomiting
- Food is regurgitated into the mouth
- Indigestion or cramping chest pain

- Weight loss

Acne Rosacea

Red rash, associated with facial flushing, caused by a problem with sebaceous glands in the skin.

SIGNS
- Rash, red in colour, which may cover much of the face
- Rash may have pustules

> NOTE
> May not resolve for years, and treatment may be ineffective.

Acne Vulgaris

Pores in the skin become blocked, particularly the face, back and upper chest, causing spots, and both blackheads and whiteheads. It is caused by an increase in the production of hormones, as experienced during adolescence.

SIGNS
- Spots, pimples and blackheads which block glands. These can become infected, causing pus-filled spots (whiteheads). The condition affects the face, as well as the back and upper chest.

- Skin can become red and inflamed
- Skin appears greasy or oily

> NOTE
> Most usually found in adolescents and young adults, and it can last for years. May be treated with antibiotics. If left, acne may cause permanent scarring. There is no evidence that acne is linked to diet.

Acoustic Neuroma

A benign and slow-growing tumour that can develop on the nerve associated with hearing.

SYMPTOMS
- Progressive deafness which affects only one ear
- Ringing in the same ear (tinnitus)
- Vertigo, giddiness and loss of balance

Later:
- Face becomes progressively numb on the affected side

> NOTE
> Very rare condition. Tests will be needed to confirm a diagnosis.

Acoustic Trauma

see LOUD NOISES

Acquired Dislocation of the Hip

The thigh bone (femur) can become displaced from the hip joint, usually as a result of a severe injury. The trauma will usually have occurred when the individual is sitting down, as in motorbike and car accidents.

SYMPTOMS & SIGNS
- Severe pain

- Head of the thigh bone (femur) may be apparent, sticking out of the leg or hip
- Leg is shortened and twisted inwards
- Leg cannot be moved
- Knee is slightly bent

> NOTE
> It is unlikely this will be the only injury, and recovery may take a very long time.

Acromegaly

The skeleton becomes larger, caused by excessive growth hormone, which is secreted by the pituitary gland.

SYMPTOMS & SIGNS
- Skeleton becomes much larger than normal
- Hands and feet become enlarged (rings need to be resized and shoe size increases)
- Face may look swollen with thicker lips and enlargement of the tongue
- Jaw becomes enlarged and protrudes
- Increased amount of body hair
- Heavy and excessive sweating

> NOTE
> Medical help should be sought.

Acute Inflammatory Polyneuropathy

see GUILLAIN-BARRE SYNDROME

Addison's Disease

Condition caused by the long-term under activity of the adrenal glands.

SYMPTOMS & SIGNS
- Weakness and fatigue
- Loss of appetite and weight loss

- Nausea and vomiting
- Diarrhoea
- Blood pressure is low
- Dehydration
- May be hair loss, including pubic hair
- Brown skin pigmentation on areas exposed to sunlight or on pressure points or old scars. Also pigmentation on lips and in mouth.
- Vitiligo, where pigment-producing cells are lacking, which will be especially noticeable in those with black or dark skins as it will leave patches of white skin
- In severe cases, may be collapse

> NOTE
> Medical help should be sought.

Adenoids

Adenoids are tissue pads at the back of the nose, and are similar to tonsils. It is thought, like tonsils, they help to fight infection, but they can grow so large that they block passages to the nose, making the individual breath through their mouth. The adenoids are also prone to infection.

SYMPTOMS
- Speech is nasal or muffled
- Mouth breathing
- Snoring
- May be recurrent ear infections
- May be loss of sense of smell
- May be a dry cough

> NOTE
> It may be necessary to have medical treatment or even surgery.

Adie's Pupil (or Holmer-Adie Pupil)

Usually one pupil (but occasionally both) of the eye is dilated, and responds only slowly to exposure to bright light.

SIGNS
- Dilated pupil of one eye, which responds only slowly to bright light
- No other symptoms

> NOTE
> More likely in young women.

Adverse Drug Reaction

Drugs, both medical and recreational, can produce a range of adverse reactions and unpleasant side-effects. Only some of the most common are listed here, and symptoms may appear singly.

SYMPTOMS & SIGNS
- Sore throat
- Inflammation of the mouth
- Fever
- Bleeding from the gums, nose, gut, rectum or vagina. There may be blood in vomit (like coffee grounds) or blood in stools causing dark and tarry faeces. Drugs which can cause bleeding include steroids, anti-inflammatory medicines such as aspirin, and drugs which reduce the body's ability to clot or thin the blood (anticoagulant therapy) such as warfarin
- Some drugs, such as 'statins', lithium, and alcohol, can cause muscle pain
- Nosebleeds can be caused by drugs which reduce the ability of the blood to clot, such as warfarin
- Deafness and ringing in the ears (tinnitus) can

be caused by several drugs, such as aspirin, particularly where an overdose has been taken, quinine, and streptomycin

■ Constipation can be caused by many drugs, including morphine, diamorphine (heroin) and codeine, as well as other pain killers

■ Some drugs can cause retention of urine, particularly individuals with problems with the prostate

■ Diuretic drugs given or taken in too high quantities can cause thirst, perhaps excessive in nature, associated with dehydration

■ Some drugs, such as those used to treat high blood pressure, tranquillisers and heroin, may make it difficult for a men to get or maintain an erection. Other drugs can reduce sperm counts and reduce a man's fertility

■ Some drugs can cause bad or unusual-smelling breath as they have characteristic smells

■ ACE inhibitors, used for high blood pressure, may cause a dry cough

■ Digoxin, used in the treatment of heart failure, can cause a range of side-effects, including very slow heart rate with extra beats, nausea and vomiting, abdominal pains, hallucinations, and fatigue. It can also make the world appear to have a green or yellow tint. Beta blockers can also cause a very slow heart rate

■ Some drugs used as cold remedies and anti asthmatic drugs may cause an increased heart rate in some individuals

■ Some drugs, especially antipsychotics and some antidepressants, can cause symptoms of Parkinson's Disease.

■ Some prescriptions drugs, such as steroids, and recreational drugs, such as amphetamines or even cannabis, can cause mania and hyperactivity

■ Some drugs can cause headache. These include glyceryl trinitrate and other nitrates (given for angina) and calcium channel blockers (given for angina or high blood pressure). If prescribed drugs cause headache, contact a doctor to see if there is an alternative medication.

■ Some drugs, particularly where the individual is allergic, can cause the development of a rash or may cause the skin to become blotchy, itchy and swollen, with the affected areas red or purple. If this does develop, the course of drugs should be discontinued until advice has been sought. In extreme cases, some drugs can cause Scalded Skin Syndrome, which can lead to large areas of the skin peeling off and can even prove fatal. Drugs such as penicillin or aspirin can also cause the skin to become red and patchy or blotchy. Adverse reactions to drugs can occur at any time, even after long-term use

■ Some drugs, such as betablockers, aspirin, and anti-rheumatic drugs such as NSAIDs (non steroidal anti-inflammatory drugs), can cause breathlessness and wheezing

■ Some drugs can cause hair loss or hair to fall out, including chemotherapy drugs given for cancers. Vitamin A toxicity can also cause hair loss.

■ Some drugs can increase development of hair on the face or body including some steroids, some epileptic drugs, such as Phenytoin, and Minoxidil, used to lower blood pressure (this is used also as a hair restorer)

■ Some drugs can cause a change in the colour of the skin. These include Amiodarone, used for heart conditions, and medications for leprosy and dermatitis, as well as some chemicals. These all colour the skin blue. Mepacrine, an antimalarial drug, can make the skin look yellow

- Some drugs can make the pupils of the eye contract, including drugs to treat Glaucoma and some narcotics, including morphine, pethidine and heroin
- Some drugs can make vision blurred, including antidepressants and drugs for controlling the function of the bladder
- Some drugs make the pupils of the eye dilate, including atropine and other drugs used for Iritis
- Steroids, when used over the long term for the eyes, can cause Cataracts and infections
- Some drugs, such as antidepressants and tranquillisers, can reduce core body temperature, making the individual more prone to hypothermia
- Some drugs, such as steroids and the contraceptive pill, may result in weight gain

NOTE
Drugs which have been prescribed by a doctor may cause problems. It is important, however, to consult a doctor before stopping taking a course of prescribed drugs.

CROSS-REFERENCED UNDER:
Drug Reaction or Side-Effect; Drug Induced

African River Blindness

see FILARIASIS

AIDS

Infection by the human immunodeficiency virus (HIV). This can lie unnoticed for years until a large variety of symptoms appear and full-blown AIDS (Acquired Immune Deficiency Syndrome) becomes apparent. Although there is currently no cure, treatments can prolong life and an early diagnosis is essential. The virus is spread through body fluids, such as semen and blood, including through sexual intercourse and drug users sharing needles. Risks can be reduced by using condoms and clean needles.

SYMPTOMS & SIGNS
- Fever
- Swollen lymph nodes
- Weight loss
- Sweating, particularly heavy at night
- Recurrent infections including thrush
- Diarrhoea with abdominal pain
- Feeling generally unwell
- Sore throat
- Skin rash
- Aching muscles and joints
- Headache
- Enlarged liver and spleen
- Kaposi's Sarcoma: malignant tumours which appear as blue-red patches on the skin
- Hair loss in later stages
- May be Dementia, even in the young

NOTE
If the possibility of infection is high, medical help should be sought immediately: a test can determine infection, although this may not be accurate for up to three months after any contact. Individuals thought to be especially at risk are homosexual men, bisexuals, and injecting drug users, although increasingly heterosexuals are not taking precautions. There is no evidence that

HIV can be contracted from day-to-day non-sexual contact with individuals who have the condition.

CROSS-REFERENCED UNDER:
HIV; Auto-Immune Deficiency Syndrome

Albinism

The individual has no pigment in the skin and other tissues, so that skin is very pale and the irises are pink. There will be associated problems with sight.

SIGNS
- Skin is fair, pale or even white
- Hair is white
- Irises of the eyes are pink: eyes are very sensitive to light

Alcohol or Narcotics

Addiction to alcohol or drugs and the ability to manage consumption varies from individual to individual. Signs of abuse may be obvious, but in many alcoholics and other drug addicts all signs of abuse may be carefully hidden, even from loved ones. Indeed, some addicts go to extreme lengths to make everything appear normal. Some drugs, such as alcohol, may be managed by the individual fairly safely, while other substances, such as solvents, are always dangerous and may cause death even after repeated use.

SYMPTOMS & SIGNS
Alcohol:
- Temporary slurring or slowness of speech
- Face may be red
- May be excessive sweating
- May be confusion

- Snoring may be worse, especially when a lot of alcohol has been consumed
- Drinking may cause increased heart rate
- Unsteadiness on walking
- May be vomiting, nausea, diarrhoea or incontinence
- May be blurred vision
- May be problems getting and maintaining an erection
- Drinking lots of alcohol (water, tea or coffee will also have the same affect) may cause increased frequency of urination
- Headache, either caused by dehydration or because of the toxic build up of chemicals in the body
- May be greater susceptibility to hypothermia as alcohol dilates blood vessels and increases heat loss. This may be a danger in cold conditions such as drinkers walking home in the winter
- May be unconsciousness and coma with deep but shallow breathing and very small pupils of eyes
- May be convulsions or fits, although this is rare except in long-term alcoholics

Long term abuse or alcoholism:
- Morning vomiting
- Noticeably red palms
- Muscle cramps
- Heart problems, such as extra beats and rhythm disorders, and excessive consumption of alcohol can lead to heart disease
- Vitamin B1 (Thiamine) deficiency: symptoms similar to Beri-Beri, such as neuropathy, congenitive heart failure, oedema
- May be Dementia, caused by above
- May be convulsions or fits

- May be alcoholic neuropathy including muscle wastage, altered sensation, including numbness, tingling, reduction in strength and stamina, limb weakness and joint damage and deformity, as well as ulcerated or infected feet
- May be problems with impotence as well as reduced sperm count and fertility
- May be Cirrhosis of the Liver
- May be hair loss, including pubic hair
- Breakdown of relationships, deteriorating work performance/unemployment

Other drugs (these signs are somewhat obvious; actual addicts may exhibit few obvious signs of their addiction):

- Appearance and many aspects of life, such as relationships, become neglected
- Mania and hyperactivity with drugs such as amphetamines
- May be hallucinations
- May be confusion
- Tram lines: needle marks on limbs on in the groin: anywhere where a vein lies close to the surface
- May be unconsciousness and coma with deep but shallow breathing and very small pupils of eyes. In severe case of overdose, the skin may have a blue tinge: medical help should be sought immediately if an overdose is suspected

Withdrawal from alcohol can cause:

- Symptoms of Anxiety (even a hangover in those who drink less may experience Anxiety)
- Tremor, often very marked
- Sweating
- May be convulsions or fits
- Stomach cramps and diarrhoea
- Insomnia

- Headache
- Palpitation
- DTs – hallucination, disorientation, tachycardia

Withdrawal from other drugs such as morphine or heroin as for alcohol, plus goose flesh and running eyes and nose

> NOTE
> Alcoholism and excessive drinking is a widespread but often ignored problem, as is the abuse of narcotics and other illegal drugs. All are dangerous. Alcohol is the most widely abused drug.

CROSS-REFERENCED UNDER:
Drugs; Narcotics

Aldosteronism

Over production of aldosterone, causing high blood pressure and muscle weakness. It is caused by a tumour on the adrenal gland.

SYMPTOMS & SIGNS
- High blood pressure
- Muscle weakness
- Low blood level of potassium
- Excessive urination
- Severe thirst
- Muscle spasms
- Often not associated with any symptoms

> NOTE
> Medical help should be sought.

CROSS-REFERENCED UNDER:
Conn's Syndrome; Primary Aldosteronism

Alkaptonuria

Urine turns black after it has been excreted, caused by the incomplete breakdown of substances in the urine, and due to a rare inherited metabolic variation between individuals. The condition is noticed in babies, as urine can stain nappies black or go black if it is left to stand.

SIGNS
- Urine turns very dark, and even black, once it has been excreted

  Sometimes the whites of the eyes, and cartilages can be pigmented
- No other symptoms

> NOTE
> Not believed to cause any major illnesses, except possibly arthritis in later life.

Allergic Alveolitis

Allergic inflammation of the small air sacs in the lung (alveoli), which allow the transfer of oxygen and carbon dioxide between the air and the blood. If these become inflamed, breathing becomes harder and harder. An attack can be precipitated by exposure to many allergens, including hay, flour or pigeons; and can involve either a sharp short episode or long-term problems. A classic form of this is 'farmer's lung' caused by inhalation of dust from mouldy hay.

SYMPTOMS
- Breathlessness and wheezing, although this may take some hours to develop fully
- Dry cough
- Generally feeling of ill health, with fever-like flu, chills and joint pains, headaches, loss of appetite and tiredness
- May develop into a chronic condition with prolonged episodes
- Clubbed fingernails are an occasional accompaniment if develops into a long-term problem

> NOTE
> An acute attack should resolve in a few days, but the best course of management is to avoid whatever causes the attack.

CROSS-REFERENCED UNDER:
Farmer's Lung

Allergic Reaction, Severe

Severe allergic reactions to nuts, insect stings or medical injections may cause body tissues to swell, including the larynx. This can block the windpipe and cause suffocation. Allergies may have less severe symptoms, such as skin rash, Hay Fever, Reddened Eyes, Rhinitis or Asthma.

SYMPTOMS & SIGNS
- Swelling of soft tissues such as throat, face, eyes, lips and limbs
- Wheezing and difficulty in breathing
- Rapid pulse
- Collapse and possible suffocation
- Coma

> NOTE
> Medical help should be sought immediately as this can be fatal. Many susceptible individuals will have an antidote with them (adrenaline is one such antidote).

CROSS-REFERENCED UNDER:
Swelling of the Larynx; Anaphylactic Shock

Allergic Rhinitis

see RHINITIS

Alopecia

Alopecia – thinning of the hair of any extent up to total baldness – is normal in men and part of the ageing process in the male: it is not an illness. The rate at which men become bald, if indeed they lose their hair at all, is likely to be down to their genes; typical male hair loss is also permanent. In females, hair also becomes thinner with age, although there should be no actual baldness. Baldness may also be caused by various diseases, discussed elsewhere, may be a side effect of some drug treatments and by hormonal disorders and occasionally after childbirth and traumatic experiences, such as bereavement or terror.

SIGNS ('male-pattern' alopecia)

- Hair recedes from the forehead and temples
- Hair becomes progressively thinner on the crown
- These areas of recession become larger and join up until hair remains on the sides and back of the head
- Alopecia can also affect body hair including pubic hair

NOTE

Treatments and remedies for baldness are available, although it remains open to question how effective they are.

CROSS-REFERENCED UNDER:
Baldness; Hair Loss

Alopecia Areata

Localised patches of complete hair loss. Occassionally extensive. Scalp may be slightly red. May run in families. Associated with eczema and other conditions including thyroid disorders.

SIGNS

- Patchy baldness or thinning, some of which may join into a larger area or areas
- Hair will usually grow back after some months, often initially grows in white

---

NOTE

In this type of baldness, hair will often grow back, at least partially.

CROSS-REFERENCED UNDER:
Baldness; Hair Loss

Altitude Sickness

see MOUNTAIN SICKNESS

Alzheimer's Disease

see DEMENTIA

Amaurosis Fugax

see CENTRAL RETINAL ARTERY BLOCKAGE

Anaemia

Disorder where there is lack of red blood cells, which affects the blood's capacity to carry oxygen around the body. It may be as a result of several conditions, although common causes are lack of iron or vitamins in the diet, very heavy menstruation with severe blood loss, any condition with severe bleeding, or problems with bone marrow (which produces red blood cells). Thalassaemia is a generally milder form of chronic anaemia, although there are more serious forms, and it runs in families.

SYMPTOMS & SIGNS

■ General fatigue, prolonged weakness and tiredness
■ Feeling short of breath
■ Skin looks abnormally pale and white, or may have a yellowish tinge
■ The normally red membranes inside the lower eye lid may be very pale
■ Feelings of dizziness or giddiness when rising to the feet
■ Noises in the ears (tinnitus)
■ May be sore tongue or cracks at the corners of the mouth
■ Fingernails may be spoon shaped

In severe cases:

■ Increased heart rate, only obvious in severe cases
■ May be Angina as the heart is not getting enough oxygen
■ May be swollen ankles because of mild heart failure

> NOTE
> Tests can confirm the diagnosis and underlying cause of Anaemia. In the case of Thalassaemia, regular blood transfusions may be needed.

CROSS-REFERENCED UNDER:

Thalassaemia

Anaemia, Pernicious

see PERNICIOUS ANAEMIA

Anal Abscess

Abscess can form in the anal canal or rectum. Faeces contain many bacteria, and the moistness of this area means that it may be prone to infection. The abscess may also be an indication of some other underlying condition, such as Diabetes or Crohn's Disease or Ulcerative Colitis.

SYMPTOMS

■ Pain localised to one area, and throbbing and persistent
■ Localised inflammation which will be very tender
■ Skin will be red if the abscess occurs near the surface
■ May be fever, chills, and general feeling of ill health with loss of appetite
■ Pulse rate may be unusually fast

> NOTE
> May resolve itself, but may need surgical assessment and treatment.

Anal Fissure

The surface of the anal canal can become torn by the passage of hard faeces or from anal intercourse.

SYMPTOMS

■ Pain localised to the tear, worse after passing faeces
■ Pain may be very severe and may dissuade the individual from opening their bowels from the discomfort: they may become constipated
■ May be bleeding from the tear: blood will be bright red
■ Anus or rectal area may be itchy

> NOTE
> The tear will usually resolve itself without treatment, although pain-relieving cream may soothe the discomfort.

Anaphylactic Shock

see ALLERGIC REACTION, SEVERE

Ancylostoma

see HOOKWORMS (HUMAN)

Angina

Chest pain, usually caused by coronary artery disease and the heart muscle not receiving enough blood and oxygen during exertion. Although it is a sign of heart disease due to narrowed coronary arteries, it is not in itself necessarily life threatening or dangerous. Often runs in families and is more likely in smokers and those with high blood pressure or high cholesterol.

SYMPTOMS

- Heavy or tight or pressure-like pain in the front of the chest behind the breast bone, which can go into the jaw or down the arms, most commonly the left arm
- Onset is usually with exertion or exercise
- Usually if the individual rests, the pain will settle
- Exacerbated by the cold, emotional stress, and following eating

NOTE
Most likely in older individuals. It is usual for an ecg to be undertaken to confirm the diagnosis of Angina. Sometimes this is followed by taking an ecg during exercise. Further tests including an angiogram (coronary) may be necessary to decide whether medical or surgical treatment is necessary. Often medical intervention is all that is needed, and the individual can lead a relatively normal life.

Angioneurotic Oedema

Swelling of the tongue, mouth, lips, throat and also at times, face, especially around the eyes and hands, most usually as the result of an allergy or adverse drug reaction, although the cause may not be clear. Substances which can cause an allergic reaction include shellfish and penicillin.

SYMPTOMS & SIGNS

- Swollen tongue, mouth, lips, throat, face. Swelling can be more extensive
- Mucous membranes can become swollen: this is particularly serious in the throat as the swelling can cause death
- Very itchy

NOTE
Medical help should be sought immediately.

CROSS-REFERENCED UNDER:
Giant Urticaria

Ankle Fracture

see BROKEN ANKLE

Ankylosing Spondylitis

Inflammation of the joints and tendons in the spine. May start as painful inflammation of the sacroiliac joints

SIGNS

- Bone and joint pain, starting with the spine
- Stiffness
- Pain and stiffness worse in early morning
- Hunched or stooped posture
- May also affect the heart, lungs and eyes

> NOTE
> Medical help should be sought. Most likely in young adult males.

Anorexia Nervosa

Eating disorders, often identified in adolescent girls but possible in any individual. The individual is convinced that they need to lose weight, even when it is obvious to others that they are already underweight. In Bulimia there are periods of dieting and bouts of binge eating, after which the individual often make themselves vomit up what they have eaten. Alternatively, they may use purgatives or laxatives. These are not trivial conditions: a significant proportion of those affected eventually die from the condition.

SYMPTOMS & SIGNS
- Gradual but persistent weight loss
- Fine body hair
- If an individual goes through a major change in body weight, menstruation will usually be disrupted or even stop (amenorrhoea). In adolescent girls who haven't started having periods the onset of the periods can be significantly held back, for the duration of the appetite disorder
- May be eating binges, followed by bouts of vomiting or purging

> NOTE
> Most common in individuals between about 11 and 30 years of age, and more likely in females than males. Medical help should be sought if body weight becomes too low, although this can be a difficult condition to tackle.

CROSS-REFERENCED UNDER:
Bulimia; Weight Change

Anxiety

Anxiety is a general term to describe feelings of over concern, arousal or worry, many of the symptoms being caused by the normal release of adrenaline into the body. Many emotions such as fear, shock or even sexual arousal, will produce a similar response. Most individuals will experience anxiety at some time, but long-term over-arousal can work on the autonomic nervous system and develop into phobias, Depression or anxiety states, and anxiety may also be a sign of other psychological or mental problems. It is, under any circumstances, very tiring.

SYMPTOMS & SIGNS
- Dry mouth
- May be rapid, over-breathing ('hyperventilation')
- Increased heart rate and extra beats: thumping of heart and palpitations
- Stiffness in the neck and into the shoulders
- Pressure, like a band, around the head or headache
- Tingling of hands, feet and around the mouth (because of hyperventilation)
- Feelings of dizziness or giddiness
- Problems thinking straight and poor memory
- Sweating, which may be severe and unrelated to exercise or to ambient temperature
- May be diarrhoea
- Tremor
- Eyes wide and staring: pupils dilated
- Deep feelings that some terrible event is about to take place
- Individual may faint if they have received a

shock or very bad news: this is not unusual and they will usually recover without problems

- It is not common, but certainly possible, that bereaved people see hallucinations of a newly deceased loved one
- It is possible, though rare, that if someone receives a shock or emotional blow they can literally be struck dumb or blind without any underlying physical cause (Hysteria). They may alternatively become quite manic
- Similarly, there may be memory loss (amnesia) and associated disorientation
- With long-term anxiety or severe stress, it is possible that menstruation can stop. This is not uncommon, but if it lasts longer than six months (and pregnancy has been excluded already), medical help should be sought to exclude disease or cancer
- In any event, Anxiety is very tiring and may result in health problems such as Depression, mental illness, weight loss and self-neglect

---

NOTE

Most individuals will experience a certain amount of Anxiety, Emotion and Stress from time to time. If this becomes difficult to cope with, there are many strategies, such as relaxation, counselling to explore the source of Anxiety, or medical treatments.

CROSS-REFERENCED UNDER:
Emotion; Stress

Aortic Aneurysm

The main artery of the body (aorta) that runs through the chest and abdomen can have a weakness in its wall that results in a local expansion and swelling of the artery. This swelling can develop very slowly, but if the swelling develops rapidly or is large it can rupture without warning. Rupture of an aortic aneurysm is very serious, and is a potentially fatal condition. An aortic aneurysm may not, however, be apparent unless it ruptures.

SYMPTOMS & SIGNS

- Pain in the abdomen or upper chest that often is also felt in the back may appear to resolve but then recur
- Abdomen can have a swollen area, which pulsates in time with the heartbeat
- Back pain
- Hoarseness (very rarely)

If the aneurysm beings to leak:

- Crushing pain similar to a Heart Attack but felt also in the back
- May be vomiting of blood (very serious)
- May cause collapse and coma

NOTE

May have very similar signs to that of a Heart Attack. Medical help should be sought immediately. Although potentially life-threatening, surgery is possible in many cases.

Aortic Stenosis

The valve that controls the outflow of blood from the heart to the main artery (aorta) of the body does not work efficiently because it is narrowed.

SYMPTOMS & SIGNS

- Angina
- Breathlessness
- May be fainting on exercise or exertion
- Palpitation or irregular heartbeat

NOTE
Most likely in older people, most commonly due to Rheumatic Heart Disease, a complication of Rheumatic Fever, in earlier life. The condition may be diagnosed as it produces a very characteristic heart murmur. Surgical treatment may be needed to replace the faulty valve, although other treatments are also used.

CROSS-REFERENCED UNDER:
Aortic Valve Disease

Aortic Valve Disease

see AORTIC STENOSIS

Aphthous Ulcer

Ulcers that may found anywhere in the mouth, either singly or in groups, including on the inside of the lips. The ulcers may be caused by injury, by biting the inside of the mouth or by dental problems, or may be caused by stress.

SYMPTOMS & SIGNS
- Very intensely painful: made worse by acids from fruit
- May be so painful that opening the mouth is difficult
- Ulcer is quite small, white or grey in colour, and oval in shape
- May be found singly or in groups
- May make eating, talking or brushing teeth difficult because of the intense pain

NOTE
Most mouth ulcers heal within a few days, and should do so within a couple of weeks. It is possible to buy pain-relieving remedies from pharmacists.

CROSS-REFERENCED UNDER:
Mouth Ulcer; Ulcer, Mouth

Appendicitis

The appendix, a now apparently redundant organ in the intestine, may become inflamed.

SYMPTOMS & SIGNS
- Pain in the right side of the lower abdomen. It often starts around the belly button (navel or umbilicus), but then moves down and to the right
- Pain exacerbated by pressing the area of the abdomen where the appendix is situated
- May be fever
- Loss of appetite: even nausea and possibly vomiting
- May be constipation, or alternatively diarrhoea (the latter is less likely)
- General feeling of being unwell
- Sometimes a lump can be felt on the right side of the abdomen, although this is not usually the appendix itself but other tissues wrapped around it (appendix mass)

NOTE
Although appendicitis may resolve itself, surgery is usually required to remove the inflamed appendix and medical help should be sought. Most likely in those between the ages of two and 30 years of age, and in developed countries.

Arcus Senilis

White circle around the cornea of the eye.

SIGNS
- White circle around the cornea of the eye

NOTE
Most likely in older individuals, such as those over 60 years of age, and is harmless. If found in younger people, it may be associated with high blood cholesterol, and should be investigated.

Arterial Disease

see PERIPHERAL VASCULAR DISEASE

Arteriosclerosis

see ARTERY DISEASE

Artery Disease

Insufficient blood flow in the body caused by blocked or partially blocked arteries. The walls of the artery may become hardened (Arteriosclerosis), or the arteries may become furred up with fatty deposits (Atheroma), particularly as an individual grows older. This condition is also associated with Heart Attacks, Angina, Strokes and Aneurysms.

SYMPTOMS & SIGNS
- Angina or Heart Attack
- Transient Ischaemic Attack of Stroke
- Aneurysms
- Peripheral Vascular Disease with cold peripheries (this can lead to loss of toes)
- Vertigo and giddiness, particularly when standing up and when the head is suddenly moved up or to the sides (vertebrobasilar insufficiency). Tinnitus. Variable deafness
- Men may have problems getting and maintaining an erection
- If an artery supplying blood to an area becomes blocked, the area may become pale or white and that area can become non-viable

NOTE
Medical help should be sought. More likely in those who smoke, those with High Blood Pressure, High Cholesterol, and Diabetes.

CROSS-REFERENCED UNDER:
Arteriosclerosis; Atheroma

Arthritis (Osteoarthritis)

see OSTEOARTHRITIS

Arthritis, Rheumatoid

see RHEUMATOID ARTHRITIS

Asbestosis

see PNEUMOCONIOSIS

Ascites, Malignant

see MALIGNANT ASCITES

Aspergillosis

Respiratory condition, caused by a fungus found in rotting vegetation and in damp places however most individuals are not affected by the fungus itself but it causes asthma-like breathlessness due to an allergic reation.

SYMPTOMS & SIGNS
- Wheezy cough
- May be fever

NOTE
Diagnosis may be confirmed by testing for an allergic reaction to the fungus.

Asthma

A potentially severe respiratory condition, characterised by excessive constriction of muscle in the airways in the lungs. This narrows the airways (bronchial tubes) is associated with wheeze and makes every breath forced and difficult. Asthma is a potentially fatal condition. It may be associated with particular occupations, such as those working in the manufacture of cotton, hemp and flax, and is associated with Dermatitis (Eczema) and allergies.

SYMPTOMS & SIGNS

■ Wheeze, particularly when exhaling, most noticeable after the individual has been exercising or exerting themselves

■ Shortness of breath

■ Breathing is shallow, noisy and may be very rapid

■ Cough, usually dry in nature, most frequent at night

■ Tightness around the chest

■ Rapid pulse

■ Sweating

■ Muscles in the neck are straining to aid breathing

■ Recurrent attacks

■ Dehydration caused by fluid being lost through breathing

■ Often associated with Hay Fever and Eczema (Dermatitis)

If the attack becomes worse or particularly acute (this may take minutes or even hours):

■ May be blue tinge to the skin 'cyanosis' (serious)

■ Distress and may not be able to speak because of alteration in breathing (serious)

■ Drowsiness, mental confusion and coma (very serious)

If linked to an occupation:

■ Asthma attack or wheezing on returning to work

■ Condition may be eased or absent by staying away from work

NOTE

Approx 1 in 10 children suffer from Asthma at some time in their lives. About half of those affected no longer have the condition in adulthood. If an attack is serious, and if existing medication for Asthma appears to be ineffective medical help should be sought immediately. Most individuals with Asthma will carry an inhaler, but may need help using it. If the inhaler does not help, or is absent, help should be sought immediately.

CROSS-REFERENCED UNDER:

Occupational Asthma

Atheriosclerosis
see PERIPHERAL VASCULAR DISEASE

Atheroma
see ARTERY DISEASE

Athlete's Foot

Irritation and itching of the feet, caused by a fungal infection.

SYMPTOMS & SIGNS

■ Itching, irritation, redness and burning pain between the toes

■ Smelly between the toes

■ Skin is blistered or flaky

■ May be opportunistic infections and crusting

■ Toenails may be affected, making them either soft or brittle

NOTE

Anti-fungal powders are available. More likely in those with sweaty feet or who wear shoes which do not allow the feet to breathe.

Auricular Appendage

A benign growth on the outer ear.

SYMPTOMS & SIGNS
- Small painless lump on the ear

NOTE
May be removed by surgery if necessary, although it is harmless.

Auto-Immune Deficiency Syndrome

see AIDS

Axillary Vein Thrombosis

Blockage of the main vein in the upper arm, usually occurs without any obvious cause.

SIGNS
- Arm becomes swollen, including the hand
- Discomfort rather than pain
- Veins in the arm and upper chest may appear swollen
- Arm becomes dusky bluish

NOTE
Medical help should be sought.

Bacillary Dysentery

see DYSENTERY

Back Strain

Back Strain can occur for a variety of reasons, including direct injury, twisting or lifting, or because of a number of such episodes having a cumulative affect.

SYMPTOMS & SIGNS
- May occur anywhere on the back, but most often the lower back
- Often severe pain to begin with, then diminishes with time
- Pain exacerbated by any movement of the spine
- Repeated episodes of pain may develop with age
- May be Sciatica, pain radiating into the buttock and leg

If caused by trauma or injury:
- Onset of pain is less severe, but becomes worse over time
- May resolve within a few days

NOTE
May resolve spontaneously, but may need painkillers or the services of a physiotherapist, chiropractor or osteopath.

CROSS-REFERENCED UNDER:
Lumbago

Balanitis

The foreskin and the penis near the foreskin can become infected. It may be associated with Diabetes.

SYMPTOMS & SIGNS
- Pain around the foreskin
- Itch
- Discharge from the foreskin (although not the opening of the penis itself)

NOTE
Medical help should be sought as the condition will require antibiotics.

Baldness

see ALOPECIA

Baldness

see ALOPECIA AREATA

Bartholin's Cyst

Cyst found on the vagina, which may be accompanied by no other symptoms. The cyst may become infected, however.

SYMPTOMS & SIGNS

- Cyst on one lip of the vagina
- No pain or other symptoms

If infected:

- Swollen and tender
- May be fever

> NOTE
> The cyst will need to be treated with surgery.

Basal Cell Carcinoma

see RODENT ULCER

Bedridden

When an individual becomes incapacitated or bedridden, muscle loss, wastage and reduction in stamina and strength can occur remarkably quickly. It is necessary to do as much exercise as possible without aggravating any underlying condition.

SIGNS

- When bedridden or incapacitated, muscles, lose strength, stamina and bulk within a week or so
- If incapacitation is long-term, bone bulk decreases and the individual may be prone to painful fractures (breaks)

> NOTE
> Other problems may also arise from being bedridden, such as bed sores and Constipation.

Behcet's Syndrome

Recurrent painful Ulcers in the mouth and/or on the genitals. Other features can arise months or even years later, such as inflammation elsewhere including the eyes and occassionally in nerves and brain, the blood vessels (vasculitis), the joints (arthritis), kidneys and gastrointestinal tract (usually as ulcers).

SYMPTOMS & SIGNS

- Ulcers in the mouth often multiple and extensive, followed a few weeks later by ulcers on the genitals
- Ulcers are painful
- Eye inflammation or Uveitis
- Skin nodules
- Arthritis in large joints
- Resolves, then recurrent episodes
- Ulcers in small or large bowel
- Mild kidney impairment

> NOTE
> Most likely in the Middle East. Rare in men from their teens to their 30s. The condition may appear to resolve, but it often recurs, and treatment is only to alleviate the symptoms.

Bell's Palsy

One side of the face becomes paralysed, caused by damage to a facial nerve, although there may be no obvious reason for the damage. The onset is sudden, and may be noticed on waking or following an attack of Shingles. Similar symptoms can be caused by damage to the face, such as knife wound, although this is more likely to be permanent.

SYMPTOMS & SIGNS
- One side of the face is paralysed: the eye on that side cannot be closed, it is impossible to smile properly or bare the teeth, and the mouth is drawn to the affected side
- Eyelid on affected side droops
- Affected side may ache
- Saliva may dribble from the affected side
- Taste may be affected as one side of the tongue is involved

> NOTE
> Will usually resolve within a week to ten days. If suspected, however, advice should be sought from a medical practitioner as they may be able to speed up resolution. Similar damage can be done by a Stroke, so this should be excluded.

CROSS-REFERENCED UNDER:
Facial Nerve Damage

Benign Tumours of the Nose
see NASAL POLYPS

Beri-Beri
see VITAMIN B1 (THIAMINE) DEFICIENCY

Bile Duct Cancer
see CANCER OF THE BILE DUCTS

Bilharzia (Schistomiasis)

Infestation by blood flukes, a kind of trematode flatworm. The flukes are found in Africa, the West Indies, Brazil and Japan, and can be caught from drinking or bathing in infested water. Liver and spleen damage can result, and it may also cause Cancer of the Bladder.

SYMPTOMS & SIGNS
Acute features
- Fever, chills, sweats, aches and pains, weakness, cough, vomiting, diarrhoea, weight loss
- Enlarged glands, liver, spleen

Chronic features
- Lower abdominal pain, need to urinate frequently, pain when urinating
- Blood in urine or cloudy urine
- Upper abdominal pain, diarrhoea, blood in the stool
- Enlarged liver or spleen

> NOTE
> May be treated by drugs, but the condition can be fatal.

CROSS-REFERENCED UNDER:
Schistosomiasis

Biliary Colic

A gall stone can temporarily block a bile duct, causing the muscle around the bile duct to go into painful spasm.

SYMPTOMS & SIGNS
- Severe pain in the upper part of the abdomen, which may also be experienced in the shoulder tip. Spasms of pain can last from minutes to many hours
- Vomiting
- Pallor and clamminess
- May be fever
- May be jaundice
- May be extreme itchiness

> NOTE
> Medical help should be sought.

Bite, Animal

Larger animals, such as dogs, can bite or maul children or adults. The wounds may be serious, or even life-threatening.

SIGNS
- Puncture wound or wounds which may penetrate deep into the flesh
- Bleeding, possibly copious
- Bruising, possibly severe

> NOTE
> If wounds or injuries or severe, medical help should be sought immediately. If possible wounds should be washed with fresh water. Direct pressure applied to a wound may staunch or reduce the bleeding, as may lifting an injured limb. A Tetanus booster may be required.

Bite, Insect

Insect bites or stings can cause areas of the body to become swollen. This can be particularly serious if an individual is allergic to the bite or sting, (*also see* Allergic Reaction, Severe).

SIGNS
- Swelling centred around the location of the bite or sting
- May be very itchy, and area around the bite may develop into a rash with reddened hard nodules
- Will usually resolve in a few days
- Unusually the area may become infected, with further swelling. The area will become red and hot. A fever may develop: if this is the case,

medical help should be sought
- Individual may have a severe allergic reaction to the sting or bite. If the larynx swells up it can block the airway and cause suffocation

> NOTE
> Most insect bites or stings will resolve, but if the individual is allergic to the sting or they have been bitten or stung in the throat, medical help should be sought. Some insects leave the sting in the skin, and this may be removed carefully using tweezers.

CROSS-REFERENCED UNDER:
Sting, Insect; Insect Bite or Sting

Black Eye

Injuries to the eyes, forehead or area above the eye can cause bruising around the eye, even when the injury has not been directly to the area around the eye.

SYMPTOMS & SIGNS
- Immediately after injury: redness and pain
- Within a few hours the skin around the eye goes black and blue
- Should resolve in just over one week: colour fades from black to blue, green and yellow

> NOTE
> Not usually a cause for concern, unless the eye itself has been damaged and there are problems with vision such as from a Detached Retina. Any severe blow may cause concussion, and medical help should be sought.

Bladder Cancer

see CANCER OF THE BLADDER

Bladder, Enlarged

see ENLARGED BLADDER

Bladder Neck Obstruction

This condition can cause similar symptoms to an Enlarged Prostate as the outlet to urethra gets blocked by muscle.

SYMPTOMS & SIGNS

- Urinary incontinence or dribbling of urine
- Increase in frequency of urination, although the quantity in each urination will not usually be excessive
- Problems starting or finishing urinating (dribbling)
- Even after urinating, the bladder still feels full
- Needing to urinate at night
- May become impossible to urinate. If this is the case, there will be severe abdominal pain

> NOTE
> May be rarely found in women. This condition is more likely in older men with Enlarged Prostate.

Bleeding

Excessive bleeding for long periods, which may be from an external wound or may be from internal organs or tissues, can cause many symptoms in itself. The cause of the bleeding may be trauma or penetrating injuries, gastric or duodenal ulcers, inflammation or bowel problems including piles (haemorrhoids), heavy periods, use of drugs to reduce the body's ability to clot such as aspirin and warfarin.

SYMPTOMS & SIGNS

- May be blood in vomit, urine or faeces. Blood in

the faeces may appear red or be altered causing black discolouration of the faeces
- May be an obvious source of bleeding, such as a penetrating wound or severe bruising
- Feeling faint when standing upright
- Heart rate increases
- Tiredness
- Sweatiness and pallor
- Thirst

If bleeding is not treated:
- Skin and face look pale
- Weakness
- Extremities feel cold
- Excessive thirst
- Dehydration
- Confusion
- Fainting
- Shock and collapse

> NOTE
> Medical help should be sought for cases of excessive bleeding. If there is copious bleeding from a wound, putting pressure with the hand may staunch or reduce the amount of bleeding. Lifting an injured limb will also reduce bleeding. Tourniquets should not be used. If the individual has anything large embedded in them, this should not be removed as this may make bleeding even worse.

CROSS-REFERENCED UNDER:
Haemorrhage; Blood Loss

Blepharitis

Inflammation of the eyelid, usually caused by a condition such as Dandruff or Dermatitis.

SIGNS
- Eyelid looks red and sore
- Skin flakes from affected area
- Area is irritated and itchy
- Crusting occurs around the skin, by the eyelashes

NOTE
The condition may resolve by itself, although antibiotic ointments or washing the eyelids regularly may help.

Blindness

Several conditions can lead to blindness or problems with the eye, including congenital disorders.

SYMPTOMS & SIGNS
- Cornea may look cloudy and become opaque
Blindness:
- Pupils may not respond to light and darkness, and may appear large
- May be 'searching' movement of the eyes, particularly when the individual has been blind from birth (nystagmus)

NOTE
If an individual becomes blind, medical help should be sought.

CROSS-REFERENCED UNDER:
Congenital Blindness; Congenital Problems of the Eye

Blisters

Blisters can be caused by a range of conditions, although the most common is damage done to the skin by heat, cold, friction, caustic substances, insect bites or stings, jelly fish stings, and some animal bites.

SYMPTOMS & SIGNS
- An area (or areas) of the skin is affected by fluid being trapped between different layers of skin
- Blisters are localised to the area of the skin that has been damaged
- The area around the blister(s) may be angry and red
- Scabs can form later at the sites of the blister(s)
- The affected areas may lose pigmentation for a time, although this will usually return

NOTE
Many blisters will resolve by themselves, if damage to the skin has been limited. Medical help should be sought if this is not the case.

Blockage of Central Retinal Artery
see CENTRAL RETINAL ARTERY BLOCKAGE

Blockage of Central Retinal Vein
see CENTRAL RETINAL VEIN BLOCKAGE

Blocked Tear Duct

Tear duct is blocked or too narrow to drain into the nose, and causes the eyes to stream with tears.

SYMPTOMS & SIGNS
- Normally only one eye is affected
- Tears run constantly, even when happy and well

NOTE
Most likely in young babies, when it may be accompanied by episodes of Conjunctivitis. Will usually resolve within the first year of life, although minor surgery may be necessary.

Blood Loss
see BLEEDING

Blood Poisoning
see SEPTICAEMIA

Blood Pressure, High
see HIGH BLOOD PRESSURE

Blood Pressure, Low
see LOW BLOOD PRESSURE

Blue Naevus
see MONGOLIAN BLUE SPOT

Boil

Skin infection around a hair follicle, where a pus-filled abscess may form.

SYMPTOMS & SIGNS
- Swollen, red area which may have a yellow middle which discharges pus
- Painful
- Affected skin feels warm
- Most likely in the buttocks, armpit and neck, or even in the ear, where it will be particularly painful

> NOTE
> Will normally resolve when the boil bursts and discharges pus. The boil can be lanced at the right time, although this should only be attempted by a health professional. Scarring can result if the operation is done poorly. Antibiotics may be needed in some cases.

CROSS-REFERENCED UNDER:
Hair Follicle Infection; Furuncle

Bone, Broken
see BROKEN BONE

Bone Cancer
see CANCER OF THE BONES

Bone Injury
see BROKEN BONE

Bottle Nose
see RHINOPHYMA

Botulism

A rare but virulent and potentially life-threatening form of food poisoning, caused by contamination with spores of Clostridium botulinum. Symptoms will manifest between 12 and 36 hours after consumption of contaminated food.

SYMPTOMS & SIGNS
- Feeling generally unwell
- Nausea and vomiting
- Diarrhoea and abdominal cramps, and may be bouts of constipation
- Dry mouth with sore throat
- Pupils of the eyes wide open and 'staring'
- Double vision or blurred vision
- Drooping of eyelids, difficulty speaking and difficulty swallowing
- Breathing difficulties, due to weakness of chest wall muscles
- Progressive limb weakness
- May be collapse and coma

> NOTE
> Medical help should be sought immediately.

Bow Legs
see KNOCK KNEES

Bowel Cancer

see CANCER OF THE COLON OR RECTUM (BOWEL)

Brain Abscess

An abscess can form in the brain, caused by infection following trauma or from nearby structures, such as from the ear, nose, throat, face, sinuses and the lungs.

SYMPTOMS & SIGNS

Signs resulting from the initial infection source

- Fever and chills
- Generally feeling very unwell
- Lack of appetite and vomiting
- Severe headache, which gets progressively worse
- Convulsions
- May be sudden paralysis
- Progressive drowsiness to unconsciousness and coma

NOTE
Medical help should be sought immediately.

Brain Cancer

see BRAIN TUMOURS

Brain Haemorrhage

see SUBARACHNOID HAEMORRHAGE

Brain Haemorrhage

see SUBDURAL HAEMORRHAGE

Brain Tumours

A 'tumour' is a swelling, which in the brain can be benign or malignant (cancerous). These tumours can arise anywhere within the brain. Tumours within the pituitary (also called pituitary adenomas) or arising in the linings around the brain (called meningiomas) are typically benign. Cancerous growths can arise within the brain by spread of 'secondary tumours' from tumours elsewhere (such as from lung, breast or bowel).

SYMPTOMS & SIGNS

- Headache, low in intensity to begin but gradually increasing in severity. May be particularly noticeable first thing in the morning
- Vomiting of stomach contents and undigested food
- May be personality change
- May be paralysis and/or altered sensation which are slowly progressive
- The tumour may press on the facial nerve and cause paralysis and symptoms similar to Bell's Palsy
- Eyes may have twitching movements (nystagmus)
- Vision may be affected, including partial loss of fields of vision
- May be deafness or tinnitus restricted to one side
- May be loss of senses, such as smell, because of pressure on the associated nerves
- May be impaired consciousness, drowsiness and confusion
- Convulsions and Epilepsy
- Pulse and respiration may become slower
- In babies under 18 months, brain tumours may lead to raised intracranial pressure and bulging fontanelles, soft places in the skull. This is not found in adults or older children

NOTE
Medical help should be sought immediately. The

tumour may be benign and able to be removed or reduced by surgery, chemotherapy or radiotherapy. Even if this is not the case, pressure symptoms and signs may be alleviated

CROSS-REFERENCED UNDER:
Cancer of the Brain; Brain Cancer

Breast Abscess

An abscess forms in the breast, usually caused by an infection through breast feeding, and most often in the first few weeks. More rarely it can be caused by a persistent infection.

SYMPTOMS & SIGNS
- May be discharge, with blood, along with the production of milk
- May be a red area in the breast which is firm to the touch
- Pain, which may be severe in intensity
- Sweating and fever
- Shivering

NOTE
Medical help should be sought as antibiotics will probably be needed.

Breast Cancer
see CANCER OF THE BREAST

Brittle Bone Disease
(Osteogenesis Imperfecta)

Problems with bones, leading to breaks (also called 'fractures'), caused by a hereditary disorder. There are severeal forms of this disease. Typically fracture risk is highest in infancy and diminishes with increasing age in those who survive. Some forms are severe and the multiple fractures that occur in infancy and childhood lead to major defects and stunt growth and development and can shorten life.

SYMPTOMS & SIGNS
- Bones break ('fracture') very easily
- Ligaments are not taut enough, allowing joints too much movement
- Whites of the eyes appear blue
- May be deafness
- Teeth may be abnormal
- May be deformity because of repeated bone breaks

NOTE
Medical help should be sought.

CROSS-REFERENCED UNDER:
Osteogenesis Imperfecta Congenita; Osteogenesis Imperfecta Tarda

Broken Ankle

The bones of the lower leg, ankle or foot can be broken, usually because of direct injury or damage sustained from a fall.

SYMPTOMS & SIGNS
- Severe pain
- Ankle cannot bear weight
- Swelling
- Bruising, although this may take some time to be apparent

NOTE
Medical help should be sought immediately, and X-ray will be needed.

CROSS-REFERENCED UNDER:
Fractures of the Ankle; Ankle Fracture

Broken Bone (also called Fractured Bone)

Trauma or injury to the body can cause broken or fractured bones. Often a fracture also affects other local structures, such as blood vessels, nerves, ligaments and may even break the overlying skin. It is not always easy to distinguish a bone break or fracture from soft tissue injuries.

SYMPTOMS & SIGNS
- Pain
- Loss of movement or function
- Unable to bear weight
- Broken bone may be apparent, leaving the limb bent or with a joint in the wrong place

When the bone heals:
- A lump of bone may develop where the bone heals because of new bone forming
- May be a hard lump left after injury, caused by a subperiosteal haematoma
- If the bone break has not been properly set or has trouble knitting, it may leave the bone or bones lumpy and deformed

NOTE
If a broken bone is suspected, medical help should be sought immediately. An X-ray will usually be required.

CROSS-REFERENCED UNDER:
Bone, Broken; Bone Injury

Broken Collar Bone

The collar bone (clavicle) can be broken by trauma resulting from a fall or other accident.

SIGNS
- Pain where the collar bone is broken

- Pain exacerbated by moving the arm: individual will attempt to keep the affected side immobile
- Break may be apparent as bone deformed
- Loss of movement

NOTE
Medical help should be sought immediately. An X-ray will usually be required.

CROSS-REFERENCED UNDER:
Collar Bone Fracture; Fracture of the Collar Bone

Broken Lower Arm Bones (Radius, Ulna and wrist)

The lower arm bones (radius, ulna and wrist) can be broken by trauma resulting from a fall, particularly with an outstretched hand, or violent blow.

SYMPTOMS & SIGNS
- Pain exacerbated by moving the arm
- Break may be apparent as bone deformed
- May be extensive bruising
- Loss of movement

NOTE
Medical help should be sought immediately. An X-ray will usually be required.

CROSS-REFERENCED UNDER:
Lower Arm Bones (Radius, Ulna and wrist) Fracture; Fracture of the Lower Arm Bones (Radius, Ulna and wrist)

Broken Upper Arm Bone (Humerus)

The upper arm bone (humerus) can be broken by trauma resulting from a fall or violent blow.

SYMPTOMS & SIGNS
- Pain exacerbated by moving the arm or shoulder
- Break may be apparent as bone deformed
- May be extensive bruising
- Loss of movement

NOTE
Medical help should be sought immediately. An X-ray will usually be required.

CROSS-REFERENCED UNDER:
Upper Arm Bone (Humerus) Fracture; Fracture of the Upper Arm Bone (Humerus)

Bronchiectasis

Widening of the bronchioles, with extensive damage to the air sacs in the lungs, usually caused by previous infection, which reduces the ability of the lung to absorb oxygen from the air. It may cause chronic and recurrent chest infections and other serious disease.

SYMPTOMS & SIGNS
- Generally feeling and looking unwell
- Recurrent chest infections
- Copious amounts of foul-smelling and purulent sputum, which is yellow or green in colour. Sputum may also include or be streaked with blood
- Bad breath, which may be extremely unpleasant
- Shortness of breath, wheeze
- Chest pain
- Fever
- Weight loss
- Clubbing of end of fingers and finger nails

NOTE
Medical help should be sought, and a chest X-ray will be needed to confirm the condition.

Bronchiolitis

Condition similar to Asthma and most commonly found in children and most likely in winter. This form is caused by a virus, and may occur in epidemics. In adults bronchiolotis can result from exposure to infections, inhaled fumes and as side effect of some drug treatments.

SYMPTOMS & SIGNS
- Onset is similar to symptoms of a Cold
- Wheezing starts, and becomes progressively worse over time
- Each breath causes a crackling noise in the chest
- Feeding of infants with bronchiolitis is difficult because of breathlessness
- Breathing becomes forced and rapid, often with sounds like grunting

If the condition is severe:
- Pallor
- Blue tinge to the lips because of cyanosis

NOTE
Medical help should be sought immediately. Children with this condition are more likely to develop Asthma in later years.

Bronchitis

Potentially severe lung condition, characterised by the inflammation of the airways (bronchial tubes) in the lung, caused by a bacteria or virus. This can partially block airways into the lungs making breathing progressively difficult. Chronic Bronchitis involves recurrent episodes of long-term duration.

SYMPTOMS & SIGNS
- Wheezing
- Persistent or smokers' cough, particularly after waking as well as in the winter
- Copious amounts if sputum, which may be white, yellow or green in colour
- Breathlessness, which becomes worse and worse as the years go on, and which may be particularly acute if the individual also develops a chest infection
- Bad breath
- Lips, finger-nail beds, earlobes and other areas of the body may appear bluish because of lack of oxygen reaching tissues (cyanosis)
- Polycythaemia: blood becomes too concentrated in trying to transfer oxygen around the body
- May be confusion, particularly in elderly individuals

NOTE
Smokers are far more likely to have recurrent episodes than non-smokers, but also common in those who have suffered from long-term exposure to dust, fumes and chemicals – and cold and damp climates. Also far more likely in men than women. The condition often cannot be cured.

CROSS-REFERENCED UNDER:
Chronic Bronchitis

Bronze Diabetes
see HAEMOCHROMATOSIS

Brucellosis

Infectious disease contracted by taking unpasturised milk, (cow's and goat's). This infection can affect any or all organ systems.

SYMPTOMS & SIGNS
- High fever often comes and goes
- Sweating, particularly heavy at night
- Feeling of malaise or ill health
- Fatigue and lack of energy
- Weight loss and loss of appetite
- Joint pain
- Low mood
- Recurrent bouts of fever

NOTE
Most likely in individuals coming into contact with milk, and the condition may resolve by itself.

Bruise

Bruising is usually caused by injury or trauma, slight or major, and is a normal reaction. The skin at the site of the injury may not have been penetrated, but the trauma causes blood to leak into tissues beneath the skin. As this blood is broken down, it changes colour from red to purple-black, then to brown, green and yellow.

SYMPTOMS & SIGNS
- An area or areas of the skin are discoloured
- This discoloration fades over time

NOTE
Minor bruising will usually not require treatment, but if from major trauma medical help should be sought.

Bulimia

see ANOREXIA NERVOSA

Bunion

see HALLUX VALGUS

Burns

Skin and the underlying tissues become severely damaged due to burning from fire, chemical exposure or electric shock.

SYMPTOMS & SIGNS
- Red area of skin
- Area usually blisters
- Superficial burns are very painful, but severe burns may have no pain as the underlying nerves may also be damaged
- If burns are extensive they can cause life-threatening shock with collapse and coma

NOTE
If burns are severe, medical help should be sought immediately. The affected area should be cooled if possible for at least ten minutes with cold running water, but lotions or ointments should not be applied, and blisters should never be burst. If the skin has been affected by a chemical burn, the area should be thoroughly and repeatedly washed with clean water. If the electrical burns are suspected, ensure that electrocution is not a possibility (by switching off any local live electricity).

Bursitis

Swelling of a sac overlying a bone or joint, caused by overuse, such as kneeling for long periods, or associated with Rheumatoid Arthritis, Tuberculosis and Gout.

SYMPTOMS & SIGNS
- Swollen joints
- Usually uncomfortable rather than severely painful, but may be very painful
- Area is red and hot to the touch

NOTE
Resting the affected area may help to resolve the condition.

CROSS-REFERENCED UNDER:
Housemaid's Knee

Cafe-Au-Lait Spots

see MOLE

Caffeine

Caffeine is a stimulant which is found in coffee, tea and fizzy drinks. Excess of Caffeine – the actual amount will vary from individual to individual – can cause anxiety, tremor and rapid heart beat

SYMPTOMS & SIGNS
- Anxiety
- Tremor and shaking
- Fast heart beat
- Extra heart beats
- Increased urination

NOTE
Any unpleasant results of taking Caffeine may be lessened by reducing the amount of tea, coffee or fizzy drinks consumed.

CROSS-REFERENCED UNDER:
Coffee; Tea

Callus

Thickening of the skin in areas where there is repeated rubbing or use.

SYMPTOMS & SIGNS
- Thickened skin (callus) is often found on the soles of the feet or palms of the hands, especially individuals who go barefoot or who have manual jobs
- If shoes rub against the toe or toes, thickened skin (corn) forms at the area
- Harmless

NOTE
Calluses or corns may be removed if necessary.

CROSS-REFERENCED UNDER:
Corn

Campbell de Morgan Spots

Very small red spots which develop on the skin, most usually on the chest and abdomen.

SYMPTOMS & SIGNS
- Very small bright-red spots, which may be raised above the surrounding skin
- Harmless

NOTE
Most usually found in older individuals.

Cancer in the Chest

Tumours, malignant or benign, primary or secondary, can affect the chest, usually in the lung.

SYMPTOMS & SIGNS
- Swollen lymph nodes on the neck which are not painful

- Prominent, symmetrical veins on the head, neck and upper chest – unchanged by body position
- Face may be rather red and swollen, along with the neck and upper chest
- Breathing may be difficult
- The cancer may also cause weight loss, lack of appetite, feeling generally ill and weakness
- Voice may be hoarse because of pressure put on the laryngeal nerve
- Clubbing of fingers
- May cause infection in adjacent lung

NOTE
Medical help should be sought immediately.

CROSS-REFERENCED UNDER:
Chest Cancer; Tumours of the Chest

Cancer of Ducts in the Breast

A tumour can develop in the ducts of the breast.

SYMPTOMS & SIGNS
- Bloody discharge from the nipple
- Uncomfortable feeling from behind the nipple

NOTE
Investigations will be needed to confirm a diagnosis.

Cancer of the Bile Ducts

SIGNS
- Progressive jaundice with pale faeces and dark urine
- Weight loss and other signs of cancer
- Ultimately liver failure
- Mass in the upper right part of the abdomen

CROSS-REFERENCED UNDER:
Bile Duct Cancer

Cancer of the Bladder

SIGNS
- General health may appear fine
- Although not painful, copious blood in urine (haematuria)
- Flow of urine may be blocked by the formation of blood clots
- Anaemia due to blood loss
- Prominent blood vessels on the abdomen
- Although unusual and may not be noticeable, the bladder may become enlarged. This may be apparent as a mass in the lower abdomen
- Fever
- Weight loss
- Anaemia
- Pain in the abdomen
- May be pain in bones because of the spread of the cancer

NOTE
Medical help should be sought immediately. Cancers are typically malignant although some are much more aggresive than others, and are most likely in those of more than 50 years of age. This cancer is particularly linked to long-term smokers.

CROSS-REFERENCED UNDER:
Haematuria; Bladder Cancer

Cancer of the Bones

Cancer of the bones may develop, usually as the result of secondary cancer spreading from another part of the body, although primary bone cancers can occur.

SIGNS
- Bone pain, potentially severe but may be isolated to one area
- May be no lump
- Bones may be more likely to fracture and break
- It is rare for this to be the first symptom of a cancer, but where there is an existing tumour or cancer, this should be considered urgently
- May be tendency to spontaneously bleed

Benign bone tumours can occur:
- Hard and smooth lumps
- Occasionally no pain, pain of present can vary from mild to severe
- Grow slowly

NOTE
Medical help should be sought immediately, even if only to exclude serious disease.

CROSS-REFERENCED UNDER:
Bone Cancer

Cancer of the Brain
see BRAIN TUMOURS

Cancer of the Breast

Tumours can form in the breast (both female and male).

SIGNS
- A lump may be felt, which stays in the same place and is irregular to touch

- Skin over the lump looks different and is dimpled
- Swollen glands in the armpit
- May be discharge which can be bloody from the nipple
- May be change in look or texture of the nipple
- Nipple may be sunk into the breast (retracted), formerly having been protruding (it should be noted that some women have naturally retracted nipples)
- May be discomfort or pain, although this is unusual as an early symptom, although much more common if advanced

> NOTE
> Medical help should be sought immediately if breast cancer is suspected. The success of treatment increases if an early diagnosis is made. The disease affects about one in 12 of females over the age of 50 years.

CROSS-REFERENCED UNDER:
Breast Cancer

Cancer of the Cervix

Cancer may develop on the cervix, the opening from the vagina into the womb (uterus).

SIGNS
- May be disturbed Menstruation
- May be heavy periods
- May be persistent and severe back or abdominal pain
- May be discharge from the vagina, with blood, which smells unpleasant
- May be a mass in the abdomen
- In advanced cases, cancer may spread to the urinary tract and cause problems urinating or may even cause inability to urinate
- May be weight loss, lack of appetite, anaemia and general feeling of ill health

> NOTE
> Medical help should be sought immediately as the success of treatment is improved by early diagnosis. This cancer should be detected by cervical smears.

CROSS-REFERENCED UNDER:
Cervical Cancer

Cancer of the Colon or Rectum (Bowel)

Cancer of the bowel, colon or rectum can block the intestine, either gradually or with a sudden onset. One of the first signs may well be a change in bowel habit. The cancer can affect any part of the colon, and a mass may be found on either side of the abdomen.

SIGNS
- Abdominal pain, like colic, possibly localised to one side
- Abdomen may become swollen because of a build up of faeces, fluid or flatulence
- A mass or lump may be present in the abdomen
- Slime or mucous in faeces
- Diarrhoea with loose or abnormal faeces
- Blood in faeces which may make or streak faeces with dark blood
- Symptoms may be intermittent
- Swollen lymph glands in the groin
- May be anaemia because of persistent blood loss
- In advanced cases, may be inability to urinate
- May be discharge from the vagina, which has an unpleasant smell

CROSS-REFERENCED UNDER:
Colorectal Cancer; Bowel Cancer

Cancer of the Ear

Cancerous tumours can form within the ear canal.

SIGNS

- Pain which is usually severe and persistent
- Discharge of pus and blood from the ear, which usually is persistent
- One side of the face may become paralysed

NOTE
Cancer of the Ear is very rare.

Cancer of the Eye

Cancerous tumours may develop on the eyeball or eye socket. In children, they condition may be inherited and tumours can occur in both eyes.

SIGNS

- Eyeball becomes swollen and enlarged
- Lens of the eye appears cloudy or opaque
- Vision is disturbed
- Loss of vision
- Pain in the eye
- Squint which suddenly appears

NOTE
Medical help should be sought immediately.

CROSS-REFERENCED UNDER:
Tumour of the Eye

Cancer of the Gall Bladder

SIGNS

- Progressive jaundice with pale faeces and dark urine
- Weight loss and other signs of cancer
- Mass in the upper right part of the abdomen
- General feeling of ill health

NOTE
Medical help should be sought immediately.

Cancer of the Kidney

SIGNS

- General health may appear fine
- Although not painful, copious blood in urine (haematuria)
- Flow of urine may be blocked by the formation of blood clots
- Anaemia due to blood loss
- Prominent blood vessels on the abdomen
- Although unusual and may not be noticeable, the kidney may become enlarged. This may be apparent as a mass on the right or left side of the abdomen

If the cancer is malignant:

- Persistent and unrelenting fever
- Inability to urinate caused by kidney failure
- Pain in the abdomen
- Weight loss
- May be pain in bones because of the spread of the cancer

NOTE
Medical help should be sought immediately. Cancers tend to be malignant, and are most likely in those individuals of more than 50 years of age.

CROSS-REFERENCED UNDER:
Haematuria; Nephritic Cancer

Cancer of the Larynx

Cancer of the larynx (which is also known as the voice box).

SIGNS
- Hoarse voice
- Speech may be muffled or altered
- May be pain when swallowing or because of ulceration
- Dry or non-productive cough
- Bad breath
- Enlarged lymph nodes which are not painful
- Feeling generally unwell
- Weight loss
- Anaemia

> NOTE
> Medical help should be sought immediately as earlier diagnosis aids the effectiveness treatment.

CROSS-REFERENCED UNDER:
Larynx Cancer

Cancer of the Liver

Cancer of the liver. Although primary tumours of the liver are unusual, the liver can also have secondary tumours from other cancers, including the breast and the lung. These cancers will usually have been discovered before spreading to the liver.

SIGNS
- SIGNS of cancer from primary tumours
- Upper abdominal pain

- Palms of hands may be unusually red
- Jaundice and the skin looks yellow
- Progressive and long-term weight loss

> NOTE
> Medical help should be sought immediately.

CROSS-REFERENCED UNDER:
Liver Cancer; Hepatoma

Cancer of the Lung

see LUNG CANCER

Cancer of the Mouth

Cancer of the mouth or throat, including the lips, tongue, and the tonsils. Cancer should be suspected if an ulcer or growth does not resolve within a few weeks.

SIGNS
- Large, irregularly shaped ulcers which do not clear up within a few weeks
- Ulcers on the surface of polyps or with raised edges
- Enlarged lymph nodes in neck
- Chronic pain in the mouth, tongue, neck or face
- Bad breath
- Voice sounds different
- Dentures no longer fit
- General feeling of ill health
- Weight loss
- Anaemia

> NOTE
> Smokers are especially at risk, particularly those who smoke pipes or chew tobacco. Most likely in those who are in their 50s or older, particularly if they have smoked for a long time.

CROSS-REFERENCED UNDER:
Cancer of the Throat; Throat Cancer

Cancer of the Nasal Fossa or Naso pharnyx

see CANCER OF THE NOSE

Cancer of the Nose

Cancer may develop within the passages or on the skin of the nose.

SIGNS

- Lump may be visible in the nose or mouth, or the cancer may produce swelling in the face
- Lump may ulcerate and bleed, causing nosebleeds
- Chronic pain, often like toothache
- Discharge of foul-smelling and blood-stained sputum
- Bad breath
- Speech may be muffled or nasal
- May be pain
- Enlarged lymph nodes in the neck

NOTE
Most likely in the elderly.

CROSS-REFERENCED UNDER:
Cancer of the Nasal Fossa or Naso pharnyx; Nose Cancer

Cancer of the Oesophagus

Cancer of the Oesophagus (gullet), the tube down which food goes into the stomach.

SIGNS

- Swallowing difficulties: worse with solid food than with liquid

- May be regurgitation of food
- Loss of appetite and loss of weight
- Fatigue
- Not usually pain, although heartburn and indigestion may be signs
- Hoarse voice: usually as one of the last signs to occur
- Possible anaemia, especially in women
- May be prone to chest infections (from regurgitation of food rather than the cancer)
- May appear to be too much saliva
- May be bad breath

NOTE
More common in those over the age of 50. If the tumour is benign, health may appear to be good and there may be little weight loss.

CROSS-REFERENCED UNDER:
Oesophageal Cancer; Gullet Cancer

Cancer of the Ovaries

Cancer may develop on the ovaries.

SIGNS

- May be male changes, such as hair growth on the face, chest or abdomen, deeper voice, and disturbed Menstruation
- May be heavy periods
- May be persistent and severe back or abdominal pain
- May be discharge from the vagina, with blood, which smells unpleasant
- May be a mass in the abdomen
- In advanced cases, cancer may spread to the urinary tract and cause problems urinating or may even cause inability to urinate

- May be weight loss, lack of appetite, anaemia and general feeling of ill health

> NOTE
> Medical help should be sought immediately as the success of treatment is improved by early diagnosis.

CROSS-REFERENCED UNDER:
Ovarian Cancer

Cancer of the Pancreas

Cancer of the pancreas. A malignant tumour can form on the organ and block the bile ducts, so that yellow bile has to be excreted through urine rather than in faeces.

SIGNS
- Pain in th abdomen and in the back
- Progressive jaundice: skin looks yellow
- May be extreme itchiness
- Pale faeces
- Dark urine, which is brown, orange or dark yellow
- Weight loss, loss of appetite, generally feeling unwell, fatigue and other signs of cancer
- Ultimately liver failure
- Mass in the upper right part of the abdomen
- May be occasional vomiting

> NOTE
> Medical help should be sought immediately.

CROSS-REFERENCED UNDER:
Pancreatic Cancer

Cancer of the Penis

Cancer can develop on the penis.

SIGNS
- Red area develops at the end of the penis or on the foreskin
- Area ulcerates
- Pain
- Discharge
- Bleeding

> NOTE
> Medical help should be sought immediately as the condition will require surgery and other treatment. This is an unusual cancer in the developed world, but is more common in the Middle East. It is less likely to occur in circumcised men.

Cancer of the Pituitary

The pituitary gland is located in the brain and controls the function of many hormone-producing glands. Most growths in the pituitary are benign and are called 'adrnomas'. These may themselves produce hormones in excess or they may compromise normal hormone secretion and may press on nearby structures. Rarely cancers can arise in or around the pituitary or can spread to the pituitary (metastasis). Cancers are likely to compromise hormone production or cause local pressure effects because they tend to grow rapidly.

SYMPTOMS & SIGNS
- Excessive hormone production. Excess growth hormone, prolactin, thyroid hormone, steroid hormones.
- May alternatively lead to lack of the above hormones, also testosterone or oestrogen deficiency (hypogonadism)
- Loss of peripheral vision, affecting both eyes

- Mild headache
- May lead to double vision if nerves beside pituitary are affected

> NOTE
> Medical help should be sought immediately.

Cancer of the Prostate

Cancer of the prostate, a gland at the base of the bladder which is only found in men. Often the individual will be treated for symptoms due to enlarged prostate (prostatism), and the diagnosis will often only become apparent after surgery.

SYMPTOMS & SIGNS

Symptoms are the same as for an Enlarged Prostate:
- Urinary incontinence or dribbling of urine
- Increase in frequency of urination, although the quantity in each urination will not usually be excessive
- Problems starting or finishing urinating
- May be blood in urine: urine may be stained red, pink or may be cloudy
- Swollen lymph glands in the groin
- In advanced cases, inability to urinate. If this is the case, there will also lower abdominal pain caused by a very full bladder
- Pain or aching between the legs or in the pelvis or back because of the spread of the cancer

> NOTE
> Enlargement of the prostate is common in elderly men, although it may cause no symptoms or problems.

Cancer of the Skin

There are several different types of skin cancers, usually caused by a prolonged overexposure to sunlight. Those with fair skins are at greater risk. Skin cancer is on the increase, perhaps because of more foreign holidays in hot climates, or perhaps because the depletion of the ozone layer means that more harmful radiation from the sun is now getting through the earth's atmosphere.

SYMPTOMS & SIGNS
- Small black area or areas, lump or lumps, similar in appearance to moles, found on the skin and more unusually on the whites of the eyes (melanoma)
- The area bleeds and/or is itchy
- Change in colour, size or shape
- Pain
- Smaller black areas may appear near the melanoma
- Skin may become ulcerated
- One form of skin cancer found usually on the face, particularly on the ear is basal cell carcinoma. The onset is a small shiny nodule spot which bleeds and crusts but does not heal. The spot becomes larger. This form of cancer is relatively benign.

> NOTE
> Medical help should be sought immediately.

CROSS-REFERENCED UNDER:
Skin Cancer; Melanoma, Malignant

Cancer of the Spinal Cord
see SPINAL CORD TUMOURS

Cancer of the Spine

A tumour can develop on the spine, either as primary cancer or having spread from another cancer elsewhere in the body. In some cases, the tumour may be benign, but investigations will be needed. Neurological problems can develop if the affected vertebra(e) collapse.

SYMPTOMS & SIGNS
- Persistent back pain, concentrated in one area or general in nature
- Pain and/or altered sensation in the arms and legs
- Occassionally weakness and even paralysis especially of the legs
- Other signs of cancer such as lack of appetite, weight loss and general ill health

NOTE
Medical help should be sought immediately.

Cancer of the Stomach

Cancer of the stomach, usually a primary tumour. The tumour may form at the outlet of the stomach, and may not be noticed itself, although other symptoms will be present.

SYMPTOMS & SIGNS
- Lack or reduction of appetite for food
- Feeling full or bloated after only eating a small amount
- Feelings of indigestion which are difficult to alleviate
- May be regurgitation of food and eventually even vomiting, sometimes with blood (which may look like coffee grounds)
- Swallowing difficulties: worse with solid food than with liquid, especially in later stages and if the entrance into the stomach or the outlet of the stomach have been blocked by the cancer

- Swollen lymph nodes in the neck
- Anaemia
- Fatigue
- Persistent loss of weight
- Not usually obvious pain, although may be abdominal pain and indigestion as mentioned above
- May be a mass in the upper part of the abdomen, although this may not be detectable
- May be fever
- May be bad breath
- In later stages, may also be jaundice and ascites as a result of the cancer having spread

NOTE
Medical help should be sought immediately. Having a family history of a stomach ulcer increases risk in family members of developing stomach cancer, although the disease is rare in those individuals under the age of 45 years. This is a relatively common cancer, and is more likely in men than women.

CROSS-REFERENCED UNDER:
Stomach Cancer; Gastric Cancer

Cancer of the Testicles

Cancer can develop on one or both of the testicles. In rare cases, this may develop before puberty and cause adolescent changes such as a deepening voice and growth of body hair.

SIGNS
- Lump felt on the testicle
- Lump is hard to the touch
- Scrotum may be swollen
- Pain is only occasionally experienced

■ Early puberty is possible in boys

> **NOTE**
> Medical help should be sought immediately as treatment is more effective the earlier it is begun. Although rare in itself, this cancer most commonly affects adolescents and men up to the age of 40. This is a serious, even life-threatening condition, although if caught early enough can usually be treated.

Cancer of the Throat

see CANCER OF THE MOUTH

Cancer of the Urethra

Cancer of the urethra, the tube which takes and expels urine from the bladder. Similar symptoms can be caused by urethral stricture which is benign.

SYMPTOMS & SIGNS

■ Little urine expelled and poor flow

■ May be quite difficult, and take some effort, to empty the bladder

■ May be urinary incontinence, such as a dribble of urine when finished

> **NOTE**
> More likely in men than women, but can affect both.

CROSS-REFERENCED UNDER:
Urethral Cancer

Cancer of the Uterus

see CANCER OF THE WOMB

Cancer of the Vagina

Tumours and growths can form in or near the vagina.

SYMPTOMS & SIGNS

■ Lump seen or felt during examination

■ Persistent discharge from the vagina, particularly after sex

■ Pain

> **NOTE**
> Medical help should be sought immediately.

CROSS-REFERENCED UNDER:
Tumour of the Vagina

Cancer of the Womb

Cancer can develop in the womb (uterus).

SYMPTOMS & SIGNS

■ Womb (uterus) become enlarged and can be felt as a mass in the abdomen

■ Mass may be an apparent mass in the vagina

■ Swollen lymph glands in the groin

■ May be heavy periods

■ May be persistent and severe back or abdominal pain

■ May be discharge from the vagina, with blood, which smells unpleasant

■ In advanced cases, cancer may spread to the urinary tract and cause problems urinating or may even cause inability to urinate

■ May be weight loss, lack of appetite, anaemia and general feeling of ill health

> **NOTE**
> Medical help should be sought immediately as the effectiveness of treatment is improved by early diagnosis.

CROSS-REFERENCED UNDER:
Cancer of the Uterus; Uterine Cancer

Cancrumoris

Conditions characterised by a very severe and general infection to all parts of the mouth, caused by bacterial infection from the gums (Vincent's Acute Ulcerative Gingivitis) or from the tonsils (Vincent's Angina). The condition is very contagious.

SYMPTOMS & SIGNS
- Fever
- Pain and sore throat
- Lymph nodes swollen in neck
- May be that only one tonsil is infected and ulcerated, with a membrane which can spread to the hard and soft palate
- May be copious production of saliva
- May be ulcers on the gums if this is the source of the infection

NOTE
Mostly likely in malnourished children. Help should be sought immediately if these conditions are suspected, and they will need to be treated with antibiotics.

Candidiasis

A fungal yeast-like infection by Candida albicans, which can affect the mouth, lips, throat, gastrointestinal tract, skin and especially the vagina. It is also known as Thrush. Other yeast-type infections can also infect the gastrointestinal tract

SYMPTOMS & SIGNS
- White patches are seen most commonly in the mouth and throat and on the lips, and the vagina
- Swallowing may be difficult and painful
- Inside of the mouth, tongue and lips may be red and painful

- Lips may crack and bleed
- It may be possible to dislodge the white patches
- Vagina may be itchy, tender or painful with white patches on the walls and a white discharge
- Anus may be itchy
- Sexual intercourse may be painful

NOTE
Most likely in the elderly and immunosuppressed, and newly born infants, but possible at any time of life. Also commonly associated with use of antibiotics. May be treated with anti-fungal creams or medication, although recurrence is common.

CROSS-REFERENCED UNDER:
Thrush; Yeast Infection

Carbon Monoxide Poisoning

Carbon Monoxide is a poisonous, odourless gas which is produced when appliances have too little oxygen to burn fuel completely. It is potentially fatal, and may give the individual no clue as to the fact they are being poisoned.

SYMPTOMS & SIGNS
- Tiredness and fatigue
- Feeling unwell
- Headache
- Nausea
- Symptoms resolve when in the fresh air
- Black out or seizures
- Possible coma and death

NOTE
This can be a tragic cause of death: gas appliances should be regularly checked and it should be ensured that there is suitable

ventilation for any fuel burning device (even a coal fire).

Carbuncle

Skin infection, where a group of boils can join beneath the skin and a pus-filled abscess forms. Several episodes of boils or carbuncles may be associated with poor personal hygiene or Diabetes Mellitus.

SYMPTOMS & SIGNS
- Swollen, red area which may have a yellow middle which discharges pus
- Painful
- Affected skin feels warm
- Most likely in the buttocks, armpit and neck

NOTE
Will normally resolve when the carbuncle bursts and discharges pus. The carbuncle may be lanced at the right time, although this should only be attempted by a health professional. Scarring can result if the operation is poorly done. Antibiotics may also be used.

Carcinoid Syndrome

A tumour can form in the gut, the lung or elsewhere, that secretes hormones, which cause many unpleasant symptoms, usually including flushing and diarrhoea. Late complications can include narrowing of the heart valves on the right side of the heart (especially tricuspid valve). The tumour may take a long time to be recognised as causing the problems. Carcinoid tumours, especially of the gut, generally behave like slow-growing cancers. Most of these will have spread by the time hormone-related symptoms start.

SYMPTOMS & SIGNS
- Persistent diarrhoea which is watery and explosive
- Abdominal pain and liver enlargement
- Flushes and sweating
- Wheezing and respiratory distress
- Weight loss
- Breathlessness and swelling of neck veins due to heart complications
- Cyanosis: lack of oxygen to the tissues of the body, causing a bluish tinge, especially noticeable on the skin, lips and under the nails

NOTE
Medical help should be sought as soon as possible.

Cardiac Failure

see HEART ATTACK AND FAILURE

Cardiomyopathy

Several conditions can damage the heart muscle and compromise its functions; causes include coronary artery disease, Alcoholism and inherited conditions including iron overload.

SYMPTOMS & SIGNS
- Breathlessness and tiredness
- Heart failure
- May be rapid heart rate, which may be either regular or irregular in rhythm
- May be slow heart rate, which may be either regular or irregular in rhythm
- May faint during any exertion or exercise

NOTE
Tests will be needed to confirm a diagnosis, and the condition may be treated with drugs.

Carotenaemia

Skin turns orange, due to a build up of carotene, caused by eating large quantities of foods, such as carrots, tomato juice, and some snacks which use it as a colouring. Generally speaking, very large quantities would need to be consumed.

SYMPTOMS & SIGNS
- Skin is orange

> NOTE
> Should resolve itself if the individual reduces the consumption of food with carotene.

Carotid Aneurysm

Swelling of the carotid artery (aneurysm) in the brain, which can press on the optic nerve(s).

SYMPTOMS & SIGNS
- Peripheral and outer field of vision becomes lost
- May begin in only one eye, but both eyes become involved
- Nerve palsies resulting in facial pain and double vision

> NOTE
> Medical help should be sought immediately.

Carpal Tunnel Syndrome

Pain, tingling, numbness and altered sensation in the hands, especially the thumb and adjacent three fingers, caused by pressure put upon the median nerve at the base of the hand. The condition is associated with fluid retention, such as during Pregnancy or during the Menstrual cycle, Rheumatoid Arthritis, Myxoedema, and growth hormone excess.

SYMPTOMS & SIGNS
- Pain in the wrists, hands and fingers: usually the thumb, index, middle and half the ring finger
- Tingling, numbness and altered sensation in the hand
- Muscle wasting and reduction in strength especially over the thumb
- Weakness in thumb and when gripping objects
- May be pain and heaviness in the rest of the arm

> NOTE
> May resolve spontaneously or with rest, but in some cases may need surgery.

CROSS-REFERENCED UNDER:
Repetitive Strain (Wrist)

Cartilage Damage (Knee)

see CARTILAGE TEAR (KNEE)

Cartilage Tear (Knee)

The cartilage of the knee may be damaged or torn, usually because of direct injury or severe trauma. The severity of the symptoms will depend on how bad the tear or damage is.

SYMPTOMS & SIGNS
- Pain
- Reduced movement and function
- Swelling, which may take some hours to develop
- Knee may lock or give way
- May also be recurrent episodes of Dislocation of the Kneecap

> NOTE
> If a tear is suspected, medical help should be sought. Once cartilage has been damaged, the knee may be become more susceptible to injury.

CROSS-REFERENCED UNDER:
Cartilage Damage (Knee); Torn Medial Meniscus

Cat Scratch Fever

Infectious disease, caught from a penetrating injury, by either a scratch or bite of a cat.

SYMPTOMS & SIGNS
- Scratch or cut
- Small red lump appears around a week later
- Swollen lymph glands near to the scratch
- May be joint pains
- Rarely can affect the brain causing confusion, unsteadiness, seizures or stroke

NOTE
The condition will usually resolve after a few weeks and may be treated with antibiotics. Can be more serious if immunity is compromised.

Cataract

Cloudy patch on the eye.

SYMPTOMS & SIGNS
- Grey, cloudy patch on the cornea
- Becomes progressively worse, making it increasingly difficult to see
- May be blurred vision or difficulty distinguishing colours, caused by the interference of light by the Cataract, or haloes appear around bright objects
- No pain and no other obvious symptoms
- May cause blindness if left untreated

NOTE
Most likely in older individuals, particularly those over 60 years of age. Treatment is to replace the affected lens of the eye with an artificial lens.

Cauda Equina Syndrome

The lower part of the spinal canal may be damaged by conditions such as trauma, vertebral collapse eg by tumour or osteoporosis or a slipped disc between the vertebrae. The nerves that leave the bottom of the spinal cord can be compressed causing the syndrome.

SYMPTOMS & SIGNS
- Back pain
- Loss of or altered sensation in a saddle distribution
- Symmetrical leg weakness
- Loss of bladder control and possible urinary incontinence
- There may be evidence of tumour elsewhere, if tumour is the cause

NOTE
Medical help should be sought immediately.

Cauliflower Ear

Large, fleshy and misshapen outer ear, caused by recurrent blows or injury. The cartilage, which makes up the external ear, becomes scarred.

SYMPTOMS & SIGNS
- Ear is large, fleshy and misshapen

NOTE
Most likely in individuals likely to damage the external ear, such as boxers or rugby players.

Cellulitis

The soft tissues of the body can become infected by bacteria through a penetrating wound. This may be widespread or localised to one part of the body.

SYMPTOMS & SIGNS

- Swelling
- Skin may be red and shiny – affected area has a distinct border with normal skin. This rapidly becomes more extensive if untreated
- May be severe pain
- Fever
- General ill health
- May be evidence of the original wound which may be as trivial as a paper cut

NOTE
Antibiotics will be needed, along with a period of rest.

CROSS-REFERENCED UNDER:
Erysipelas

Central Retinal Artery Blockage

Complete sudden blindness, caused by the artery which supplies the eye being blocked by a blood clot or because it is constricted.

SYMPTOMS & SIGNS

- Complete blindness in one eye
- Sudden onset, usually painless
- May resolve in a fairly short time, or may be permanent

NOTE
Medical help should be sought immediately.

CROSS-REFERENCED UNDER:
Blockage of Central Retinal Artery; Amaurosis Fugax

Central Retinal Vein Blockage

Condition characterised by sudden blurring of vision typically on awakening as this often occurs during the night, caused by the vein which supplies the retina, becoming blocked with blood clot.

SYMPTOMS & SIGNS

- Blurring of vision in affected eye (usually affects one eye)
- Happens quickly
- May resolve in a few weeks, or may be permanent

NOTE
Most likely in the elderly, those individuals with high blood pressure, diabetics and those with blood disorders. Medical help should be sought immediately.

CROSS-REFERENCED UNDER:
Blockage of Central Retinal Vein

Cerebral Palsy

Condition caused by injury or infection of the brain and nerve centres of a baby during pregnancy or in early infancy. It may be caused by Rubella or other infections contracted during pregnancy.

SYMPTOMS & SIGNS

- Limbs floppy, ultimately, if walking is possible, walking is slow to start and will be compromised
- Failure to thrive
- Limbs have spasmodic movements
- Walking is stiff and jerky to compensate for the weakness or paralysis
- For some the severity of weakness prevents walking completely
- May be mental impairment, but this is by no means always the case

> NOTE
> Medical help should be sought.

CROSS-REFERENCED UNDER:
Little's Disease

Cervical Cancer
see CANCER OF THE CERVIX

Cervical Erosion
see EROSION OF THE CERVIX

Cervical Polyp

A fleshy growth can develop on the cervix or in the vagina.

SYMPTOMS & SIGNS
- Fleshy lump may be felt
- Discharge of blood
- May be an unpleasant copious discharge

> NOTE
> Medical help should be sought as investigations will be needed to exclude cancer or other serious disease.

CROSS-REFERENCED UNDER:
Vaginal Polyp

Cervical Rib

Some people have an extra rib or possibly fibrous material in the neck which can press on nerves or arteries. Alternatively, there may be no symptoms at all.

SYMPTOMS & SIGNS
- Lump can be felt in the neck
- Although the neck is not usually painful, pain can be experienced behind the collar bone or up

the inner side of the arm. This especially noticeable after carrying or exercising.
- Finger may turn blue or feel cold

> NOTE
> Although this extra rib is present from birth symptoms are most likely to appear in individuals in their late 20s.

Cervical Spine Infection

Infection of the spine in the neck, caused by bacterial infection of the bone – osteomyelitits. This can be caused by a number of bacteria including tuberculosis. Paralysis caused by infection of the spinal cord is possible if the affected vertebra collapses.

SIGNS
- Mild to severe pain in neck, but much worse with movement
- Stiffness in the neck and movement curtailed
- Fever
- General feeling of illness, malaise
- Lethargy, fatigue
- Loss of appetite
- Collapse of affected vertebra can cause spinal cord compression

> NOTE
> Medical help should be sought

CROSS-REFERENCED UNDER:
Infection of the Spine (Cervical)

Cervical Spondylosis

Degeneration of cervical (neck) vertebral discs is associated with development of arthritis (spondylosis) as the edges of the bone tend to rub together.

SYMPTOMS & SIGNS
- Pain located in the neck and back
- Pain worse when waking up
- Movement may be slightly curtailed
- Movement worsens pain

Also present may be:
- Pain going down the arms
- Weakness in the muscles of the arms
- Numbness in arms

NOTE
Most likely in middle-aged individuals.

Chagas' Disease

Acute or chronic disease caused by a parasite introduced by the bite of an infected insect. Chronic disease (gullet may dilate) damages the nerves that control the gullet and bowel.

SYMPTOMS & SIGNS
- Often no symptoms
- Initially may be fever, swollen face or eyelids, conjunctivitis, lymph node enlargement
- Swallowing difficulties
- Undigested food regurgitated into mouth
- Vomiting
- Weight loss
- Can cause confusion and convulsions
- Heart involvement damages the heart muscle and can cause heart failure or rhythm disturbance

NOTE
Common in South America.

Chancre
see SYPHILIS

Chancroid

Sexually transmitted diseases, common in tropical areas, but rare in developed countries

SYMPTOMS & SIGNS
- Genital ulcer develops some days after sexual contact. Starts as red spot that becomes a blister which bursts to become an ulcer
- Varies in size but normally painful
- Lymph nodes in the groin are enlarged and may burst, discharging pus

NOTE
Medical help should be sought, and treatment is with antibiotics.

CROSS-REFERENCED UNDER:
Lymphogranuloma Venerium; Granuloma Inguinale

Change in Breast Size

Several normal factors can cause an increase in breast size, such as Pregnancy, changes during menstrual cycle, the Contraceptive Pill and hormone replacement therapy (HRT).

SYMPTOMS & SIGNS
- Both breasts change size
- No other abnormal signs

NOTE
Medical help should be sought if change occurs in only one breast or if lumps are discovered.

Charcot's Joints

Swollen, deformed and disrupted joints, caused by

conditions such as Diabetic neuropathy, long-term Alcohol misuse, Spina Bifida, and Syphilis. The loss of sensation due to nerve damage in these conditions leads to repeated joint damage that destroys the joint completely.

SYMPTOMS & SIGNS
- Joints are swollen and deformed
- Bits of bone and fluid can be felt
- No pain
- Dislocation likely
- May become infected – bone infection can be very deep rooted

NOTE
Medical help should be sought.

Chest Cancer
see CANCER IN THE CHEST

Chest Infection

Chest infections can be caused by different viruses and bacteria, and are normally preceded by a Cold or sore throat. If serious, may develop into Pneumonia.

SYMPTOMS & SIGNS
- Production and coughing up of yellow or green sputum, which may be tinged with blood
- Wheezing
- Fever, with chills and shivers, and generally feeling ill
- May be difficulty in breathing for high-risk groups such as the elderly and those with Bronchitis or cardiovascular problems
- Bad breath and unpleasant taste in mouth
- May be rapid breathing and flaring nostrils
- May be pain in the chest and Pleurisy
- May be blue tinge to the lips caused by cyanosis

- May be mental confusion

NOTE
Smokers and elderly people stand a greater risk of getting Chest Infections. Chronic Chest Infections may be very serious, and may be need to be treated with antibiotics in high-risk groups.

CROSS-REFERENCED UNDER:
Infection of the Chest

Chest Injury

Severe injuries to the chest can break ribs and puncture the lungs, causing both internal and external injuries.

SYMPTOMS & SIGNS
- Cutting or stabbing pain in the chest
- Pain is exacerbated by inhaling
- Cough brings up blood
- May be difficulty breathing
- May be copious bleeding from a wound
- Confusion
- Unconsciousness and shock
- May be blue tinge to lips and skin

NOTE
Medical help should be sought immediately if severe injury is suspected. If an injury is bleeding copiously, pressure should be applied to staunch the bleeding.

CROSS-REFERENCED UNDER:
Chest Wound

Chest Wound
see CHEST INJURY

Chickenpox

Infectious illness, caused by the same virus (Herpes Zoster) which causes Shingles. Typically infects children but can infect non-immune adults. Tends to be more serious in adults. If the immune system is compromised the infection can be life threatening. Incubation period about two weeks.

SYMPTOMS & SIGNS
- Fever often with feeling of malaise or sore throat
- Within 1–2 days following fever, widespread blistering rash with red spots, including in the mouth and on the scalp
- The rash is very itchy and appears in crops over the next 3–4 days
- These blisters can burst and crust over, forming scabs
- Rash lasts over the next two weeks
- Generally feeling unwell
- Rarely complications such as inflammation of the brain (encephalitis) or development of a severe pneumonia

NOTE
The condition will usually resolve in a few weeks, and this is usually a fairly mild illness.

CROSS-REFERENCED UNDER:
Varicella

Chilblains

Blood vessels in the skin become damaged, caused by the cold.

SYMPTOMS & SIGNS
Onset:
- Itching and burning pain in the fingers and toes

Then:
- Digits become swollen
- Area affected becomes purple or red
- Blisters

NOTE
Treatment is by gently warming the affected area.

Child Abuse
see SEXUAL ABUSE

Childbirth
see PREGNANCY

Chlamydia

Bacterial infection of the vagina and penis, which may be passed by sexual contact. Currently this is the commonest sexually transmitted disease. Many infected people do not have symptoms of this disease, but can infect others. Women are more likely not to have symptoms.

SYMPTOMS & SIGNS
- Discharge from the vagina, persistent in nature
- May be tenderness and pain
- Discharge from penis (urethritis)
- May be pain on passing urine, and frequency of passing urine
- May result in infertility if left untreated
- Women may develop pelvic inflammatory disease

NOTE
Medical help should be sought as antibiotics will be needed.

CROSS-REFERENCED UNDER:
Non-Specific Urethritis

Choking

Food or any object can get trapped in the gullet or in the windpipe (trachea). If the airway is blocked this results in choking. Inhaled objects may become lodged in the lungs.

SYMPTOMS & SIGNS

If the foreign body blocks the airway (medical emergency):

- Choking
- Clawing at throat
- Breathing may be rasping and forced (stridor)
- May be blue tinge to the lips, ear lobes, under the fingernails and elsewhere caused by a lack of oxygen reaching tissues (cyanosis)
- Unconsciousness and coma

In children:

- Body may be inhaled into the lungs
- Initially a coughing fit, although symptoms may pass
- Later, may become fatigued and may develop symptoms of a Chest Infection or Lung Abscess as the foreign body becomes a focus for the body's defences
- An x-ray will be needed to confirm if a foreign body has been inhaled

NOTE

Medical help should be sought immediately as the foreign body may get caught in the wind pipe. The Heimlich Manoeuvre can be employed should there be difficulty in breathing: it is very important to carry out this manoeuvre quickly and efficiently or the individual may choke to death.

CROSS-REFERENCED UNDER:

Foreign Body in Airway; Inhaled Foreign Body

Cholecystitis

see GALL STONES

Cholera

Potentially severe infectious disease, caused by a micro-organism, which may cause epidemics of infection. Spread by contaminated water and insanitary conditions, especially where there is severe overcrowding.

SYMPTOMS & SIGNS

- Vomiting (either before or after diarrhoea starts)
- Diarrhoea with copious and watery faeces, although may start quite mildly
- Abdominal pain and colic
- Thirst
- Muscle cramps
- Low-grade fever

NOTE

Most likely in tropical countries, although outbreaks are not as severe as epidemics around the turn of the 20th century. Dehydration is a severe problem with Cholera and should be addressed as it may lead to death.

Cholesteatoma

Development of a lump of inflammation in the ear, which can destroy surrounding tissues, usually caused by recurrent ear infections.

SYMPTOMS & SIGNS

- Discharge from ear
- Deafness
- Vertigo, dizziness and feelings of falling

Chondritis

Cartilage in the chest becomes inflamed and painful, caused by injury or infection, or without apparent cause.

SYMPTOMS & SIGNS

- Takes a few hours to develop
- Pain on both side of the breast bone in the middle of the chest, which may be severe in intensity
- Worse with movement or inhaling or exhaling
- Swollen joints which may be tender to the touch
- May be mild fever
- May last for several weeks

NOTE

Although not life-threatening, the pressing symptom may be severe pain.

Choroiditis

Inflammation of part of the retina, which may be caused by infections such as Toxoplasmosis or Syphilis, although the cause is not fully understood. The inflammation causes a blind spot at the site.

SYMPTOMS & SIGNS

- Affects one eye usually
- Onset may be disturbed vision in that eye
- Blind spot develops gradually, although it remains constant in size and in its position

NOTE

Medical help should be sought.

Chronic Bronchitis

see BRONCHITIS

Chronic Mastitis

see FIBROCYSTIC DISEASE

Chronic Otitis Media

see INNER EAR INFECTION

Chronic Pelvic Inflammatory Disease

see SALPINGITIS

Cigarettes

Sticks of tobacco which when smoked can lead to addiction in particular to the nicotine that is present in tobacco products. Smoking over a number of years damages the circulation, causes angina, heart attacks, limb amputation, bronchitis as well as cancers especially of lung, throat, gullet and stomach.

SYMPTOMS & SIGNS

- Heart rate increased, may be with extra beats
- Many other problems from long-term use

NOTE

Smoking during pregnancy may damage the developing baby.

CROSS-REFERENCED UNDER:

Nicotine

Cirrhosis of the Liver

Irreversible, progressive replacement of normal liver cells by scar tissue which can be caused by several conditions, such as viruses, bacteria, toxic substances, chronic Hepatitis, chronic Cardiac Failure and Wilson's Disease, as well as Alcohol abuse. The function of the liver is progressively compromised resulting in liver failure.

SYMPTOMS & SIGNS

- Generally feeling unwell, weak and fatigued
- Weight loss
- Ankles swollen
- Abdomen swollen because of retention of fluid (ascites)
- May be prominent blood vessels in the abdomen
- Nausea and vomiting, possibly including blood
- Blood in faeces
- Jaundice, including skin looking yellow
- Spleen enlarged
- Bruising happens very easily
- Mental facilities impaired
- Red vascular marks on the skin (spider naevi)
- Clubbing of finger and toe nails
- Breath may smell sweet and of faeces
- Loss of hair, including pubic hair

In men:

- Testes shrink and breasts enlarged

NOTE
Medical help should be sought immediately.

Clap
see GONORRHOEA

Claw Toes
see PES CAVUS

Cleft Lip and Palate

Lip and palate do not develop normally in the infant while in the womb. This leaves a gap, a cleft lip and palate, on one side, or even on both, sides of the nose.

SYMPTOMS & SIGNS

- Cleft palate and lip
- Nose is distorted on one side of the face
- Will be difficulty in feeding and speaking if not treated

NOTE
Occurs in about one in every 750 births. Usually treated by reconstructive surgery.

Cluster Headache

Headaches which resolve and recur, often over a relatively short period of time. The headache may be very severe in intensity, but is rarely a cause for concern, other than because of the underlying stresses or emotional distress.

SYMPTOMS & SIGNS

- More often one-sided pain centred behind an eye
- May be very severe and stabbing pain
- Recurs often within a relatively short space of time
- Eye on side of pain may look red and may be watery
- Resolves, but within a short time recurs

NOTE
May resolve as long as the underlying stresses are dealt with. More common in men, and often occur at night or during periods of relaxation.

CROSS-REFERENCED UNDER:
Headache, Cluster

Coccydynia

The coccyx, the small bones at the end of the spine

and all that remains of a tail, can become damaged by injury or trauma.

Symptoms & Signs
- Lower back pain following a fall or injury
- Pressing the sore area or sitting exacerbates the pain

> Note
> Medical help should be sought.

Coeliac Disease

Intolerance to gluten, a protein which is found in wheat and rye, and food made from them, such as bread and pasta. The condition causes malabsorption of food and a failure to thrive.

Symptoms & Signs
- May be very mild or no symptoms
- Fatigue
- Anaemia
- Weight loss
- Diarrhoea often with pale malodorous, floating faeces
- May be dermatitis herpetiformis
- Can affect children or adults of any age

> Note
> Symptoms become apparent when the baby is between three and six months old. Treatment involves a gluten-free diet.

Cross-referenced under:
Gluten Intolerance; Wheat Intolerance

Coffee
see Caffeine

Cold, Common

Common illness, caused by many strains of viral infections, and characterised by a cough with phlegm.

Symptoms & Signs
- Sore throat and cough
- Mild fever, which usually only lasts a couple of days, with shivers or chills
- Lymph nodes in neck may be inflamed and tender
- General feeling of being unwell and giddiness
- Nose running with phlegm, which may be clear, yellow or green
- Blocked nose and loss of sense of smell
- May be nosebleeds, caused by inflammation of the inside of the nose and blowing the nose
- May have speech which is hoarse, nasal or muffled
- May be earache
- May be pain in and around the eyes caused by nasal congestion
- May be muscle and joint pain
- Bad breath and unpleasant taste in mouth
- May be difficult to open the mouth because of pain or swelling
- May develop into Chest Infections, Ear Infections or related areas

> Note
> Will normally resolve itself. Smoking exacerbates symptoms, and smokers may suffer from associated infections of the chest.

Cross-referenced under:
Upper Respiratory Tract Infections; Common Cold

Cold Sore
see Herpes Simplex

Collarbone Fracture

see BROKEN COLLARBONE

Colorectal Cancer

see CANCER OF THE COLON OR RECTUM (BOWEL)

Colour Blindness

Inability to distinguish between various colours, usually red-green, but sometimes blue-green. This is usually a normal variation, and of little importance except in occupations such as, drivers, pilots or train drivers.

SYMPTOMS & SIGNS

- Inability to distinguish between various colours, usually red-green, but sometimes blue-green
- No other symptoms

> NOTE
> Most common in males, but also found in females.

Coma

Coma is a state of deep unconsciousness, which can be caused by various conditions that compromise brain function such as Stroke, systemic infection, Head Injury or drug excess or overdose.

SYMPTOMS & SIGNS

- Dilated or constricted pupils, which do not react to changes in light
- Unconsciousness
- Irregular and shallow breathing
- No response to stimulus, even if very painful

> NOTE
> Medical help should be sought immediately.

Common Cold

see COLD, COMMON

Concussion

see HEAD INJURY

Congenital Adrenal Hyperplasia

Inborn error of adrenal steroid hormone production present from birth that causes excessive androgen (male hormone) production and reduces production of aldosterone (that regulates salt control and blood pressure) and cortisol (hormone has many actions including regulation of metabolism). Both adrenal glands are enlarged. Requires life-long replacement usually with hormones that are equivalent to cortisol and aldosterone.

SYMPTOMS & SIGNS

- Excessive body hair, although can be mild
- Fused labia
- Clitoris is enlarged
- Infant girls can be virilised and may rarely be thought to be male, initially
- Severe forms may present in first 2 weeks of life with vomiting, diarrhoea, salt loss dehydration and shock

Later in life:

- Acne
- Early apparent puberty
- Menstruation is occasional or absent

> NOTE
> Medical help should be sought.

Congenital Atresia of the Oesophagus

New born infants cannot swallow properly and have problems breathing when being fed because the gullet has not opened up properly during development.

SYMPTOMS & SIGNS

- Feeds regurgitated
- Mouth may be full of frothy saliva
- Baby may appear blue tinged (cyanosis)
- Problems breathing when feeding
- Pneumonia

NOTE
Medical help should be sought immediately.

Congenital Blindness

see BLINDNESS

Congenital Dislocation of the Hip (CDH)

The thigh bone (femur) can become displaced from the hip joint, caused by congenital problems with the socket of the hip bone being unusually shaped.

SYMPTOMS & SIGNS

- Congenital problem with the hip, exacerbated if baby is delivered as a breech birth. The condition tends to run in families
- May affect both hips, but one is more likely
- Hips look different
- Legs do not part properly
- Baby may take longer than normal to start walking
- When baby finally walks, limps and legs look as if they are different lengths
- If both hips are affected, baby walks with a waddling movement
- In later life, hip joint is severely deformed and severe Osteoarthritis will develop if left untreated

NOTE
More likely in girls than boys. Care should be taken to identify this condition as soon as possible as it can be treated.

CROSS-REFERENCED UNDER:
Dislocated Hip

Congenital Heart Disease

see HEART DISEASE

Congenital Problems of the Eye

see BLINDNESS

Conjunctivitis

Inflammation of the white area of the eye, leading to visible blood vessels, usually caused by a bacterial infection. This can be a very contagious condition. It may affect one or both of the eyes.

SYMPTOMS & SIGNS

- Eyes (or one eye) becomes itchy or are mildly painful with a prickling sensation: may feel as if something is stuck in the eye
- Eyes sore and red, most noticeable around the outside of the white of the eye
- Bright light can be painful or cause discomfort
- Crusty eyeballs and a small discharge from the corner of the eyes, yellow in colour
- Eyelids stuck together in the morning

NOTE
Individuals wearing contact lenses are far more likely to get Conjunctivitis. Treatment for serious bouts of the condition is with antibiotic eyedrops.

Conn's Syndrome

see ALDOSTERONISM

Constipation

A symptom as well as a condition. Constipation can have several causes, although the regularity of any particular individual's bowel can vary from several times a day to once a week or less. There is no 'correct' regularity, only what is normal for the individual. More important is a change in bowel habit. An alteration in life-style or diet, or long periods of immobility due to being bed-bound, may result in constipation, especially in the young. Causes can also be drinking too little fluids or a diet too low in roughage, as well as medical conditions such as Stroke, Head Injury or some neurological conditions.

Constipation with a sudden onset or change in bowel habit with constipation and bleeding and without even passing wind, particularly in the elderly, may be signs of serious underlying disease and should be investigated as soon as possible.

SYMPTOMS & SIGNS
■ A change in bowel habit, involving the infrequent and difficult evacuation of the bowel
■ If passing hard, dry or pellet-like faeces, the cause may be a change in life-style or an alteration in diet such as eating less or drinking too little fluids
■ If no stools or wind are being passed at all (acute constipation), then it may be the indication of a serious underlying problem
■ In young children, particularly during potty training, there may a psychological component to constipation. Forcing a child into potty training before they are ready, may, in some circumstances, cause problems in later life
■ Old people may become so constipated that

diarrhoea passes the compacted mass of faeces and leaks out of the rectum – giving the impression that they actually have diarrhoea.

NOTE
If Constipation cannot be resolved with eating more roughage or drinking more fluids, and persists, medical help should be sought to exclude serious illness.

Constrictive Pericarditis

The sac around the heart becomes progressively inflamed and rigid. Caused by infections, such as Tuberculosis, or injury, although it may take several years to become apparent. The function of the heart may be compromised due to constriction.

SYMPTOMS & SIGNS
■ Rapid, possibly irregular, pulse
■ Low blood pressure
■ Excessive fatigue and weakness
■ Prominent veins in the neck: more so when inhaling
■ Liver is enlarged
■ Fluid collects in the abdomen
■ Ankle swelling
■ Chest pain

NOTE
Medical help should be sought immediately.

Consumption
see TUBERCULOSIS

Contraceptive Pill

The contraceptive pill prevents women from ovulating and unwanted pregnancy.

SYMPTOMS & SIGNS
- May be no periods
- May be significant weight gain
- Breasts may become larger
- Slight increase risk of Deep Vein Thrombosis
- If coming off the pill, may take some months for periods to return. If it is more than six months, medical help should be sought, although it may still be possible to get pregnant during this time
- May be some bleeding between periods of a normal cycle, caused by hormones. If this does occur, the pill should still be taken as normal, although if it does persist for six months or more, it may be necessary to use a different kind of contraceptive pill

Corn
see CALLUS

Corneal Damage
see CORNEAL ULCER

Corneal Ulcer

An ulcer can form on the cornea of the eye, caused by an infection, such as Herpes, or from trauma.

SYMPTOMS & SIGNS
- Only one eye is affected
- Eye is itchy and has a feeling as if there is a foreign body in it
- Eye is severely painful, made worse by bright light
- Eye is red, usually around the coloured part of the eye

NOTE
Medical help should be sought.

CROSS-REFERENCED UNDER:
Corneal Damage

Crab Lice
see SCABIES

Cramp
see MUSCLE CRAMP

Crohn's Disease

A form of inflammatory bowel disease caused by areas of inflamation and ulceration.

SYMPTOMS & SIGNS
- Chronic and recurrent diarrhoea. Faeces may be normal if somewhat loose, but may be abnormal with blood and mucus
- Intermittent colicky pain, accompanying diarrhoea or occurring by itself
- Sometimes constipation
- May be intermittent fever
- May be pain experienced in the back
- May be pain in joints
- Aphthous (mouth) ulcers
- Possible weight loss
- May feel ill and unwell
- May come and go
- May be mistaken for a grumbling appendix
- May be anal abscess with localised throbbing pain and tenderness in the rectum
- May be clubbing of end of fingers and finger nails
- May be collapse in severe cases

NOTE
Most likely in young adults between about 20 and 40 years of age, and tests will be need to confirm a diagnosis. Treatment with drugs or surgery may be necessary.

Croup

Condition with a very distinctive cough, caused by inflammation of the larynx and a viral or bacterial infection.

SYMPTOMS & SIGNS
- Distinctive, dry cough
- Breathing is harsh and noisy
- Heavy sticky phlegm
- May be difficulty breathing and even suffocation

NOTE
Medical help should be sought immediately.

CROSS-REFERENCED UNDER:
Laryngotracheo-bronchitis

Cushing's Disease

see CUSHING'S SYNDROME

Cushing's Syndrome

Obesity of the trunk and face (with thin limbs), excess sugar in the blood, high blood pressure caused by excess production of steriod hormones and steroid use. Steriod hormone excess within the body may arise from lumps in the pituitary and adrenal.

SIGNS
- Puffy face which looks round ('moon face')
- Obesity and weight gain
- Fat is deposited on the trunk, although not the legs and arms, and especially on the back, which can cause a hump
- Muscle fatigue and weakness
- Stretch marks on abdomen, thighs and shoulders
- Skin is easily bruised and is thinner and more fragile

- Bone pain
- Diabetes
- Excessive urination
- High blood pressure
- May be psychiatric problems including depression

In women, also:
- Absence of menstruation
- Excessive body hair
- Clitoris becomes enlarged

In men, also:
- Impotence
- Acne

NOTE
More likely in females.

CROSS-REFERENCED UNDER:
Cushing's Disease

Cystic Fibrosis

A hereditary disease, characterised by abnormal body secretions, that leads to recurrent, severe pulmonary infections. It begins to affect the child noticeably later in infancy.

SYMPTOMS & SIGNS
- Failure to thrive, although may eat normally
- Thin in build, but with a swollen abdomen
- Persistent chest infections and bad breath. Copious phlegm
- Diarrhoea due to poor absorption with especially unpleasant faeces (pale and may float)
- Weight loss
- Clubbing of end of fingers and finger nails
- May be rectal prolapse, where the intestine pops out through the anus

> NOTE
> Affects about one child in 2500. There is currently no cure.

Cystitis

Inflammation of the bladder, usually caused by bacterial infection. Although blood in urine should always be treated seriously, it is a much more urgent symptom in children, and should be properly investigated.

SYMPTOMS & SIGNS
- Urine passed frequently, with need to get up at night to pass urine
- Urine may be dark, cloudy or stained with blood: this can be the colour of blood, but may only appear to be slightly pinkish
- Passing urine causes searing or burning pain
- Very urgent feeling of needing to urinate or having a very full bladder, but little urine actually produced
- Ache in the lower part of the abdomen, which can be persistent or worse after urination
- Backache
- Fever
- May be general feeling of being unwell

> NOTE
> More likely in females, because the urethra is shorter than in males. Mild cases may resolve without intervention, although may need antibiotics. Urinary infections in children are very unusual, and should always be thoroughly investigated by a doctor.

Cystocele

see STRESS INCONTINENCE

Dacryocystitis

Inflammation of the glands which produce tears, which are found at the corners of the eyes, caused by an infection.

SYMPTOMS & SIGNS
- Pain and swollen area by the bridge of the nose
- Red and tender skin
- May be discharge of pus
- May be mild pain in or around the eye

> NOTE
> Medical help should be sought as soon as possible, as probably needs treated with antibiotics.

Damage to Testicles

Testicles, which produce sperm, can be damaged by several conditions or problems. These can be injury to the testicles, if a testicle is undescended, Mumps, as well as treatments for cancer. These can reduce sperm count and a man's fertility. Behavioural factors can also affect fertility, including drinking too much alcohol, smoking, and the testicles being too warm. Hormone disorders in men can also produce fertility problems, as can chromosomal disorders.

SYMPTOMS & SIGNS
- May be no obvious physical symptoms
- Testicles may be small and soft

If a hormone disorder is present, also:
- Little or no body hair
- Breasts in men
- Individual may be unusually small or tall in height
- Obesity

> **NOTE**
> Medical help should be sought.

CROSS-REFERENCED UNDER:
Small Testicles

Damage to the Retina
see DETACHED RETINA

Dandruff

Skin flaking from the scalp. The causes are not clear, although it has been associated with skin disease, infection and even general ill health, it is, however, a very common condition among the fit and healthy.

SYMPTOMS & SIGNS
- Skin of the scalp is dry and flakes
- Scalp can be very itchy

> **NOTE**
> Treatment is by anti-dandruff shampoos.

Decreased Fluid Intake
see DEHYDRATION

Deep Vein Thrombosis

The veins of the leg become blocked by a blood clot, caused by immobility due to surgery, lack of movement such as when bedridden or on an aeroplane for a long time'economy class syndrome', or for no apparent reason.

SYMPTOMS & SIGNS
- Calf and ankle become swollen; as the thigh may also be swollen if blood clot includes pelvic veins
- Onset is sudden
- Mild pain or discomfort and tenderness
- Swelling may recur long after DVT has gone

- Tenderness
- Affected leg is reddened

> **NOTE**
> Most likely in individuals who smoke, are obese or elderly, or have cancer, and there is a small increased risk for those on the Contraceptive Pill. Medical help should be sought immediately as the clot can dislodge and get stuck in the brain, lungs or heart, possibly causing death.

CROSS-REFERENCED UNDER:
Venous Thrombosis

Deficiency in Potassium
see POTASSIUM DEFICIENCY

Dehydration

A symptom and a condition. If the individual has been undergoing strenuous exercise or been spending time in a hot environment, they can become dehydrated through losing fluid by sweat. Salt can be lost in the same manner, and the individual may end up suffering from heat exhaustion. Dehydration can also be the result of many other conditions, such as vomiting, diarrhoea, blood loss, and moisture loss through breathing as in Asthma. Dehydration is particularly serious in babies and children, and in old people.

SYMPTOMS & SIGNS
- Urine very dark in hue and strong smelling, but not passed in large quantities
- Thirst
- Dry tongue and mouth
- Dry and lax skin
- Eyes may be sunken
- Red face

- May be painful, swollen and protruding eyes with restricted movement caused by blood clots in the tissues behind the eyes
- In extreme cases may be confusion, Shock, torpor, collapse and even death

In babies and children:

- Babies' heads have soft gaps (fontanelles) where the skull bones have not yet fused together. These become sunken when they are dehydrated
- Sunken eyes
- Skin loses elasticity
- Dry lips and mouth
- Baby becomes listless and unresponsive

NOTE

May be resolved, usually within a day or so, by drinking more fluids or staying in cooler conditions. It may also be necessary to replace lost salt. If dehydration is suspected in children or babies, medical help should be sought immediately: the condition kills thousands of infants, especially in poorer parts of the world.

CROSS-REFERENCED UNDER:
Decreased Fluid Intake

Dementia

As individuals get older, may become prone to confusion resulting from memory loss (usually for recent events). This confusion is mild and can be managed by making lists or developing a routine, but the extent of memory loss may progress, usually slowly.

SYMPTOMS & SIGNS

- Confusion, caused or exacerbated by a change in routine
- Short-term memory loss; old memories, such as of childhood, are often preserved
- Delusions caused by the above and the individual 'filling in gaps' that they cannot remember
- Change in personality and progressive mental impairment
- Anxiety and mania
- Depression
- Self-neglect
- Health otherwise normal for an individual of that age
- Reversal of night-day sleep pattern – tends to be up, wandering at night

---

NOTE

There is currently no treatment for severe Dementia.

CROSS-REFERENCED UNDER:
Senile Confusion; Alzheimer's Disease

Dengue

Infectious disease caused by virus, spread by mosquitoes.

SIGNS

- Sudden onset of high fever
- Facial flushing
- Aches
- Headache
- Severe pain in the bones
- Loss of appetite, vomiting
- Rash

- Disease appears to improve, but then worsens again, including a more widespread rash
- May be complicated by bleeding and shock

> NOTE
> May resolve after several weeks of illness.

Dental Caries
see TOOTH DECAY AND ABSCESS

Dental Infections

Infection of the teeth and gums, caused by dental caries and abscesses, poor dental hygiene, and even pregnancy when bleeding gums can occur because of hormone changes.

SYMPTOMS & SIGNS
- Toothache
- Facial pain and apparent earache, especially if problems are with molar teeth
- May be difficult to open the mouth because of the pain or swelling
- Bad breath
- Gingivitis (gums which are inflamed and bleed) - gums are particularly prone to bleeding after brushing teeth
- Damaged teeth and dental abscesses
- Enlarged and tender lymph nodes near affected teeth

> NOTE
> Any serious or long-term problems with the teeth, gums or mouth should prompt a visit to the dentist.

CROSS-REFERENCED UNDER:
Infections of the Teeth; Infections of the Gums

Dentures

If dentures are not cleaned either thoroughly or regularly, food and saliva can become trapped in them. This may give the individual bad breath. It should stop when the dentures are properly cleaned.

SYMPTOMS & SIGNS
- Bad breath
- Dentures are not properly cleaned
- No other symptoms

Depression and Manic Depression

General feelings of lowness, fatigue and weariness, physical, mental and spiritual, and loss of or reduction in interest and enjoyment of life. This may be caused by external factors such as stress or bereavement (neurotic) or may arise apparently spontaneously with no underlying cause (psychotic); or may be a mixture of both. Sometimes may follow pregnancy, post-natal depression. The severity can vary from mild to severe, and suicide may be a real risk.

Manic Depression may be seen as bouts of Depression, followed by bouts of Mania and hyperactivity.

SYMPTOMS & SIGNS
The depressed individual may exhibit the following:
- Difficulty sleeping with early morning awakening
- Headaches and general aches and pain
- Lethargy, tiredness and apathy
- Sadness and weeping
- Loss of appetite, which in the long-term may result in weight loss
- Lack of emotion: face may appear expressionless

- Lack of interest and concentration
- Lack of interest in sex or sexual contact: women may appear to be frigid, while men cannot get or maintain an erection
- May be Anxiety
- General dark or suicidal thoughts
- May be complete feelings of hopelessness and a complete lack of self worth
- May be delusions and hallucinations in severe Depression, and it is possible that these may move the individual to harm themselves or others or they hear voices

Manic Depression:
- Periods of Depression as above
- Periods of Mania, such as frantic and frenetic actions, rapid speech, unrealistic plans, sudden changes in direction of thought, restlessness, hyperactivity and even hallucinations

---

NOTE

Severe depression and Manic Depression will usually need to be treated with drugs, therapy, or even hospitalisation, particularly if the individual is feeling suicidal.

CROSS-REFERENCED UNDER:
Manic Depression

Dermatitis

The skin becomes irritated, red and inflamed. This can be caused by allergy to various triggers, such as soap or cosmetics, but may also be associated with stress. It is also often worse in folds of the skin, such as at the elbow and knee, and sensitive parts of the skin, like the eyelid, the skin below the eye, and the skin around the groin.

Dermatitis Herpetiformis is a form of the condition caused by auto-immune disease and associated with Coeliac Disease.

SYMPTOMS & SIGNS
- Skin becomes angry and red
- Affected areas become itchy and sore
- Skin may flake, scale or weep, and blisters, crusts and dry skin may form
- May be hair loss from the affected area
- The area may be raised above the unaffected skin
- May affect the eyes, making them particularly sensitive to light – and there may be a feeling as if something is in the eye
- Transverse ridges on fingernails
- Condition may spread progressively over the body

NOTE

Dermatitis Herpetiformis is treated with drugs, and skin symptoms will improve with medication.

CROSS-REFERENCED UNDER:
Eczema; Dermatitis Herpetiformis

Dermatitis Herpetiformis

see DERMATITIS

Dermatomyositis

Muscle inflammation, and skin rash occassionally, associated with cancer.

SYMPTOMS & SIGNS
- Muscle weakness and pain especially muscles of upper arms and legs
- Widespread rash on face, limbs and trunk
- Fluid retention (oedema)
- Feeling unwell

- Fever

> **NOTE**
> Most likely in individuals over 40 years of age.

Dermoid Cysts

Benign cysts that can develop in the head and neck, back, testicles or elsewhere.

SYMPTOMS & SIGNS
- Cysts develop on the head, neck and elsewhere, but are particularly likely to grow near the eyebrow
- Cysts are benign
- No other symptoms
- Although cystic they can occasionally contain skin, hair, teeth or cartilage

> **NOTE**
> Medical help should be sought to exclude a more serious underlying cause.

Detached Retina

The retina, the light sensitive part of the eye at the back of the organ, can be come detached or damaged, caused by trauma, bleeding, inflammation or tumours. The retina is not actually attached to the back of the eye but is held in place by the pressure of fluid within the eye itself.

SYMPTOMS & SIGNS
- Heralded by numerous floaters in the eye and/or flashing lights
- Blurred vision
- Problems seeing or even blindness
- May be problems distinguishing colours

If the retina is distorted:

- Partial or complete loss of vision often with the sense of a curtain coming down
- If long standing, the lens of the eye may become white in colour

> **NOTE**
> Medical help should be sought immediately as surgery may be able to return the retina to the correct position.

CROSS-REFERENCED UNDER:
Distortion of the Retina; Damage to the Retina

Diabetes Insipidus

Diabetes Insipidus, which is not due to insulin problems and is caused by problems with the pituitary gland in the skull, may be congenital or caused by head trauma, infection or tumours, arising within or above the pituitary.

SYMPTOMS & SIGNS
- Thirst and excessive drinking
- Excessive urination
- Needs to get up overnight for urination
- May be symptoms and signs of lack of thyroid hormone, steriod hormone testosterone or oestrogen (leading to lack of periods)
- May be symptoms of hormone excess including thyroid hormone, Cushing's syndrome, acromegaly

> **NOTE**
> Onset in elderly people is slower, and the most obvious signs may be problems with feet and eyesight.

Diabetes Mellitus

Diabetes Mellitus too much sugar in the blood (hyperglycaemia) caused by problems with carbohydrate metabolism and either too little insulin being produced in the pancreas or the body becomes resistant to the effect of insulin.

SYMPTOMS & SIGNS

- Frequent urination (polyuria): urine is very pale and contains a lot of sugar – it may smell of apples
- Need to get up overnight to pass urine
- Increased thirst
- Severe and progressive weight loss
- Generally feeling unwell and fatigued
- May be periods of blurred vision, which resolve within a short time
- Itch around genitals or anus
- Increased tendency to develop abscesses

If diabetes is very poorly controlled, in the short term there may be:

- Breath may smell sweet or sickly, caused by excessive sugar in the blood (ketoacidosis)
- May be vomiting
- May be abdominal pain
- May be muscle cramps
- If untreated, may be coma and ultimately death

If diabetes is poorly controlled over the long term there can be a number of complications:

- May be eye, nerve, foot and kidney damage
- In the long term, may be loss of vision and even blindness caused by degeneration in the blood vessels which supply the eye
- Increased risk of Cataracts in later life
- Diabetic neuropathy including muscle wastage, altered sensation and numbness, reduction in strength and stamina and joint damage and deformity
- Other symptoms may be feelings of pain, impotence or maintaining an erection, inability to orgasm, postural hypotension, loss of sweating in the lower limbs and ulcerated feet
- Kidney damage including proteinuria nephrotic syndrome and kidney failure
- Damage to the peripheral arteries with peripheral vascular disease and gangrene
- Greatly increased risk of ischaemic heart disease
- If individual is suffering from low blood sugar during treatment with diabetes the following symptoms may develop:
- Hunger
- Feeling light-headed or giddy
- Anxiety
- Sweating
- Nausea
- Dehydration with an intense thirst and dry mouth
- Fast heart beat
- Confusion
- Unconsciousness and coma
- Death is possible

Diffuse Thyroid Gland Enlargement

Swelling of the thyroid gland (which is on both sides of the neck below the Adam's apple). It is associated with an over- or under-active thyroid gland. It is typically benign, occasionally can be malignant.

SYMPTOMS & SIGNS

- Feeling of swelling that moves up and down when swallowing
- Swelling may not be symmetrical

If malignant (which is more unusual), the following will also be present:

- The wind pipe (trachea) may be pressed upon, making breathing difficult
- Pain over enlarged thyroid
- Lymph glands enlarged. Occasionally solitary or multpile nodules can develop in the thyroid. If large they may give rise to symptoms as above. Occasionally they can also produce too much thyroid hormone. Occasionally they are malignant

NOTE
Medical help should be sought.

Diphtheria

A serious bacterial infectious disease, characterised by the formation of a false grey membrane at the back of the throat or on the respiratory tract, which can block the windpipe and cause suffocation. The illness also involves the releasing of toxic substances into the body which affect the nervous system, as well as the heart muscle.

SYMPTOMS & SIGNS
- Initially appears to be a sore throat
- Feeling unwell with fever
- Loose cough
- False grey membrane, caused by the infection, forms on the mucous membrane of the respiratory tract, often at the back of the throat. This may cause suffocation
- Lymph nodes enlarged in the neck
- Breathlessness and blue tinge to the skin, especially the lips (cyanosis)
- Heart muscle may be involved (myocarditis) causing altered heart rhythm and heart failure.

Nervous system can also be involved with development of nerve damage especially to nerves of head and neck

NOTE
Due to immunisation, this is a very rare condition in developed countries. It can be treated, and help should be sought immediately if it is suspected.

Dislocated Hip
see ACQUIRED DISLOCATION OF THE HIP

Dislocated Hip
see CONGENITAL DISLOCATION OF THE HIP (CDH)

Dislocated Hip
see INFECTIVE DISLOCATION OF THE HIP

Dislocation of the Knee

The knee joint can be dislocated, although a violent injury will have been sustained. This will normally cause damage both to the joint itself, and the associated nerves and blood vessels.

SYMPTOMS & SIGNS
- Pain, severe in intensity
- Severe bruising
- Joint looks deformed

NOTE
Medical help should be sought immediately.

CROSS-REFERENCED UNDER:
Knee Dislocation

Dislocation of the Knee Cap

The kneecap (patella) may be dislocated, caused by direct damage, trauma, or because of anatomical problems with the structures of the knee.

SYMPTOMS & SIGNS
- Pain in the knee
- Kneecap may move in the joint
- Knee cannot be moved from the bent position, which may make the individual fall
- May be in both knees
- May resolve by itself but recurrent episodes

> NOTE
> Medical help should be sought.

CROSS-REFERENCED UNDER:
Dislocation of the Patella

Dislocation of the Patella
see DISLOCATION OF THE KNEE CAP

Dislocation of the Shoulder
see SHOULDER DISLOCATION

Disorders of Blood Clotting

Several conditions, such as Haemophilia or taking warfarin, reduce or stop the blood's ability to clot. This means that wound or cuts continue to bleed without stop, both externally and internally.

SYMPTOMS & SIGNS
- Persistent bleeding, even from minor cuts
- Extensive bruising, even after minor injury
- Bleeding gums and copious bleeding after tooth extraction
- May be spontaneous bleeding with no obvious cause
- May be nosebleeds with no obvious cause
- May be problems with joints cause by bleeding
- May be heavy periods
- May be blood in vomit, urine or from the bowels

> NOTE
> Tests will be needed to confirm a diagnosis of conditions such as Haemophilia.

Distortion of the Retina
see DETACHED RETINA

Diuretics

Diuretics are substances which increase the flow and quantity of urine, (and include alcohol, coffee and tea). Diuretic drugs are used to reduce blood pressure and heart failure: one symptom of the latter is the retention of fluid (oedema). Diuretics reduce the amount of fluid in the body and reduce tension in blood vessels. It is possible that individuals taking diuretics may have their sleep disturbed as they wake up to make frequent trips to urinate.

SYMPTOMS & SIGNS
- Increased frequency of urinating (the expected effect)

If used in too high doses:
- Dehydration
- Thirst
- Increasing weakness and fatigue which becomes worse with time
- Constipation
- May be vomiting
- May be apathy

> NOTE
> Medical help should be sought if excessive doses of diuretics are being taken.

Diverticular Disease
see DIVERTICULITIS

Diverticular Disease (Jejunal)

see JEJUNAL DIVERTICULITIS

Diverticulitis

The wall of the intestine can develop pouches (diverticula). These can exist without symptoms, but they may become inflamed, caused by an infection.

SYMPTOMS & SIGNS
- Change of bowel habit
- Colicky or persistent abdominal pain, often on the right side
- Swollen abdomen
- Faeces may contain blood, either bright red or dark and tarry
- Blood may be passed from the anus

If badly inflamed:
- Fever
- Severe pain
- Tender area in the abdomen

> NOTE
> May resolve itself or may need antibiotic treatment

CROSS-REFERENCED UNDER:
Diverticular Disease

Drowning

Water gets into the lungs and stops them functioning properly. This is extremely serious and life threatening, and drowning may cause death. It should be noted that children may drown in only a few inches of water.

SYMPTOMS & SIGNS
- Unconsciousness
- Difficulty breathing (if at all)
- Blue tinge to lips, finger nails and skin
- May be signs of Hypothermia

> NOTE
> Medical help should be sought immediately. The lungs may have become full of water: this should be expelled by putting the individual on their front and lifting them from the lower back.

Drug Induced

see ADVERSE DRUG REACTION

Drug Reaction or Side-Effect

see ADVERSE DRUG REACTION

Drugs

see ALCOHOL OR NARCOTICS

Duchenne's Dystrophy

see MUSCULAR DYSTROPHY

Duct Ectasia

Enlarged ducts in the breast allow the build up of normal secretions in the duct, which are then discharged through the nipple.

SIGNS
- Green or brown discharge from the nipple, which is very viscous

> NOTE
> Investigations will be needed to confirm a diagnosis.

Duct Papilloma

A warty benign tumour develops on one of the ducts of the nipple.

- Yellow or clear discharge from the nipple, but often with blood
- Lump near or behind the nipple may be felt

NOTE
Investigations will be needed to confirm a diagnosis and exclude Breast Cancer.

Dupuytren's Contracture

Little finger and ring finger become bent towards the palm and are not able to be straightened. The cause is not certain, although it has been associated with alcoholism and drugs, but it is associated with thickening and shortening of tendons in the palm of the hand

SYMPTOMS & SIGNS

- Little finger and ring finger cannot be straightened
- Finger may be very bent and pressed against the hand
- In the palm the tendons causing the contracture are thickened

NOTE
Medical help should be sought.

Dysentery

Infectious disease causing inflammation of the bowel. Dysentery is caused by micro-organisms in contaminated food, and spread by house flies (or people) from faeces to food.

SYMPTOMS & SIGNS

- Profuse diarrhoea with loose faeces and mucous, blood and pus

- Abdominal pain
- Fever
- Dehydration, thirst

NOTE
In healthy individuals, most cases will resolve, although a course of antibiotics may be needed.

CROSS-REFERENCED UNDER:
Bacillary Dysentery

Dyspepsia, Non-Ulcer

Indigestion or heartburn, but which may be due to excess acid possibly caused by a bacterium called Helicobacter pylori (which can also cause ulcers) – a peptic or stomach ulcer having been ruled out. Of course, occasional indigestion can occur in any individual, especially if unusual or spicy food or too much alcohol has been consumed.

SIGNS

- Nausea
- Flatulence and burping
- Pain in the upper abdomen
- Some individuals may lose their appetite, while others eat more to relieve discomfort from acid

NOTE
Indigestion remedies are widely available.

CROSS-REFERENCED UNDER:
Indigestion; Heartburn

Ear Infection

Infection of the middle ear and inflammation of the ear drum, caused by viruses such as the Common Cold or by bacteria The ear drum may burst, although it will normally heal.

SYMPTOMS & SIGNS
- Pain in the ear and may be tenderness behind the ear
- Followed by a blood-stained discharge which smells unpleasant and lasts for a few days
- Pain resolves

Alternatively:
- Mild pain, discomfort, pressure and mild deafness

NOTE
Most likely in children, and less often older individuals. Will usually resolve by itself but treatment may be needed.

CROSS-REFERENCED UNDER:
Middle Ear Infection; Otitis Media

Ear Infection

see INNER EAR INFECTION

Ear Polyp

Fleshy growths can occur within the ear, particularly if there has been persistent or recurrent infection. It may be associated with Cholesteatoma.

SYMPTOMS & SIGNS
- Fleshy growth in the ear
- Discharge from ear
- May be bleeding from ear
- Not usually any pain

CROSS-REFERENCED UNDER:
Polyp in Ear

Ear Wax

Wax produced in the ear can build up and form a hard mass.

SYMPTOMS & SIGNS
- May be pain in the ear
- Hearing may be impaired and sounds are muffled
- Pressure in ear
- Giddiness and vertigo

NOTE
Will usually resolve by itself as mechanisms in the ear keep it clean. Cleaning the inside of ears with cotton buds is not recommended, and may cause problems. If ear wax is persistently a problems, ears may need to be syringed, although this should be done professionally.

Eardrum, Ruptured

see RUPTURED EARDRUM

Ectopic Testicle

A testicle fails to migrate down to scrotum during development and remains in the abdomen.

SYMPTOMS & SIGNS
- Testicle inside the groin or abdomen rather than the scrotum
- If left untreated, may damage fertility and is more likely to develop cancerous growths

NOTE
Medical help should be sought as surgery may be needed.

CROSS-REFERENCED UNDER:
Testicle, Ectopic

Ectropion

Lower eyelid sags and turns outwards.

SYMPTOMS & SIGNS

- Lower eyelid turned outwards, exposing the red part of the lid
- Tears stream out of the eye
- More likely to develop Conjunctivitis

> NOTE
>
> Most likely in elderly individuals. Will not usually require treatment, but can be managed with surgery should the condition become a problem or too unsightly.

Eczema

see DERMATITIS

Electrical Conduction Disorders of the Heart

see HEART DISEASE

Elephantiasis

see FILARIASIS

Emotion

see ANXIETY

Emphysema

Formation of holes in the lungs, which reduces the effectiveness of the lung in transferring oxygen and carbon dioxide, leading to a lack of oxygen reaching body tissues. Often associated with chronic bronchitis.

SYMPTOMS & SIGNS

- Difficulty in breathing or shortness of breath
- Chest appears expanded as if the individual is always inhaling: individual may be barrel-chested
- Often accompanies Bronchitis
- Respiratory infections

- Blue tinge to the lips, ear lobes, under the fingernails and elsewhere caused by a lack of oxygen reaching tissues (cyanosis)
- Progressive respiratory failure
- May be confusion, particularly in elderly individuals
- Polycythaemia: blood becomes too concentrated in trying to transfer oxygen around the body

> NOTE
>
> Condition cannot be reversed, but symptoms can be alleviated by stopping smoking, fresh and clean air, and treating Bronchitis. A chest X-ray is needed to confirm diagnosis.

Encephalitis

see MENINGITIS

Endocarditis

Inflammation of the inner lining of the heart (endocardium), often caused by infection of valves damaged previously by Rheumatic Fever. This is a serious condition and the individual will be very ill.

SYMPTOMS & SIGNS

- Fever and sweats, particularly at night
- General feeling of being unwell
- Loss of appetite, weight loss
- Lines under the nails so called 'splinter haemorrhages'
- Rash
- Blood in urine
- Clubbing of end of fingers and finger nails
- Pain in the joints
- Chest pain
- Anaemia
- Affected heart valves can be damaged or rupture

■ Heart failure

NOTE
Medical help should be sought immediately, and treatment is with antibiotics.

Endometriosis

Womb tissue grows outside the womb, causing a range of problems.

SYMPTOMS & SIGNS
■ Severe pain, deep inside, during sexual intercourse
■ Menstruation may be heavy, irregular and painful
■ Severe abdominal, pelvic or back pain around menstruation
■ Infertility

NOTE
Most likely in women between about 20 and 40 years of age. Medical help should be sought as treatments are available.

Enlarged Bladder

The bladder becomes swollen and enlarged, usually caused by problems with the prostate gland (see separate entry).

SYMPTOMS & SIGNS
■ Lower abdomen is swollen
■ Persistent pain
■ Cannot urinate
■ May dribble urine, perhaps constantly

NOTE
Medical help should be sought to determine the cause.

CROSS-REFERENCED UNDER:
Bladder, Enlarged

Enlarged Prostate

The prostate, a gland below the bladder which is only found in men, can become enlarged, especially as males grow older. If severe, it may be difficult or impossible to urinate, and the individual may suffer from urine retention. The symptoms are similar to cancer of the prostate. Over time, the bladder may become larger to compensate for the Enlarged Prostate. The individual may not notice this growth, but may experience urinary incontinence. The bladder does not empty properly and there will be leakage of urine (overflow incontinence).

SYMPTOMS & SIGNS
■ Urinary incontinence or dribbling of urine
■ Increase in frequency of urination, although the quantity in each urination will not usually be excessive
■ Problems starting or finishing urinating
■ Even after urinating, the bladder still feels full
■ Needing to urinate at night
■ May be blood in urine: urine may be stained red, pink or may be cloudy
■ As the prostate becomes larger, it can obstruct the outflow of the bladder and it will become impossible to urinate. If this is the case, there will be severe abdominal pain - an enlarged prostate in the most common cause for this condition

If the individual has a malignant cancer:
■ Back pain or ache between the legs
■ Pain in the bones

NOTE
Medical help should be sought should this condition become a problem, and particularly in cancer is suspected.

Epidermolysis Bullosa

Inherited condition characterised by the formation of blisters on the skin, even when only minimal damage or irritation has occurred.

SYMPTOMS & SIGNS
- Blisters can form, even although there has been only very minor injuries, usually caused by friction 'burns'

NOTE
The condition is passed down through families.

Epididymal Cyst

Cysts can develop in the scrotum. These are harmless, but more serious disease should be excluded.

SYMPTOMS & SIGNS
- Lumps felt in the scrotum
- Lumps are discreet from the testicles
- No other symptoms

NOTE
Most likely in elderly men. The cysts are harmless but may cause pain and discomfort. In young men and boys Torsion should be considered more likely than this condition.

Epididymitis

The epididymis, a body in the scrotum which conveys sperm from the testicles, can become inflamed. This may be because of an infection, or there may be no obvious cause. If there is also a discharge from the penis, medical help should be sought to investigate for sexually transmitted disease.

SYMPTOMS & SIGNS
- Pain, experienced from behind the testicle
- Becomes more severe
- Scrotum and testicle become swollen
- Very sensitive and tender to touch
- Fever
- Nausea

NOTE
Medical help should be sought as antibiotics will be required to resolve this condition.

Epiglottitis

Inflammation of a leaf-shaped flap of cartilage (epiglottis), located behind the tongue. It covers the windpipe when swallowing.

SYMPTOMS & SIGNS
- Throat is very sore
- Pain when swallowing
- May be stridor with difficulty indrawing breath
- Voice may be hoarse
- Harsh barking cough
- Lymph nodes may be enlarged
- Fever and high temperature
- Blue tinge to the skin, particularly the lips, caused by a lack of oxygen (cyanosis)

NOTE
Medical help should be sought if a child has this condition as it can block the airway, causing suffocation. It may make the situation worse to examine the child's throat.

Epilepsy

Seizures during which the individual can have convulsions and fits with spasmodic movements and periods of unconsciousness, caused by electrical disturbances in the brain. Some forms of epilepsy don't lead to visible convulsions but can result in brief 'absences' where there is an episode of loss of awareness but not loss of conciousness.

SYMPTOMS & SIGNS

■ Fits may start with warning symptoms or aura that can include face looking flushed, visual disturbance, headache or acute awareness of smells
■ Periods of unconsciousness and fainting
■ Spasmodic movements and convulsions
■ Clenched jaw
■ May bite tongue
■ Frothing at the mouth
■ Urinary incontinence: the bladder empties due to the seizure
■ May fall into a coma, although this will usually resolve in a few minutes
■ Individual comes round though they may be initially confused and drowsy

NOTE
Medical help should be sought if this is a first attack or if unconsciousness lasts for more than ten minutes. Medication can help to control the symptoms. The individual should not be restrained in any way during a fit, although sharp or dangerous objects should be removed from the vicinity and the mouth should be cleared of any objects including false teeth if possible.

Erosion of the Cervix

An area on the cervix becomes prone to bleeding, caused by 'wear and tear', which is will not affect general health but may still cause problems.

SYMPTOMS & SIGNS

■ Vaginal discharge which is copious, heavy but usually clear
■ Bleeding following sexual intercourse
■ Bleeding between periods

NOTE
Surgery may be required.

CROSS-REFERENCED UNDER:
Cervical Erosion

Erysipelas

Bacterial skin infection which also affects underlying tissues. It is usually caused by an infection passing into body tissues through a cut or graze. Can occur anywhere, classically the face but commonly on the legs.

SYMPTOMS & SIGNS

■ Skin is very red, hot, shiny and thickened
■ May be blisters
■ Pain
■ Fever
■ Feeling generally unwell

NOTE
Will need to be treated by a course of antibiotics.

Erysipelas

see CELLULITIS

Erythema Multiforme

Widespread irregular red marks, rash often resembling targets or blotches anywhere on body, including in the mouth, and usually caused by infection, allergy, or because of a drug reaction. Stevens-Johnson Syndrome is a severe form of Erythema Multiforme.

SYMPTOMS & SIGNS
- Itchy rash and weals, similar to that found in measles: raised angry blisters may occur

Stevens-Johnson Syndrome may also include:
- Painful ulcers in the mouth
- Lips may have crusty and bloody sores
- Inflammation of the gums
- Sore throat
- Headache
- Fever and general ill-health
- Inflammation of the lung
- Damage to the kidneys

NOTE
Most likely to be found in young women and children. May indicate other conditions such as Tuberculosis, acute Rheumatism or Septicaemia, and the attack may last for around three weeks. Treatment is for the underlying infection or drug reaction.

CROSS-REFERENCED UNDER:
Stevens-Johnson Syndrome

Erythrasma

Bacterial infection, particularly affecting areas such as the groin, breasts and armpits, as well as other areas where there are skin folds.

SYMPTOMS & SIGNS
- The skin becomes discoloured, and looks red or brown
- Dry skin: scaly and irregular

NOTE
Medical help should be sought.

Eustachian Catarrh

Build-up of fluid in the ear, usually caused by a condition such as Colds. It can persist for weeks.

SYMPTOMS & SIGNS
- Hearing is impaired and things sound muffled
- Pressure in the ear, which may be relieved by yawning or swallowing
- Popping and crackling noises within the ear

NOTE
Will usually resolve in adults, but children may need medical help. In severe cases, adult individuals may need decongestants.

CROSS-REFERENCED UNDER:
Eustachian Tube Dysfunction

Eustachian Tube Dysfunction

see EUSTACHIAN CATARRH

Excess of Prolactin

Pituitary gland produces too much prolactin, a hormone which controls the reproductive system in women. Prolactin rises normally in pregnancy and is essential for breast milk production. In non-pregnant or non-recently pregnant, usually arises from a benign growth from within the pituitary gland. Excess production can occur in association with use of some drug treatments especially antidepressants.

SYMPTOMS & SIGNS
- Menstruation ceases
- Production of milk from both breasts for many months when not pregnant
- Although typically small, occasionally pituitary growths can be large causing headache and interference with vision.
- May be features occasionally of deficiency of other hormones eg hypothyroidism, Addison's Disease or Diabetes Insipidus
- Occasionally associated with excess of other hormones eg acromegaly

> NOTE
> Medical help will be needed and tests to diagnose the condition.

CROSS-REFERENCED UNDER:
Pituitary Gland Disease; Hormone Disturbance

Exercise

Exercise, especially if repetitive for long periods, causes changes in the body, such as increased heart rate and sweating, as well as dehydration if not enough fluids are taken. Even light exertion will raise the heart rate. If heart rate is very fast with exercise then the individual may be very unfit. If there is chest pain with exercise, this should be investigated. Those who are extremely fit, however, may have an unusually slow heart rate when at rest.

SYMPTOMS & SIGNS
- Increased heart rate to meet increased demands for oxygen
- Prolonged or vigorous exercise causes an increase in body temperature. Sweating is the body's way of reducing temperature by the evaporation of fluid from the skin's surface, and mostly affects the forehead, armpits and back. When exercise ceases, should quickly return to normal, although how heavily an individual sweats varies with such factors as fitness and obesity. The individual may become dehydrated if they do not replace fluid lost through sweating
- Muscle ache and pain when exercise is strenuous. In some cases, if water and salt are not replaced, may lead to muscle cramps, particularly in the calf muscle
- In very extreme conditions with sustained exercise: blood in urine: urine may appear blood stained, pinkish or cloudy

In the long-term:
- Menstruation may cease in very fit women if there is a substantial commitment to exercise and especially if underweight

> NOTE
> The importance of exercising cannot be overemphasised in an age when individuals seem to be married to the motor car. Exercise helps both physical and mental well-being, although it should be remembered that periods of relaxation are just as important.

CROSS-REFERENCED UNDER:
Fitness; Sweating

Extra Heart Beats

Extra heart beats can happen from time to time. These may be the signs of an underlying condition, but more often it is a normal variation in the heart rhythm there is no explanation, except perhaps fluttering from nerves or Anxiety, and not usually any disease.

SYMPTOMS & SIGNS
- Extra heart beats, experienced occasionally, feels as if the heart beat jumps
- No other signs or symptoms

NOTE
Frequent extra heart beats may give the impression of an irregular heart beat: it may be necessary to have tests to confirm the cause.

Extrinsic Allergic Alveolitis

Recurrent allergic reactions in the lung to environmental factors, such as small particles, dust, feathers or even flour.

SYMPTOMS & SIGNS
Initially, attacks may be of brief duration (lasting up to a couple of days) when exposed to the allergen:
- Shortness of breath and difficulty breathing
- Cough
- Feeling generally unwell with loss of appetite and weight loss
- Fatigue
- May be fever
- Resolves itself as long as there is not further exposure to allergen

If long-term exposure occurs, condition may become chronic:
- Progressive and increased difficulty breathing and shortness of breath
- Finger and toe clubbing
- Blue tinge to the lips, ear lobes, under the fingernails and elsewhere caused by a lack of oxygen reaching tissues (cyanosis)
- Respiratory failure
- Heart failure

NOTE
Most likely in occupations, such as farm workers, but may also be found in individuals with hobbies such as pigeon keeping.

Eye Strain

Common condition where the eyes feel tired and sore, caused by concentrating on objects such as a VDU for hours on end. This is exacerbated where the light is bad or there is a lot of glare, such as from fluorescent lights, or where the individual is short sighted.

SYMPTOMS & SIGNS
- Pain about the eyes
- Resolves if the eyes are rested
- Vision is not affected
- Resolves if the individual takes rests from whatever they are doing

NOTE
Taking frequent breaks will help to ease eye strain. Eyes may need to be tested if this persists, or it may be necessary to reorganise the working area.

Facial Nerve Damage
see BELL'S PALSY

Factitious Diarrhoea
see LAXATIVES

Failure to Orgasm

Many women may find it difficult to reach orgasm during sexual intercourse.

SYMPTOMS & SIGNS
- May be worry about getting pregnant
- May be poor technique by their partner

- May be inadequate foreplay
- May be pain during sexual intercourse
- May be that the sexual act does not last long enough
- May be psychological problems
- May be relationship problems or insecurities

> NOTE
> Experimentation and discussion may resolve the situation. If not, counselling may help.

Farmer's Lung

see ALLERGIC ALVEOLITIS

Farting

see FLATULENCE

Fat Necrosis in Breast

Injury to the breast can make a firm lump develop, although this is a rarer condition that Breast Cancer.

SYMPTOMS & SIGNS
- Similar lump to that found in Breast Cancer
- Fixed in one area
- Skin over the lump may be dimpled

> NOTE
> In itself this is not a serious condition, but medical help should be sought so that investigations can exclude Breast Cancer.

Femoral Artery Aneurysm

Weakness in the wall of the femoral artery, which brings blood to the leg. The artery can bulge, and be felt as a large lump in the groin. Occasionally can result from medical procedures performed by putting plastic tubes (catheters) into the artery to investigate whether arterial disease is present.

SIGNS
- Lump usually in groin
- Lump pulsates with the heart
- May be tender

> NOTE
> Medical help should be sought as surgery will be needed.

Fever

Fever is a sign that the body is fighting off infection or disease, and is a normal response. The fever in itself causes many symptoms, not least sweating and increased heart rate, although the latter sign can also be caused by many infections. There may be cause for concern if combined with drenching sweats, weight loss, general ill health and enlarged glands, and if persistent.

SYMPTOMS & SIGNS
- Chills and rigor
- Sweating
- Headache
- Muscle pain
- Fatigue, drowsiness and inability to concentrate
- Lack of appetite
- Heart rate is increased by about ten beats for every 0.5 degrees centigrade raise in body temperature
- May be extra beats
- May be reddened eyes and slight pain in or around the eye
- Children suffering from fevers may have delirium and convulsions: this may not mean that they will develop Epilepsy, but medical help should be sought to exclude this
- Any feverish illness is likely to result in

dehydration if fluids lost through sweating, diarrhoea, vomiting or blood loss are not replaced

■ Any long-term feverish illness is likely to result in weight loss

> NOTE
> Should resolve with the underlying cause, but should be investigated if persists, especially if the individual has been travelling in tropical countries or might have had exposure to infection in their occupation.

Fibreglass

Fibreglass has many slivers of glass which can penetrate the skin.

SYMPTOMS & SIGNS
■ Extreme itchiness

> NOTE
> Protective clothing and facemasks should always been worn.

Fibroadenoma

Moveable lumps can form in the breast. Benign but may cause concern about risk of cancer.

SYMPTOMS & SIGNS
■ Lump in the breast, which is firm to the touch
■ No pain from lump
■ Lump can be moved slightly within breast

> NOTE
> Most likely in women around 20 to 40 years old. A definite diagnosis is needed to exclude cancer so medical help should be sought.

Fibrocystic Disease

Breast tissue may be lumpy to the touch, and larger lumps can form in the breast, often cysts. Benign condition but the lumps may cause concern because of worries that they might be cancerous.

SYMPTOMS & SIGNS
■ Breasts feel lumpy, more noticeably at times during the menstrual cycle
■ Pain or discomfort in both breasts, often before menstruation
■ Specific areas may be particularly tender
■ May be discharge from the nipple

> NOTE
> Most likely in women around 30 to 50 years of age. Investigations will be needed to exclude cancer so medical help should be sought. Larger cysts may need drained, but other than this treatment should not be needed for this condition.

CROSS-REFERENCED UNDER:
Chronic Mastitis

Fibroids

Muscular growths of varying sizes, causing swelling in the womb, which are benign.

SYMPTOMS & SIGNS
■ Pain during menstruation
■ Heavy periods
■ Periods may be irregular
■ Abdomen may become swollen if the fibroids are very large
■ Fibroids may cause abdominal pain

NOTE
Most likely in women between about 30 to 55 years of age. In many cases no treatment is needed, but surgery may be required.

Fibrosing Alveolitis

Inflammation of the small sacs in the lung (alveoli) which allow the transfer of oxygen and carbon dioxide between the air and the blood. May occur as recurrent attacks but can become chronic and progressive. An attack may be precipitated by exposure to many allergens, including hay, flour or pigeons.

SYMPTOMS & SIGNS
- Progressive difficulty in breathing and increasing shortness of breath
- Dry cough
- Finger and toe clubbing
- Blue tinge to the lips, ear lobes, under the fingernails and elsewhere caused by a lack of oxygen reaching tissues (cyanosis)

NOTE
Medical help should be sought, and tests and a chest X-ray will be needed to confirm diagnosis.

Filariasis

Parasitic infestations prevents the free drainage of fluids from tissue. African River Blindness is caused by a similar parasite, transmitted through the bite of the blackfly.

SYMPTOMS & SIGNS
- Parts of the body become swollen as lymph cannot drain away
- Part develops thickened skin
- Elephantiasis
- Blindness
- Some types have dry cough, shortness of breath
- Fever

NOTE
Most likely in the Far East. Medical help should be sought.

CROSS-REFERENCED UNDER:
Elephantiasis; African River Blindness

Fistula-In-Ano

An abscess may burst, creating a passage through the bowel and skin. May occur in association with inflammatory bowel discease, especially Crohn's Disease

SYMPTOMS & SIGNS
- Faeces appearing on the skin near the anus through the new passage
Symptoms of an abscess, such as:
- Pain localised to one area, and throbbing and persistent
- Localised inflammation which will be tender and possibly itchy
- Skin will be red if the abscess occurs near the surface
- May be fever and general feeling of ill health
- Pulse rate may be unusually fast

NOTE
Medical help should be sought immediately.

Fitness

see EXERCISE

Flashing Lights

When standing upright from squatting or sitting, it is possible that flashing lights before the eyes will be experienced. This is not unusual. Flashing lights can also appear as an aura heralding a Migraine.

SYMPTOMS & SIGNS
- Flashing lights before both eyes
- Momentary feeling of giddiness
- Resolves within a short time
- No other symptoms
- In migraine the flashing lights may appear as a flickering arc of lights

Flatulence

Flatulence is caused by gas produced from the fermentation of food in the gastrointestinal tract. It may be made worse by eating certain foods or when the individual is nervous.

SYMPTOMS & SIGNS
- Swollen abdomen
- Passing wind
- No other symptoms

NOTE
Flatulence in itself, without other symptoms, is not anything to worry about, and is an indication that the bowel is functioning normally.

CROSS-REFERENCED UNDER:
Wind; Farting

Flexor Sheath Infection

Infection of the tendons of the fingers (Flexor tendons).

SYMPTOMS & SIGNS
- Finger is red and swollen, and looks crooked
- Pain, exacerbated by attempting to move the finger
- Loss of movement

NOTE
Medical help should be sought immediately as the infection may permanently affect the fingers and may spread.

Floaters

Spots before the eyes, which move in and out of vision (if there is a 'blind spot', other than the normal area at the back of the retina, this is a cause for concern). These spots are known as floaters, and are usually harmless as long as there are only a few, and vision and the eye are otherwise normal

SYMPTOMS & SIGNS
- Floating spots before the eye
- No other symptoms

NOTE
If Floaters appear suddenly, or become suddenly worse, medical help should be sought to exclude any underlying problem.

Flu

Viral illness, of which there are many strains.

SYMPTOMS & SIGNS
- Headache
- Fever with shivers and chills
- Heavy sweating at night
- Severe lethargy
- Muscle and joint pain

- Lightheadedness
- May be mild pain in and around the eyes with redness
- May be sore throat and cough and a running nose
- May be problems with the heart, causing a fast heart beat
- May develop into symptoms of the Common Cold or Upper Respiratory Tract Infection
- May lead to severe pneumonia

NOTE
If most healthy adults, Flu will make the individual extremely unwell, but will resolve with rest. Some individuals are at risk, however, including the elderly and those with pre-existing heart or chest problems, including Asthma. People in high-risk groups should consider getting vaccinated.

CROSS-REFERENCED UNDER:
Influenza; Viral Illness

Food Poisoning
see GASTROENTERITIS

Foreign Body in Airway
see CHOKING

Foreign Body in Eye

Foreign bodies can get lodged in the eye. Normally this will be something like a grain of dust or sand, or an in-growing eye lash, but it is important to wear eye protection when undertaking work where fragments of material are shed at high speed, such as when drilling, cutting or machining.

SYMPTOMS & SIGNS
- Feeling as if there is something in the eye
- Onset is sudden
- One eye is affected
- Eye waters, which may make it appear as if vision is blurred
- Intense pain in affected eye, made worse by bright light. Feeling of grittiness in the eye.
- Vision is not affected

NOTE
Will usually resolve itself, or it may be possible to easily remove the foreign body. However, it is possible that the foreign body may have penetrated into the eye. If this is suspected, medical help should be sought immediately.

Foreign Body in Nose

A foreign body can get lodged inside the nose: young children may be prone to this, as they are more likely to push things up their nose. It may not be apparent for some time that this is the cause.

SYMPTOMS & SIGNS
- Foul-smelling phlegm which may be streaked with blood
- Centred on the foreign body
- Affects one side of the nose
- May be blocked nostril or nose, and loss of sense of smell
- Inflammation
- Nosebleeds
- Speech may sound nasal

NOTE
The foreign body may need to be surgically removed.

Foreign Body in Vagina

It is possible to get objects such as tampons, condoms, or contraceptive sponges stuck in the vagina.

SYMPTOMS & SIGNS
- Brown discharge from the vagina
- Unpleasant smell from the vagina
- No pain
- No other symptoms

NOTE
It may be necessary to get medical help to remove objects.

Fracture of the Collarbone (Clavicle)

see BROKEN COLLARBONE

Fracture of the Lower Arm Bones (Radius, Ulna and wrist)

see BROKEN LOWER ARM BONES (RADIUS, ULNA AND WRIST)

Fracture of the Upper Arm Bone (Humerus)

see BROKEN UPPER ARM BONE (HUMERUS)

Fractures of the Ankle

see BROKEN ANKLE

Fractures of the Knee Cap (Patella)

The knee cap (patella) can be fractured, most usually caused by direct injury or damage sustained from a fall.

SYMPTOMS & SIGNS
- Swelling
- Pain
- Knee is bent and cannot be straightened because of the pain

- Complete lack of movement

NOTE
Medical help should be sought immediately.

Fractures of the Lower Leg (femur, tibia and fibula)

The bones of the lower leg – the thigh bone (femur) and the lower leg (tibia and fibula) – may be fractured or broken, most usually because of violent injury or trauma. Fractures of the femur in the elderly are common in association with osteoporosis.

SYMPTOMS & SIGNS
- Severe pain worsened by movement, prevents weight bearing
- Leg looks deformed at the site of the break
- Bruising and inflammation
- In fractures of femur leg often looks shorter and is rotated

NOTE
Medical help should be sought immediately.

CROSS-REFERENCED UNDER:
Lower Leg (femur, tibia and fibula) Fractures

Freckles

see MOLE

Friedreich's Ataxia

Problems with the brain, spinal cord and nerves, caused by an inherited disorder.

SYMPTOMS & SIGNS
- Trembling hands when trying to undertake a task using the hands
- Progressive unsteadiness on feet, and loss of

sense of distance and position

- Clumsiness
- Problems with speech
- The progressive unsteadiness may lead to need for wheelchair
- Curvature of spine
- High arch in foot
- Disturbance of heart rhythm
- Diabetes mellitus is common

> NOTE
> Symptoms become apparent in childhood or young adulthood, typically under the age of 25.

Frigidity

see LOW OR ABSENT SEXUAL DRIVE

Frost Bite

Severe damage to the skin and underlying tissue caused by exposure to extreme cold for a prolonged period. The damaged tissues wither and die. Areas most at risk are extremities of the body, such as the ears, nose, fingers and toes, and even the male genitals.

SYMPTOMS & SIGNS
Onset:

- Pain, tingling and altered sensation in the affected area
- Area becomes purple or red

Later:

- May be no pain, which may mean that severe damage has occurred
- Affected area turns white

If left untreated:

- Affected areas may develop gangrene (black putrid areas) and may need to be amputated

- Ulceration

> NOTE
> Although this condition can affect any individual, those at especial risk include the elderly, children and those with poor circulation. Medical help should be sought immediately as affected areas need to be warmed over time and with care to reduce damage.

Frozen Shoulder

Severe, even disabling, pain and restricted movement in the shoulder.

SYMPTOMS & SIGNS

- Onset may be injury to the shoulder
- Severe pain and stiffness in the shoulder, which may restrict movement

> NOTE
> Most likely in older individuals, and often will resolve without treatment.

Fungal Infection of the Ear

see OTITIS EXTERNA

Fungal Infections of the Skin

Inflammation of the skin, caused by fungal infections. Can occur anywhere but most commonly occurs between toes (althete's foot).

SYMPTOMS & SIGNS

- Affected skin becomes red, scaly and extremely itchy
- Skin may become cracked and thickened
- Skin can rub off and blister
- Skin can look and feel very dry
- May be an unpleasant smell from the area

- Fingernail may be affected, making it thick, irregular, and creamy or opaque in colour

NOTE

May be resolved using anti-fungal preparations.

Funny Bone

see ULNAR NERVE

Furuncle

see BOIL

Gall Bladder Disease

see GALL BLADDER INFECTION

Gall Bladder Infection

Gall bladder can become infected, inflamed or enlarged. This can be precipitated by eating certain foods, particularly where there is a lot of fat in the diet.

SYMPTOMS & SIGNS

- Pain in the upper right abdominal area which may spread into the chest or even the tip of the shoulder
- Pain may take some minutes to build in intensity but is persistent in nature
- Inhaling may make the pain worse
- May be a mass just below the rib cage on the right side, which is tender to the touch
- Fever
- Feeling generally unwell
- May be nausea and vomiting
- May be recurrent episode of illness, followed by periods with fewer symptoms
- May be long-term weight loss
- May be collapse

NOTE

Most likely in older women.

CROSS-REFERENCED UNDER:

Gall Bladder Disease

Gall Stones

Inflammation of the gall bladder (cholecystitis), usually caused by the formation of gall stones, which may block the bile ducts causing pain, back pressure in the gall bladder and result in severe inflammation.

SYMPTOMS & SIGNS

- Abdominal pain usually in spasms in the upper part of the abdomen, on the right hand side, which may spread into the chest and even the tip of the shoulder
- Nausea, vomiting, loss of appetite
- Tender area on the right side of the abdomen, just below the ribs
- Pain may be exacerbated by inhaling
- Fever
- Generally feeling unwell
- If jaundiced, faeces are pale
- Vomiting
- May be jaundice if the gall stones block the biliary tract
- Urine may be darker
- May recurr

NOTE

Occasionally cholecystitis can result in perforation of the gall bladder which is life threatening because of severe infection and peritonitis. Most likely in older women. Medical help should be sought immediately.

CROSS-REFERENCED UNDER:
Cholecystitis; Inflammation of the Gall Bladder

Ganglion

Benign lump, often found over joints, usually on the back of the wrist, caused by degeneration of fibrous tissue. It is a small sac of joint fluid that pokes through overlying tissues.

SYMPTOMS & SIGNS
- Small lump, firm to the touch
- Most likely to be found near joints and tendons, including on the back of the wrist
- Usually no pain, but may be sore or uncomfortable if knocked
- Light can be shone through the lump

NOTE
Often no treatment is required, although surgery can be used to remove the ganglion should it become a problem.

Gangrene

Loss of blood supply to an area, causing it to die. Causes can be frostbite (particularly of extremities such as toes, ears and fingers), injury or trauma, nerve damages (such as in Leprosy) or circulation problems. The dead tissue withers (dry gangrene) but it may become infected (wet gangrene).

SYMPTOMS & SIGNS
- Affected area becomes black and withers (dry gangrene)
- If infected – moist, smelly, leaks pus.

NOTE
Medical help should be sought immediately.

Gardnerella

Infection of the vagina, caused by a bacteria, which may be sexually transmitted.

SYMPTOMS & SIGNS
- May be no symptoms
- Discharge from the vagina, grey in colour and with a fishy smell
- Itchy
- May be tenderness and pain, particularly during sexual intercourse

NOTE
Medical help should be sought as antibiotics will be needed.

CROSS-REFERENCED UNDER:
Vaginal Infection

Gastrectomy
see POST-GASTRECTOMY SYNDROME

Gastric Cancer
see CANCER OF THE STOMACH

Gastritis

Inflammation of the stomach lining, which can be caused by anything which can irritate the stomach, such as gastric flu, excessive alcohol, stress, drugs such as aspirin, foods, and infections.

SYMPTOMS & SIGNS
- Vomiting: both undigested stomach contents, then green, less viscous fluid with mucus and slime. There may be blood in the vomit, either as a brown staining or appearing as coffee grains (gastric acids alter the colour of blood)
- Indigestion

- May be abdominal pain

> **NOTE**
> Medical help should be sought should Gastritis persist.

Gastroenteritis

Food poisoning, or more severely Gastroenteritis, can cause mild to severe symptoms, which occasionally in vulnerable groups, such as babies, infants and the elderly, can be potentially severe and even fatal. Caused by bacteria or viruses from poorly prepared, contaminated, rotten or badly cleaned food.

SYMPTOMS & SIGNS

- Vomiting: starts with usual stomach contents of undigested food but if vomiting persists may become green and less viscous, with mucous and clear slime
- Skin looks pale, particularly before vomiting or diarrhoea
- Abdominal pain and cramps
- Diarrhoea with faeces which are runny, watery and loose: these above two symptoms are actually far more common in bouts of food poisoning than vomiting
- May be headache
- May be joint and muscle pain
- May be an associated fever
- In severe cases, may be collapse caused by dehydration

> **NOTE**
> Most bouts of food poisoning and gastroenteritis will resolve in the young healthy adults, usually in 24 to 36 hours.

CROSS-REFERENCED UNDER:
Food Poisoning

German Measles
see RUBELLA

Giant Urticaria
see ANGIONEUROTIC OEDEMA

Glandular Fever

Contagious viral disease, passed by direct contact (such as kissing, hence also known as 'kissing disease'). The disease is characterised by swollen glands, fever and possibly skin eruptions.

SYMPTOMS & SIGNS

- Fever which may last for weeks
- Lymph nodes are enlarged and tender
- Lymph nodes at the back of the head may be most severely affected
- May be difficult to open the mouth because of the swelling
- Excessive production of saliva in the mouth
- Sore throat often with discharge on the tonsils
- Generally feeling unwell
- Spleen may also be affected and enlarged
- Resultant fatigue may last for months
- May occasionally be associated with generalised rash
- Occasionally can affect other organs including the lungs, heart and brain.

> **NOTE**
> Most likely in infants (3-5 years old) and young adults (15-25 years old). Diagnosis can be confirmed by a blood test, and it will usually take up to a few weeks to resolve. It is possible that residual fatigue can last for months.

CROSS-REFERENCED UNDER:
Infectious Mononucleosis

Glaucoma

Increased pressure of the fluid within the eye. This may have a very slow development, and the individual may not be aware it is happening. It is possible for Glaucoma to develop quickly, caused by a blockage or by drugs used to constrict the pupils. The condition can be congenital, and may develop in children.

SYMPTOMS & SIGNS
- May be no signs or symptoms
- May be slight or vague pain in or around the eye, or in acute cases the pain may be severe
- May be haloes around bright objects at night or when it is dark
- May be tunnel vision

If an acute episode develops:
- Severe pain in the eye
- May be vomiting because of the pain
- Redness of the coloured part of the eye
- Cornea may look hazy and cloudy
- Problems with vision, which may be severely affected, even blindness developing

If congenital:
- Large protruding eyes
- Eyes appear to bulge

> NOTE
> Glaucoma can be detected by visiting an optician, and is most common in older individuals and in those who have a family history of the condition. If acute Glaucoma is suspected, medical help should be sought immediately.

Gluten Intolerance

see COELIAC DISEASE

Gonorrhoea

Infectious sexually-transmitted disease in adults, which takes two to five days to incubate. Children can also accidentally catch Gonorrhoea, usually not connected to sexual contact. There may be no or few symptoms, and women are more likely to show no symptoms.

SYMPTOMS & SIGNS
In women:
- May be no symptoms
- Vaginal discharge, which may be yellow in colour
- Pain when urinating, burning in intensity
- Urine may be cloudy
- Itchiness
- Pelvic inflammatory disease or infection
- May be joint pain and inflammation
- May cause infertility

In men:
- May be no symptoms
- Purulent discharge from the penis (urethritis)
- Pain when urinating
- Urine cloudy
- Reddening and pain around the end and tip of the penis
- Unilateral testicular pain (epididymitis)
- Lymph nodes may be enlarged in groin
- May be joint pain and inflammation
- Where infection associated with rectal intercourse there can be proctitis with rectal discharge, pain and sensation of need to keep moving the bowel

In new-born babies:
- May be copious amounts of pus, yellow in colour,

from the eyes and under the eyelids

- May be swollen eyelids, which makes it difficult to open the eyes
- Cornea of eyes may become cloudy, leading to blindness

> NOTE
> Medical help should be sought. In new-born babies, Gonorrhoea may be aquired from infected mother and if left untreated can make the child blind.

CROSS-REFERENCED UNDER:

Clap

Gout

Deposit of monosodium urate crystals in the joints, in the kidneys and ears, caused by a metabolic disorder where there is too much uric acid in the blood. The big toe can become particularly swollen and painful. Attacks of gout are associated with alcohol excess, over-indulgence with food and with some drug treatments eg diuretics.

SYMPTOMS & SIGNS

- Severe pain and swelling of joints, typically the big toe, but also the joints of the fingers, hands, feet and other toes
- Recurrent bouts of arthritis
- Sudden onset
- Nodules can appear on the face, including on the ear, and on or by joints, caused by yellow crystals of uric acid
- Nodules are severely painful
- Fever
- Generally feeling of ill health
- May be kidney stones and kidney failure if left untreated

> NOTE
> Medical help should be sought immediately as drugs can control the symptoms.

Granuloma Inguinale

see CHANCROID

Graves' Disease

see HYPERTHYROIDISM

Guillain-Barre Syndrome

Weakness or paralysis of muscles, caused by a problems with the neurological system following an acute viral infection. Symptoms can be mild to very severe, and even life threatening. Typically the muscle paralysis progresses and becomes more extensive; paralysis may affect all muscles incluing those of respiration.

SYMPTOMS & SIGNS

- Altered sensation, numbness and tingling in limbs especially toes and fingers
- Pain in the back and shoulders
- Weakness in or paralysis of the limbs especially initially in the legs
- Progression and spread of weakness
- Weakness or paralysis of facial muscles
- Weakness or paralysis of muscles used for respiration: artificial respiration may be needed
- Weakness or paralysis of muscles used for swallowing: artificial feeding may be needed
- May be high or low blood pressure or abnormal sweating

> NOTE
> Needs medical attention. Will usually resolve slowly over time, but this may be over a period of months.

CROSS-REFERENCED UNDER:
Acute Inflammatory Polyneuropathy

Gullet Cancer

see CANCER OF THE OESOPHAGUS

HIV

see AIDS

Haemoglobinuria

Break down of red blood cells which are excreted in urine, making it dark brown in colour. Haemoglobinuria can be caused by several illnesses, such as Malaria, Septicaemia, valve replacement and Haemolytic Anaemia.

SYMPTOMS & SIGNS
- Urine is dark brown in colour
- Other signs and symptoms, depending on the condition: dark-brown urine is unlikely to be the most obvious or pressing of symptoms

NOTE
Medical help should be sought immediately.

Haematuria

see CANCER OF THE BLADDER

Haematuria

see CANCER OF THE KIDNEY

Haemochromatosis

Genetic abnormality in iron metabolism, and also known as Bronze Diabetes.

SYMPTOMS & SIGNS
- Skin is bronze in colour
- Liver disease including cirrhosis
- Symptoms of Diabetes Mellitus

- Testicles are greatly reduced in size, and the individual has a reduced libido
- Joints become inflamed
- Abnormalities in the functioning of the heart and in the rhythm of the heart

NOTE
Medical help should be sought, but extremely unlikely that this would not have been discovered at an early stage.

CROSS-REFERENCED UNDER:
Bronze Diabetes

Haemophilia

Blood fails to clot, due to a genetic condition. This is a potentially life-threatening problem, as even minor injuries can cause copious bleeding and bruising.

SYMPTOMS & SIGNS
- Blood does not clot so that fairly mild injury can result in severe bleeding and bruising
- Joint pain and swelling due to bleeding into joints
- Bleeding from gums and mouth, from nose and from bowel and bladder
- Trauma to head can cause haemorrhage around the brain

NOTE
Almost exclusively found in males, although females can pass the condition on to their male children.

Haemorrhage

see BLEEDING

Haemorrhoids

see PILES

Hair Follicle Infection

see BOIL

Hair Loss

see ALOPECIA

Hair Loss

see ALOPECIA AREATA

Hallux Rigidus

Joint in the big toe becomes painful and enlarged, caused by Osteoarthritis.

SYMPTOMS & SIGNS

- Pain when moving toe
- Movement may become restricted due to pain
- Joint may develop bony growths
- Skin becomes thickened

> NOTE
> Medical help should be sought.

Hallux Valgus

Big toe becomes deformed and distorted, caused by wearing shoes which are too tight.

SYMPTOMS & SIGNS

- Big toe points outwards
- Base of toe is larger
- Lump of bone can be felt at base of big toe; bone becomes thickened and painful (Bunion)
- May become infected and swollen

> NOTE
> Most likely in older women who wear ill-fitting shoes, and may need surgery.

CROSS-REFERENCED UNDER:

Bunion

Halo Naevus

Some moles, and the area around them, lose their pigment and become pale. Vitiligo may develop.

SYMPTOMS & SIGNS

- White or pale patches of skin

Hanging

see SUFFOCATION

Hansen's Disease

see LEPROSY

Hay Fever

Inflammation of the mucous membranes in the nose and ears. It usually produces a lot of phlegm, precipitated by an allergy to pollen or some other substance in the air. As it is usually a reaction to pollen in the air, it is very seasonal and the individual may not be affected during times of low pollen. Individuals can also be susceptible to other allergens, such as mould spores.

SYMPTOMS & SIGNS

- Difficulty breathing through nose
- Sneezing, wheezing
- Clear discharge running from the nose
- Eyes may be reddened and there may be a feeling as if something is in the eye
- Watering eyes

> NOTE
> Hay Fever is associated with Asthma and Dermatitis, and symptoms may be alleviated with antihistamines.

Head Injury

Injury or trauma to the head can be caused by many things such as a blow, fall or even whiplash injury. Trauma to the head can damage the contents, the brain, and cause concussion, bleeding or brain damage, as well as damage to other structures such as the eyes and ears.

SYMPTOMS & SIGNS
- Headache
- Double vision
- Flashing lights
- Dizziness and vertigo
- May be blindness, caused either by a blow to the part of the brain associated with vision or because of a Detached Retina
- May be loss of sense of smell because of damage to the nerve associated with smell. If this is the case, the loss is permanent
- May be deafness as a result of damage to the nerve associated with hearing
- May be memory loss (amnesia), permanent in some cases, although it will sometimes return completely
- May be mental impairment following the trauma
- May be bleeding from the ear as the blow may burst the eardrum if the trauma occurs on that part of the head. The fluid which surrounds the brain may leak into the ear if trauma is severe: this is clear, watery but persistent.
- Similarly, the fluid which surrounds the brain (cerebro-spinal fluid) may leak into nose: this is clear and watery but persistent.
- May be sudden onset of Dementia, confusion, drowsiness, unconsciousness and coma if damage is severe: this is also possible a long time after the initial injury should a clot get lodged in the brain
- May be paralysis

> NOTE
> If blow or trauma is severe, medical help should be sought immediately.

CROSS-REFERENCED UNDER:
Concussion; Skull Fracture

Headache, Cluster
see CLUSTER HEADACHE

Headache, Tension
see TENSION HEADACHE

Headlice
see LICE

Heart Attack and Failure

The heart is seriously damaged, usually by a heart attack, and cannot pump sufficient blood around the body to supply tissues with oxygen.

SYMPTOMS & SIGNS
Heart failure:
- Shortness of breath when walking or exercising, often progressive and with a slow and even unnoticed onset
- Shortness of breath exacerbated by lying flat
- May wake from sleep because of feeling as if suffocating: often symptoms will resolve quickly if the individual sits up for a while
- Weakness and lethargy
- Prominent symmetrical veins on the neck, which become larger when lying flat
- Heart murmur
- Skin looks pale

- Increased heart rate
- Reduced or lack of appetite for food
- Face may have a bluey tinge, as may lips, ear lobes, underneath the fingernails and other parts of the body
- Ankles, legs, abdomen and other part of the body are swollen because of the accumulation of fluid (oedema) due to kidney problems
- Confusion

Suspect a Heart Attack if:
- Sudden onset of severe crushing vice-like pain in the middle of the chest
- Sudden onset, usually when at rest
- Pain also up to the jaw and/or into the left arm
- It is possible that the attack goes virtually unnoticed, particularly in an elderly individual
- Breathlessness
- Sweating
- Confusion
- Blue tinge to the lips and skin (cyanosis)
- Unconsciousness or coma

NOTE

Most likely in older individuals. If heart attack, failure or disease is suspected, help should be sought immediately as time is of the essence.

CROSS-REFERENCED UNDER:
Cardiac Failure; Heart Disease

Heart Disease

The heart is damaged, abnormal or has a disturbed rhythm, and cannot pump sufficient blood around the body to supply tissues with oxygen. Can occur at any age but is common in middle age and older. In new-born infants it may well accompany conditions such as Down's syndrome or may be a result of the mother having Rubella when pregnant. Electrical conduction disorders of the heart disrupt the normal beating of the heart, and can lead to bouts of extremely fast or slow heart beats. These attacks may be precipitated by caffeine or alcohol.

SYMPTOMS & SIGNS
Adults:
- Difficulty breathing and shortness of breath
- Malaise and general fatigue and tiredness
- Blue tinge to lips or ear lobes, fingers due to lack of oxygen reaching tissues (cyanosis)
- Chest pain
- May be red discoloration in the half moons in the nails
- Faint or slow pulse
- May be tendency to faint or exercise
- May look pale

Children:
- Failure to thrive
- Difficulty breathing and shortness of breath
- Finger and toe clubbing
- Malaise and general fatigue and tiredness
- Blue tinge to lips or ear lobes, fingers due to lack of oxygen reaching tissues (cyanosis)
- Increased production of haemoglobin to increase oxygen carrying potential of blood
- Heart murmur

Heart rhythm problems:
- Heart either beats very slowly or very quickly
- Palpitations and heart thumping in the chest
- Sudden onset of weakness
- Feeling light-headed
- May feel as if about to faint
- Attack may cease abruptly

> **NOTE**
> The commonest alteration of heart rhythm is the occurrence of isolated extra beats called actopics. These are of no significance. An irregularly irregular pulse, called atrial fibrillation, is a common abnormality that requires medical attention.
> Medical examination necessary to confirm diagnosis of heart disease. Electrical conduction disorders will need tests to confirm a diagnosis, and may be treated medically or surgically.

CROSS-REFERENCED UNDER:

Congenital Heart Disease; Electrical Conduction Disorders of the Heart

Heart Disease

see HEART ATTACK AND FAILURE

Heartburn

see DYSPEPSIA, NON-ULCER

Heat Exhaustion

The core temperature of the body becomes raised, either because of the very high ambient temperature, particularly where there is high humidity, and/or from exercising in these conditions. The individual suffers from collapse, caused by loss of water and salt through sweating. This can develop into Sun Stroke.

SYMPTOMS & SIGNS
- Sweating and clammy skin
- Difficulty breathing
- Headache
- Feeling dizzy and faint
- Muscle cramps
- Rapid pulse, which grows progressively weaker

- Individual may look pale
- Nausea
- Collapse

> **NOTE**
> Most likely in the very young and very old. Ways of avoiding Heat Exhaustion include drinking lots of water, wearing a hat, using suntan lotion, and keeping out of the sun during the hottest part of the day. If this condition is suspected, medical help should be sought immediately. It is possible to cool the individual using a damp towel or sheet. Water, with a little salt, should also be given to the individual if they can consume it without vomiting.

Heat Stroke

The final stage of Heat Exhaustion. The core temperature of the body becomes raised, either because of the very high ambient temperature (not just from hot climates, but from working in plants such as steel mills or boiler rooms), particularly where there is also high humidity, and/or from exercising or strenuously working in these conditions, may cause several serious health problems. Symptoms of Heat Stroke can develop very quickly, and, if left untreated, may even be fatal.

SYMPTOMS & SIGNS
- Very high temperature
- Sweating ceases
- Dry flushed skin which feels very hot
- Face is reddened
- Weakness
- May be nausea and vomiting
- Headache
- Thirst

- Rapid pulse
- Dizziness
- Mental confusion
- Excessive bleeding
- Breathlessness
- Unconsciousness and collapse
- Seizures
- May lead to liver and kidney failure

NOTE
This is a serious conditions, and about 1 in 5 individuals with this condition may die. Most likely in the very young and very old. Ways of avoiding Heat Stroke in hot climates include drinking lots of water, taking salt tablets, wearing a hat, using suntan lotion, and keeping out of the sun during the hottest part of the day. If this condition is suspected, medical help should be sought immediately. It is possible to cool the individual using a damp towel or sheet or a bath of cool water.

CROSS-REFERENCED UNDER:
Sun Stroke

Henoch-Schonlein

Generalised inflammatory condition affecting blood vessels that affects children more often than adults. May follow upper respiratory infection.

SYMPTOMS & SIGNS
- Rash with purple spots or areas
- Joints are painful especially knees and ankles
- Abdominal pain often with vomiting
- Blood in urine and diarrhoea
- Kidney disease including nephrotic syndrome or even acute renal failure

NOTE
Will usually resolve by itself, although in some cases steroids may be needed. The condition may have complications involving the kidney.

Hepatitis

Inflammation of the liver, which can be caused by various conditions, including alcohol excess, viral infections such as hepatitis A, B and C, and as a side effect of drug therapy or because of an overdose of Paracetamol. Hepatitis may range from extremely serious, even life-threatening, to mild.

SYMPTOMS & SIGNS
- Fatigue, tiredness, weakness and lethargy
- May be jaundice
- Loss of appetite
- Nausea
- Reduced desire for alcohol and even cigarettes
- May be extreme itchiness
- May be dark urine – brown, dark yellow or orange – after a few days
- May be pale faeces
- Liver may be swollen and tender to the touch
- Fever, possibly intermittent in nature, and sweating
- Diarrhoea
- May be a rash
- Abdominal pain on the right side
- Pain in joints
- Breath may smell sweet or of faeces
- Drowsiness and confusion
- Unconsciousness and coma

NOTE
Medical help should be sought immediately.

CROSS-REFERENCED UNDER:
Liver Disease and Infection

Hepatolenticular Degeneration (Wilson's Disease)

Symptoms associated with Parkinson's Disease and liver damage, caused by an inherited problem with copper elimination, leading to a build up of copper in the body, especially in liver, nervous tissue, bone marrow and kidneys.

SYMPTOMS & SIGNS
- Liver damage which can lead to Cirrhosis and Jaundice and liver failure
- Eyes have a yellow-brown or green ring, known as a copper ring or Kayser-Fleischer ring
- Symptoms of Parkinson's Disease including clumsy walking and slurring of speech
- Trembling hands
- Personality change, depression

NOTE
Found in children and young adults, and can be treated with drugs.

CROSS-REFERENCED UNDER:
Wilson's Disease

Hepatoma
see CANCER OF THE LIVER

Hernia, Femoral
see HERNIA, INGUINAL

Hernia, Hiatus

Part of the stomach slides up through the diaphragm at the oesophageal opening in the chest. Common in people who are overweight.

SYMPTOMS & SIGNS
- Burning pain when swallowing, often behind the breast bone in the middle of the chest
- Heartburn
- Pain in the centre of the chest, either at the front or back, and down the arms
- Stomach contents regurgitated into the throat and mouth especially on lying down
- Acid or bitter taste
- Burping
- May be vomiting, sometimes with blood (which may look like coffee grounds)
- May be long-term weight loss

NOTE
Symptoms may be alleviated with antacids, and treatment can be medical, behavioural, or occasionally surgical.

CROSS-REFERENCED UNDER:
Hiatus Hernia

Hernia, Inguinal

A hernia is a protrusion through an aperture of one organ or part of an organ into neighbouring structures, usually an abdominal organ through the abdominal wall. In the case of Inguinal and Femoral hernias, these will be noticed as lumps in the groin. Areas of bowel can get trapped. This may cause intestinal blockage, or the blood supply may get cut off and tissue, starved of its oxygen supply, can die. If either of these are the case, surgery will be required.

SYMPTOMS & SIGNS
- Usually may be inserted back into the abdomen
- May not be apparent when lying down, only

appearing when back on the feet
- May be a gurgling sound
- Hernia can enlarge over time and in men extend into the scrotum, causing an aching pain in the scrotum and testicles

If the hernia becomes trapped:
- Pain: the hernia itself, although may be intermittent abdominal pain
- Hernia cannot be pushed back within the abdominal wall
- May be vomiting and intestinal blockage
- Peritonitis can develop

> NOTE
> As mentioned above, if the hernia becomes trapped or strangulated, surgery will be needed.

CROSS-REFERENCED UNDER:
Hernia, Femoral

Hernia, Umbilical

A hernia is a protrusion through an aperture of one organ or part of an organ into neighbouring structures, usually an abdominal organ through the abdominal wall. In the case of Umbilical hernias, these will be noticed as lumps in the abdomen, although they are most usually found in the very young.

SYMPTOMS & SIGNS
- Usually can be inserted back into the abdomen
- May not be apparent when lying down, only reappearing when back on the feet
- May be a gurgling sound
- More unusual than Inguinal and Femoral hernias in adults, and less likely to block the intestine

If the hernia becomes trapped:

- Intermittent abdominal pain
- Hernia cannot be pushed back within the abdominal wall
- May be vomiting

> NOTE
> Most likely in babies and infants, especially if they are black. As mentioned above, if the hernia becomes trapped or strangulated, surgery will be needed, although the hernia may resolve itself as the baby grows up and the abdominal muscles develop.

Herpes Simplex

Viral infection characterised by pain and ulcers and fluid-filled spots or blisters (vesicles), often associated with the final phase of a Cold or Flu, hence the name. These may be found in the mouth, lips, throat, gullet, and even the genitals, and can be found singly on the mouth or face when known as a Cold Sore. Herpes simplex is associated with upper respiratory tract infections, but may also be more prevalent when the individual is run down. Pregnant women with Herpes should report the condition as there is a small chance it may be passed to the new-born infant.

SYMPTOMS & SIGNS
- Vesicles, blisters and sores in the mouth, throat or gullet, the ear or even the genitals. These can form scabs
- Severe pain associated with the herpes sore, which can appear singly
- These sores recur in a predictable pattern eg after colds
- Sexual intercourse may be painful
- In extreme cases, fever and general ill health

■ Area affected may lose pigmentation for a time, although this will usually return

> **NOTE**
> Cold sores will normally resolve within a couple of weeks. A tingling in the affected area often precedes an attack, and if this is suspected anti-viral medication may be used.

CROSS-REFERENCED UNDER:
Cold Sore

Herpes Zoster
see SHINGLES

Hiatus Hernia
see HERNIA, HIATUS

High Blood Calcium
see HYPERCALCAEMIA

High Blood Pressure (hypertension)

Blood pressure is maintained by the body for efficient working. Blood pressure can become raised beyond normal values for a variety of reasons, although mild to moderately elevated blood pressure will normally have no symptoms. High blood pressure can lead to heart strain and failure and to stroke. May run in families. Cause of high blood pressure typically unknown, although occasionally can result from excess of blood pressure-regulating hormones or because of kidney disease or narrowed kidney arteries.

SYMPTOMS & SIGNS
If the individual has mild to moderate high blood pressure:
■ Typically no symptoms
■ May increase risk of Macular Degeneration

If the individual has very high blood pressure:
■ Headaches
■ May be nosebleeds
■ Symptoms of Heart Disease or damage, such as chest pain, palpitations, breathlessness and swollen ankles
■ Increased risk of heart attack and stroke

> **NOTE**
> Medical help should be sought if high blood pressure is suspected as it may lead to a range of problems and illnesses.

CROSS-REFERENCED UNDER:
Hypertension; Blood Pressure, High

Hirschsprung's Disease

Congenital condition when part of the young child's bowel does not work correctly due to the non-development of nervous tissue.

SYMPTOMS & SIGNS
■ Distended and swollen stomach and abdomen, caused by the build up of faeces in the bowel
■ Constipation acute or chronic
■ Obstruction of bowel
■ Vomiting that may be bilious or faecal

> **NOTE**
> Treated by surgery.

Hives
see URTICARIA

Hodgkin's Disease

Type of cancer of the lymph glands.

SYMPTOMS & SIGNS

- Glands in the neck, armpits or groin are swollen, very often large. The glands feel quite rubbery, but are painless
- May be no symptoms apart from enlarged glands
- May be Fever
- May be night sweats
- May be anaemia
- May be extreme itchiness particularly after hot baths or shower
- May be weight loss
- Fatigue and lethargy

NOTE
Medical helps should be sought immediately as this increases the chances of a cure. Most likely in individuals between 15 and 30 years of age.

Hookworms (human)

Infestation by hookworms, which live in the small bowel and survive by sucking blood from their host. They can infect through walking with bare feet on infected soil. Eggs are passed in faeces, which can then hatch in soil and infest further hosts. Serious if infestation is severe.

SYMPTOMS & SIGNS

- May be no symptoms
- May be itchy rash where the parasite enters the skin
- Cough
- Nausea, vomiting, abdominal pain
- Diarrhoea
- General feeling of being unwell
- May be Anaemia because of blood loss
- Serious infestation can cause chronic bleeding from the small intestine

NOTE
Worms are found in southern Europe, Middle and Far East, areas of tropical Africa and the Americas. If suspected medical help should be sought and drug treatment needed. Should not be caught if shoes are worn.

CROSS-REFERENCED UNDER:
Ancylostoma

Hormone Disturbance
see EXCESS OF PROLACTIN

Horner's Syndrome

Irritation of the nerve which controls the pupil, the black opening into the eye. This nerve goes from the brain, through the chest, and then to the eye. The irritation may be caused by conditions such as a Lung Tumour or enlarged glands in the chest, brain disease, and Multiple Sclerosis.

SYMPTOMS & SIGNS

- The pupil in the affected eye is very small
- Lid of affected eye droops
- Eye is slightly retracted
- Affected side of the face sweats less than the other side

NOTE
Medical help should be sought as investigations will be necessary.

CROSS-REFERENCED UNDER:
Irritation of Nerves to Eye

Housemaid's Knee
see BURSITIS

Huntington's Chorea

Very unpleasant progressive degenerative condition of the nervous system, which runs in families.

SYMPTOMS & SIGNS
- Limb jerkiness, tremor and twitching
- Personality change
- Changes in mood including depression
- Poor memory leading to dementia
- Progressive and relentless physical and mental deterioration
- Paralysis
- Epilepsy

NOTE
Onset of the condition is in the 30s or 40s.

Hydatid Disease

see TAPEWORMS

Hydrocele

Fluid accumulates in the scrotum around a testicle.

SYMPTOMS & SIGNS
- Testicle becomes swollen and tender: in severe cases, very swollen
- May be pain

NOTE
In young boys this may be caused by a hernia, and it is possible in babies.

Hydrocephalus

Overly large head in babies and very young infants. The condition is progressive, and caused by the failure of fluid to drain from the head, causing pressure within the head to increase. Babies' heads have soft gaps (fontanelles) where the skull bones have not yet fused together. Because of the increased pressure in the head, these soft areas can bulge.

SYMPTOMS & SIGNS
- Head is overly large, and the condition is progressive
- Fontanelles bulge

Increased pressure within the skull can also cause:
- Epilepsy
- Mental and physical impairment, such as Dementia
- Increased vulnerability to infection
- Clumsiness and unsteadiness on feet
- Urinary incontinence

NOTE
Medical help should be sought. The excess fluid can be drained to the abdomen by a catheter set into the skull.

CROSS-REFERENCED UNDER:
Water on the Brain

Hyper Parathyroidism

see HYPERCALCAEMIA

Hypercalcaemia

Excessive amounts of calcium in the blood. It may be caused by various conditions, including problems with parathyroid gland, too much vitamin D, bone tumours, sarcoidosis and the thyroid producing too much hormone (thyrotoxicosis). May cause serious illness.

SYMPTOMS & SIGNS
- Excessive thirst
- Frequent and excessive urination with need to get up overnight to pass urine
- Nausea and vomiting
- Loss of appetite
- Constipation and abdominal pain
- Muscle fatigue
- Weakness
- General feeling of ill health
- Kidney stones
- Bone pain
- Drowsiness
- Depression
- Hypercalcaemia due to parathyroid hormone excess may cause osteoporosis

NOTE
Medical help should be sought.

CROSS-REFERENCED UNDER:
Hyper Parathyroidism; High Blood Calcium

Hypertension

see HIGH BLOOD PRESSURE

Hyperthyroidism (thyrotoxicosis)

Over-active thyroid gland. The thyroid regulates body metabolism and overproduction from it may cause a range of problems. Most commonly due to autoimmune inflammation, but can be caused by overproduction of thyroid hormone by a benign nodule in the thyroid. Occasionally short lived hyperthyroidism can be caused by a viral infection of the thyroid gland.

SYMPTOMS & SIGNS
- Tiredness, prolonged weakness and fatigue

- Sweating and hot flushes
- Intolerance of heat
- Tremor
- Appetite increased, possibly excessive craving for food, but loss of weight
- Symptoms of Anxiety
- Hyperactivity and Mania
- May be fast heart rate or extra heart beats
- Shortness of breath
- May be absent or irregular menstruation or may be very heavy periods
- Diarrhoea with loose but normal faeces
- May be protruding eyes, occasionally double vision

NOTE
Medical help should be sought, and treatment involves trying to reduce the amount of thyroid hormones.

CROSS-REFERENCED UNDER:
Graves' Disease; Overactive Thyroid Gland

Hyperventilation

Hyperventilation is caused by over breathing, by inhaling too much oxygen. Although it is very distressing for the individual, it is not usually a sign of any physical illness. Often results from anxiety or panic.

SYMPTOMS & SIGNS
- Gulping in air
- Rapid and deep breathing
- Dizziness
- Altered sensation in hands and around face with tingling
- Confusion and inability to think straight

NOTE

Most attacks of Hyperventilation will resolve by themselves, and they are not usually a cause for concern, although there may be an underlying problems with worry, fear, phobias or Anxiety. If an attack does not resolve quickly, the individual should be invited to breathe into a paper bag (never anything else). This restores the carbon dioxide balance in the blood, and breathing should return to normal. No other type of object should be used for this purpose as it may cause suffocation.

CROSS-REFERENCED UNDER:
Over Breathing

Hypoglycaemia

see LOW BLOOD SUGAR

Hypopituitarism

The pituitary gland is underactive. May be due to benign lumps (adenomas) or occasionally inflammation or as a consequence of surgery to the pituitary.

SYMPTOMS & SIGNS

- Low sex drive
- Menstruation ceases in women
- Skin looks white or pale
- Loss of hair, including pubic hair
- Problems with eyesight – blindspots or restriction of visual fields
- Weight increase
- Fatigue and excessive tiredness
- Symptoms of Hypothyroidism
- Symptoms of Addison's Disease
- Occasionally Diabetes Insipidus

NOTE
Treatment is with hormone replacement.

CROSS-REFERENCED UNDER:
Pituitary Gland Disease

Hypotension
see LOW BLOOD PRESSURE

Hypothalmic Disease

Problems with the hypothalmus, which secretes several hormones, many of which control hormone production from the pituitary. Most commonly hypothalmic disease results in deficiency of hormones – such as of thyroid or of adrenal of testicles or ovaries. Occasionally there can be hormone excess.

SYMPTOMS & SIGNS

- Excessive appetite and craving for food
- Copious amounts of urine
- Thirst
- Drowsiness
- Visual field restricted
- Changes such as deepening voice and growth of body hair before normal onset of puberty
- Unusual stature: abnormally short or tall
- May be hypothyroidism
- May be adrenal steriod deficiency (see Addison's Disease)
- May be deficiency of testosterone or oestrogen

NOTE
Medical help should be sought as soon as possible.

Hypothermia

Temperature within the body falls below normal. This can be caused by extremely low ambient temperature. Elderly people are particularly susceptible, as they may not be aware that they are cold, as are the very young. Babies do not shiver and do not have effective ways of maintaining core temperature, so extra special care should be taken with infants. Can occur also in association with hypothyrodism.

SYMPTOMS & SIGNS

- Listlessness, confusion and difficulty thinking straight
- Decreased movement
- May be shivering, but this is not always the case, particularly with babies and elderly individuals
- Extreme cold and pallor
- Pulse is slow
- Breathing is slow
- May be blue tinge to lips
- Fingers, toes, nose and ears may look pale or have a bluish tinge
- May be unconsciousness and coma

NOTE
Elderly people are more at risk of contracting this condition. They should be warmed slowly with blankets (including covering the head, where a lot of heat is lost) and warming drinks: individuals with Hypothermia should not be exposed to high temperatures as they may go into shock. Alcohol should always be avoided as it increases heat loss. Medical help, if available, should be sought immediately.

Hypothyroidism

Weight gain and other changes caused by too little (thyroid) hormone being produced by the thyroid gland, which regulates metabolism. The condition may take a long time to develop and may therefore be missed both by the individual suffering from Hypothyroidism and those who are close to them. The condition occurs usually because of autoimmune inflammation of the gland or occasionally because of a viral infection. May run in families. *Also see* Myxoedema.

SYMPTOMS & SIGNS

- Weight gain
- Face may appear puffy
- Skin is dry and coarse to the touch
- Hair may be thin and dry
- Sensitivity to the cold, and in severe cases individual may have hypothermia
- Voice sounds gruff
- Fatigue, tiredness, prolonged weakness and lethargy
- May be absent or irregular menstruation or very heavy periods
- May be mental impairment, confusion, slowness and Dementia
- Slow pulse
- May be Carpal Tunnel Syndrome
- Reflexes are slower
- In severe cases, may be collapse even coma

In the new-born infant:

- Enlarged tongue
- Hoarse cry
- Crude features
- Deafness

NOTE
Requires medical attention. All the symptoms and signs can be reversed by giving thyroid hormone replacement. Medical help should be sought immediately. Most likely in older individuals. Treatment is with hormones, normally produced by the thyroid gland, and will need to be taken for the rest of the individual's life.

Hysteria

Paralysis, loss of speech and even blindness, caused by a psychological problem, rather than underlying physical illness. There is not usually any intention of the individual to deceive: they genuinely believe they are suffering from a physical problem.

SYMPTOMS & SIGNS
- Paralysis with no discernible cause and no neurological abnormality otherwise
- Loss of speech with no discernible cause
- Blindness with no discernible cause
- Emotional reaction of the individual may be somewhat unusual and inappropriate, considering this would normally be a very traumatic event
- Any symptom may be complained of in the absence of any diverse or true physical cause

NOTE
Most likely in those with a previous history of psychological or psychiatric problems. It should be said that physical illness as a cause for the condition should be investigated before making a diagnosis of Hysteria, however unlikely underlying illness may seem.

Ichthyosis

Skin becomes thick, dry and flaky, usually caused by an inherited disorder but very occasionally associated with malignant disease.

SYMPTOMS & SIGNS
- Scaly, flaky, thickened and dry skin
- May not appear in the inner side of joints such as the elbow, armpit and knee

Impacted Wisdom Teeth
see WISDOM TEETH

Impetigo

Unpleasant and extremely infectious skin condition, with inflammation and pustules, caused by a bacterial infection. Contagious. Most usually affects the face and scalp, hands and knees first.

SYMPTOMS & SIGNS
- Onset is angry, red areas on the skin
- Fluid-filled sacs (vesicles), blisters and pustules form on the affected area.
- Sacs and blisters burst and crust over: crust is yellow or honey-coloured
- Will probably spread if not treated
- May be mistaken at onset for a cold sore

NOTE
Most likely in children, although can occur in adults. Treatment is with antibiotics, either ointment or by tablets if condition is severe.

Indigestion
see DYSPEPSIA, NON-ULCER

Infected Meibomian Cyst

Swelling of the meibomian glands, caused by an

infection. The glands produce an oily substance, which is used as a lubricant for the eyelashes.

SYMPTOMS & SIGNS

- Similar to a Stye
- May be a pea-sized lump or lumps on the flat part of the eyelid at the foot of an eyelash
- Eyelid is red and painful

NOTE
The affected hair may need to be removed to aid draining of pus, and antibiotics may be needed.

Infection of the Chest

see CHEST INFECTION

Infection of the Larynx

see LARYNGITIS

Infection of the Spine (Cervical)

see CERVICAL SPINE INFECTION

Infections of the Gums

see DENTAL INFECTIONS

Infections of the Teeth

see DENTAL INFECTIONS

Infectious Mononucleosis

see GLANDULAR FEVER

Infectious Parotitis

see MUMPS

Infective Dislocation of the Hip

Thigh bone (femur) may become displaced from the hip joint, caused by infections such as Tuberculosis.

SYMPTOMS & SIGNS

- Pain, which may be mild or severe
- Loss of movement
- Limp
- Fever
- General feeling of ill health
- Loss of appetite, weight loss due to underlying infection

NOTE
Medical help should be sought as if left untreated this condition may require major surgery.

CROSS-REFERENCED UNDER:
Dislocated Hip

Infertility

Infertility in couples can be caused by several conditions such as failure of egg production, blocked Fallopian tubes, womb abnormalities, low sperm count, systemic disease – but often there is no identifiable cause.

SYMPTOMS & SIGNS
Some indications of problems may be:

- Irregular or absent menstruation
- Persistent pelvic pain
- Unpleasant vaginal discharge
- Pain during sexual intercourse

NOTE
In all cases investigations will be needed to determine any physical problem in conceiving. Help is available to improve fertility, but some couples cannot conceive.

Inflammation of the Gall Bladder

see GALL STONES

Inflammation of the Vagina

The vagina can become inflamed, caused either by

infection or because of changes in skin after the Menopause.

SYMPTOMS & SIGNS
- Vagina is dry
- Itchy
- Discharge which is watery but may be tinged with blood
- Painful intercourse

> NOTE
> Medical help should be sought to get rid of any infection.

Influenza
see FLU

Ingrown Eyelash

Eyelashes can grow in on themselves.

SYMPTOMS & SIGNS
- Feeling as if there is something is in the eye
- May become infected

> NOTE
> The affected hair may need to be removed.

Ingrown Toenail

Toenail grows inwards, cutting into the skin of the toe, and possibly causing infection. It can be caused by badly fitting shoes or cutting the toenail too short.

SYMPTOMS & SIGNS
- Usually the outside part of the big toe is the area affected
- May be both feet
- Pain
- May be infection, with pain, swelling, redness

and pus at the outer or inner edge of the nail

> NOTE
> Surgery may be needed.

Inhaled Foreign Body
see CHOKING

Injury to the Ankle

Damage to the ankle, caused by injury or trauma.

SYMPTOMS & SIGNS
- Pain if weight is put on the ankle
- Unable to bear weight
- Swollen ankle, although this may take some time to develop
- Bruising around ankle
- Ankle may have become affected by an injury some time before, and there are recurrent episodes

> NOTE
> Medical help should be sought if problems persist.

CROSS-REFERENCED UNDER:
Sprained Ankle

Injury to the Eye

Eye becomes damaged by a blow, trauma or injury.

SYMPTOMS & SIGNS
- Area around the eye normally bruised
- Blurred vision
- Flashing lights
- Pupil of the eye may be dilated and enlarged, and does not react to changes in light
- Eye may be very sensitive to light making bright

light very painful

- Damage to the cornea can leave an opaque area or Cataract in the eye, which may affect vision depending where it occurs in the eye and how large the area is
- Damage to the eye can leave spots which float across the field of vision and are known as floaters

---

NOTE

If serious injury of the eye has occurred, medical help should be sought immediately.

Injury to the Lower Chest or Pelvis

Injuries to this area can cause several problems, not least damage to organs and tissues by stabbing or penetrating injuries or trauma, such as car accidents or even being kicked in the groin.

SYMPTOMS & SIGNS

- Pain, bruising and swelling
- Peritonitis
- Blood in urine following an injury or accident: urine may be pink, red or cloudy
- If there is damage to the urethra, may have problems or not be able to urinate

---

NOTE

Medical help should be sought immediately.

CROSS-REFERENCED UNDER:

Abdominal Injury; Pelvic Injury

Injury to the Nails

Nails can be damaged by injury or trauma, and may develop abscesses or other problems.

SYMPTOMS & SIGNS

Injury:

- Nail becomes discoloured, through blue, purple, brown and black
- May be very painful
- Blood may build up behind the nail, and form a sub-ungual haematoma. The pressure from this can be relieved by piercing the haematoma using a heated needle
- May be a whitlow (paronychia), an abscess in the finger which is throbbing, painful and tender. This can be caused by any penetrative injury becoming infected, and it may need antibiotics or surgical treatment

In elderly individuals:

- Toe nails, and especially the large toe, may become extremely thick (onychogryphosis)

CROSS-REFERENCED UNDER:

Whitlow; Paronychia

Injury to the Nose

Trauma to the nose can make it misshapen, crooked or flattened because of damage to the bone or cartilage in the nose. This will normally be accompanied by swelling and bleeding, and it may take some time for swelling to subside and to know if the damage to the nose is permanent.

SYMPTOMS & SIGNS

- Nose may be flattened
- Nose may be crooked or misshapen in appearance
- Nose looks swollen
- Bleeding
- If a serious injury has been sustained, may also be clear or pale fluid: medical help should be

sought
- Nose may be blocked and the individual has to breathe through their mouth
- May be loss of sense of smell

> **NOTE**
> Surgery may be necessary. If there is a nosebleed with clear or pale fluid as well as blood, the individual may have sustained a serious head injury, and medical help should be sought immediately.

Injury to the Penis

Rarely the penis may be damaged by trauma to the groin.

SYMPTOMS & SIGNS
- Bleeding from the penis

> **NOTE**
> Medical help should be sought immediately.

Injury to the Spine

see SPINAL CORD INJURY

Inner Ear Infection

Inner part of the ear may become inflamed and discharges pus, caused by an infection and associated with recurrent ear infections.

SYMPTOMS & SIGNS
- Discharge from ear, yellow in colour, which comes from a hole in the ear drum
- Discharge may become less or more in quantity, but is persistent
- Deafness or hearing impairment, particularly if there are recurrent ear infections
- Crackling and popping noises within the ear

- Giddiness and vertigo

NOTE
Medical help should be sought as treatment may be needed to eradicate the infection and repair the ear drum.

CROSS-REFERENCED UNDER:
Chronic Otitis Media; Ear Infection

Insect Bite or Sting

see BITE, INSECT

Intestinal Ischaemia

Blood clot becomes lodged in and blocks the blood supply to the intestines.

SYMPTOMS & SIGNS
- Abdominal pain, severe in nature and with a sudden onset
- Diarrhoea with blood in faeces
- Vomiting
- Peritonitas
- Quickly leads to shock and collapse

> **NOTE**
> Medical help should be sought immediately as surgery will be needed to remove the clot. Most likely in elderly individuals with heart conditions.

Intestinal Obstruction

Obstruction blocks the intestine, caused by a hernia, cancer, inflammation, the bowel twisting on itself, or by a gallstone blocking the bowel.

SYMPTOMS & SIGNS
- Intermittent colicky pain in the abdomen, sometimes very severe in intensity, although the location will depend on the underlying problem

- No faeces or flatus (wind) passed from the rectum
- Abdomen becomes swollen
- May be fever
- Vomiting, both stomach contents and undigested food, and bile and green fluid with mucous, as well as sometimes vomit like diarrhoea
- May develop shock
- May be collapse in severe cases

> NOTE
> Medical help should be sought immediately.

CROSS-REFERENCED UNDER:
Obstruction of the Intestine

Intestinal Polyps

Growths can develop from the tissue in the intestine, which – at least to begin with – are not harmful. As they grow, they may become cancerous. *Also see* Cancer of the Colon.

SYMPTOMS & SIGNS
- Bleeding from the rectum
- Anaemia

> NOTE
> Medical help should be sought.

Intussusception

Part of the bowel pushes back or protrudes into another part (invaginates). This causes intestinal obstruction. Commoner in children.

SYMPTOMS & SIGNS
- Severe abdominal pain like colic
- Faeces stained with blood and mucous
- Vomiting

- Swollen abdomen

> NOTE
> Medical help should be sought immediately.

Iritis (Uveitis)

Inflammation of the coloured part of the eye (iris), which can be caused by several conditions, including arthritic problems eg Reiter's syndrome, also inflammatory bowel disease and connective tissue disorders. Can be due to infection including bacterial, viral. Normally only one eye is affected.

SYMPTOMS & SIGNS
- Usually only affects one eye
- Eye is painful and red
- Redness is most noticeable around the coloured part of the eye
- The pupil is noticeably smaller in the affected eye
- Vision is affected and may be blurred
- Eye is overly sensitive to light (photophobia) and bright light may be painful

If there are repeated episodes:
- Pupil may appear irregular

> NOTE
> Eyedrops can be used to reduce inflammation and to dilate the pupil.

Iron Ring

Brown ring in the eye. This is usually caused when a piece of iron has got into the eye, and then has been removed, leaving the ring.

SYMPTOMS & SIGNS
- Brown ring in the eye

- A piece of iron has been removed from the cornea

> **NOTE**
> If a piece of metal has got into the eye, great care should be taken removing it and medical help may be needed to prevent damage to the eye.

Irritable Bladder

Nerves becoming irritated in the bladder, although infection causing inflammation needs to be ruled out.

SYMPTOMS & SIGNS
Symptoms and signs may include:
- Need to urinate very frequently
- Urinary incontinence
- Problems urinating, only excreting small amounts despite the bladder still feeling as if it is full
- Retention of urine
- Pain in the lower abdomen
- Needing to urinate at night

> **NOTE**
> Medical help should be sought to investigate the cause.

Irritable Bowel Syndrome

Bowel problems which do not appear to have any specific cause when investigated or to be the result of any disease. Symptoms may come and go, and the condition may be affected by stress and diet. NOT associated with passage of blood in faeces.

SYMPTOMS & SIGNS
- Intermittent abdominal pain

- Periods of diarrhoea (although faeces are normal apart from being somewhat loose) and constipation
- Passage of mucous
- Swollen abdomen
- Flatulence

> **NOTE**
> Medical help should be sought to rule out other bowel conditions. It may help to investigate food intolerances or allergies, make sure there is enough roughage in the diet, or look for therapies which improve relaxation.

Irritable Hip

Pain, limp and restricted movement of the hip, although the cause cannot be identified.

SYMPTOMS & SIGNS
- Pain in groin or front of the leg down to the knee
- Movement restricted by the pain
- May limp when walking

> **NOTE**
> Will usually resolve with rest, although investigations should be undertaken to exclude more serious underlying disease.

Irritant Atmosphere
see POISONING

Irritation of Nerves to Eye
see HORNER'S SYNDROME

Ischaemic Contracture

Wasting of the muscle of the forearm, caused by insufficient blood supply to the area.

SYMPTOMS & SIGNS
- Forearm is thin and the muscle atrophied
- Skin of the hand looks pale
- Reduced sensation in the hand
- Problems gripping: the fingers can only be straightened by flexing the wrist

> NOTE
> Medical help should be sought.

CROSS-REFERENCED UNDER:
Volkmann's Contracture

Ischaemic Heart Disease

The vessels which supply the heart with blood become progressively blocked and the supply of blood to the heart is reduced. This may have no symptoms – or may be mild to severe and life threatening if the narrowed arteries to the heart become blocked, causing a heart attack with permanent damage to the heart muscle.

SYMPTOMS & SIGNS
- May be no symptoms
- May be Angina, typically on exertion but can occur at rest or at night
- May be heart attack
- Shortness of breath on exertion
- May be heart failure
- Tiredness, weakness

> NOTE
> Medical help should be sought.

Isolated Thyroid Nodule

Lump within the thyroid gland (which is on both sides of the neck below the Adam's apple). Lumps can be usually benign but can be malignant. May be associated with either an over- or under-active thyroid gland but usually thyroid works normally.

SYMPTOMS & SIGNS
- Lump which can be felt usually on one, occasionally both sides of the front of the neck below the Adam's apple
- Lump moves up and down on swallowing
- Usually painless

If malignant (which is more unusual), the following may also be present:
- Voice is hoarse
- One eyelid droops (known as Horner's syndrome) because of paralysis of nerves in the neck
- Pain
- Lymph glands may be enlarged

> NOTE
> Medical help should be sought.

Jejunal, Diverticular Disease
see JEJUNAL DIVERTICULITIS

Jejunal Diverticulitis

Wall of part of the small intestine can develop pouches (diverticula). These can exist without symptoms, but they can become inflamed.

SYMPTOMS & SIGNS
- Change of bowel habit
- Colicky or persistent abdominal pain
- Swollen abdomen
- Faeces may contain blood, either bright red or dark and tarry
- Blood may be passed from the anus
- May be diarrhoea

If badly inflamed:

- Fever
- Severe pain
- Tender area in the abdomen

> NOTE
> May resolve itself or many need antibiotic treatment

CROSS-REFERENCED UNDER:

Diverticular Disease (Jejunal); Jejunal, Diverticular Disease

Kala-azar

Infectious parasitic disease, spread by sand flies. Long incubation period of 2–8 months

SYMPTOMS & SIGNS

- Spleen is greatly enlarged, and can be felt as a mass under the rib cage on the left hand side of the abdomen but may extend to right, lower abdomen
- Liver is also enlarged
- Lymph glands enlarged
- Fever
- Sweating
- Anaemia
- Wasting
- Increased pigmentation of face, hands, feet, abdomen

> NOTE
> Tropical disease most common in middle East, Asia and Far East.

Kaposi's Sarcoma

Malignant skin tumours.

SYMPTOMS & SIGNS

- Blue-red areas on the skin

> NOTE
> Now most commonly associated with AIDS.

Keloid Scarring

Severe thickening of a scar after an injury or surgery. The scar becomes thickened, is reddened and is raised above the surrounding skin. Although not serious in itself, it can be very disfiguring.

SYMPTOMS & SIGNS

- Site of the wound develops raised hard skin with a red, rough, scarred texture, even if the original injury has not been great

> NOTE
> More likely in black people.

Keratitis

Condition of the outer membrane of the eye (cornea), caused by injury or conditions such as an ulcer or the Herpes virus.

SYMPTOMS & SIGNS

- Onset of symptoms is sudden
- Vision not affected
- Only one of the eyes is affected
- Light causes pain or discomfort
- Profuse watery discharge from the eye

> NOTE
> Medical help should be sought immediately, and treatment will be with anti-viral drugs if it has been caused by the Herpes virus

Keratoconjuctivitis Sicca

see SJOGREN'S SYNDROME

Keratomalacia

see VITAMIN A DEFICIENCY

Kidney Disease (may lead to Kidney Failure)

Disease of the kidney may result from a variety of causes including chronic inflammation (glomerulonephritis) or scarring sometimes because of abnormalities that are present from birth. Where infection is the cause there may be symptoms also of cystitis. Where there are symptoms of infection (pyelonephritis) there may be vomiting, nausea, malaise and pain in the abdomen or in the loin. These latter symptoms may not be so obvious at the onset of the infection; more pressing may be vomiting, nausea and pain in the upper part of the abdomen. Severe cases of infection may produce severe inflammation and kidney failure (acute nephritis), and may cause death.

SYMPTOMS & SIGNS
Symptoms for Cystitis, and in addition the following maybe present:
- Severe fever
- Generally feeling unwell
- Vomiting and nausea, especially at onset when the following signs may not be so apparent
- May be excessive and frequent urination
- Pain in the loins
- The side of the abdomen and loins may be tender and sensitive to the touch
- Fatigue, weakness
- Chills (rigors)
- Confusion, drowsiness
- May be brown discoloration in the half moons in the nails

The following will also be Kidney Failure:
- Severe tiredness and weakness
  Loss of appetite
  Nausea, vomiting
- Itching
- Dry and furry tongue
- Anaemia and pallid skin
- May be dehydrated
- Deep sighing breathing
- Reduced amount of urine
- May stop urinating completely
- Headache
- Retention of fluid (oedema), causing the face, ankles and other parts of the body to become swollen
- High blood pressure
- Weak pulse
- Convulsions
- Unconsciousness and coma

> NOTE
> Medical help should be sought immediately.

CROSS-REFERENCED UNDER:
Pyelonephritis; Nephritis

Kidney Stones

Formation of stones (calculus) in the kidney or urinary tract, which may then cause severe pain, blocked ducts and hamper function, even making it impossible to urinate.

SYMPTOMS & SIGNS
- Severe colicky spasms of abdominal pain centred on one side of the abdomen and over the kidney. Intermittent in nature, but very severe.

Pain usually migrates and spreads from the back to the front of the abdomen, then into the groin to the end of the penis

- Recurrent episodes of pain
- Vomiting
- Sweating
- May be blood in urine, making urine cloudy, dark or blood stained
- Stone can block the urethra or the opening of the bladder and may make it impossible to urinate. If this is the case, there will also be lower abdominal pain because of a very full bladder.
- It is possible that stones in the urinary tract may be passed through the urethra

> NOTE
> Medical help should be sought.

CROSS-REFERENCED UNDER:
Stones in the Urinary System

Knee Dislocation
see DISLOCATION OF THE KNEE

Knock Knees

Knees press against each other and the feet are splayed. This is most commonly a normal variant in children, and will resolve with age, although it can be a sign of Rickets, Osteomalacia, Paget's Disease or Charcot's joints.

SYMPTOMS & SIGNS
- Knees touch
- Feet are splayed
- Usually no other symptoms

> NOTE
> Unusually anything to be concerned about, but may need investigations to exclude any underlying condition.

CROSS-REFERENCED UNDER:
Bow Legs

Kwashiorkor

Malnutrition, caused by there being too little nutrition in the diet.

SYMPTOMS & SIGNS
- Generally unhappy child
- Swollen stomach and abdomen
- Face and limbs also swollen
- Thin and dry hair
- Areas of skin are unusually pigmented
- May be bouts of diarrhoea with loose but otherwise normal faeces
- Limbs, upper trunk and face emaciated

> NOTE
> Most likely in children from poor areas in developing countries.

CROSS-REFERENCED UNDER:
Malnutrition

Kyphosis

Deformity of the spine, caused by vertebral fracture and osteoporosis but also inherited diseases, Ankylosing Spondylitis, or even bad posture.

SYMPTOMS & SIGNS
- Spine is curved, most noticeable from the side
- Hump-back
- Back pain

- Height loss

> NOTE
> May be an indicator of the presence of osteoporosis

Laryngeal Oedema

Inflammation of the larynx, possibly blocking the airway and making breathing difficult or impossible. It can be caused by an allergic reaction or by infections, such as Diphtheria.

SYMPTOMS & SIGNS
- Blue tinge to the lips, ear lobes, under the fingernails and elsewhere caused by a lack of oxygen reaching tissues (cyanosis)
- Air being forced through the airways may cause a loud and harsh noise
- Distress caused by choking or difficulty breathing

> NOTE
> Medical help should be sought immediately.

Laryngitis

Inflammation of the larynx (located in the neck and commonly called the voice box), caused by infection or from shouting or being in dry and smoky atmospheres.

SYMPTOMS & SIGNS
- Difficulty when speaking
- Hoarse voice
- May not be possible to speak as too hoarse or painful
- Fever
- Pain in throat when swallowing, although not as severe as with tonsillitis
- Bad breath and unpleasant taste in mouth
- May be headache
- May develop into a chest infection

In particularly severe conditions:
- Inflammation may be so severe as to block the windpipe
- Laboured and forced breathing
- Bluish tinge to the skin, especially the lips, caused by a lack of oxygen (cyanosis)

> NOTE
> Smoking exacerbates symptoms, and smokers may suffer from associated infections of the chest. If unexplained hoarseness persists for a long time, it may be worth seeking medical help to exclude serious disease.

CROSS-REFERENCED UNDER:
Infection of the Larynx

Laryngotracheo-bronchitis
see CROUP

Larynx Cancer
see CANCER OF THE LARYNX

Laxatives

Laxatives are substances, some of them drugs, others natural, which cause emptying of the bowel, sometimes urgently and violently.

SYMPTOMS & SIGNS
- Diarrhoea, often with intestinal urgency, although faeces are normal if somewhat loose
- Swollen abdomen with discomfort
- No other symptoms

NOTE

Some people take laxatives on a daily or regular basis, yet may still complain of diarrhoea.

CROSS-REFERENCED UNDER:

Factitious Diarrhoea

Leprosy

Progressive condition which causes growths on nerves and on skin. The individual has no sensation, such as pain, in the affected part of the body, which may lead to the area becoming damaged and even gangrenous without the individual being aware of the damage. The disease is contagious through repeated exposure over a long time, although the actual method of transmission is not clear.

SYMPTOMS & SIGNS

- Altered or lack of sensation, particularly in the extremities of the limbs, ie the fingers and toes
- Cartilage of the nose may become ulcerated and the nose collapses
- Growths on the skin
- Patchy pigmentation of skin
- Danger of developing gangrene if affected areas become damaged through injury or 'wear and tear'
- Fingers, hands, toes and feet may become eroded by repeated trauma

NOTE

Most likely in developing countries, although once common in Britain and Europe. Drugs can control the spread of the condition and treat the infection.

CROSS-REFERENCED UNDER:

Hansen's Disease

Leptospirosis

see WEIL'S DISEASE

Leukaemia

Cancer of the blood, which may take several different forms. White blood cells may be abnormal in type and number. The condition may be fatal if not treated.

SYMPTOMS & SIGNS

Symptoms can include all or some of the following:

- Lymph nodes are swollen but not painful
- General feeling of being unwell
- May be extreme itchiness
- Mouth ulcers
- Persistent fatigue
- Weakness
- Weight loss
- Night sweats
- Fever
- Anaemia
- Looking pallid (due to anaemia)
- Shortness of breath
- Easily bruised or may spontaneously bleed from the nose, gums, stomach, rectum or vagina
- May be prolonged and unwanted erections
- Spleen and liver enlarged and felt as a mass under the rib cage on the left side of the abdomen
- Associated with increased susceptibility to a wide range of infections including bacterial, viral and fungal
- Bone pain and tenderness

NOTE

Medical help should be sought and tests will be needed to confirm underlying cause.

CROSS-REFERENCED UNDER:

Myeloid Leukaemia

Leukoplakia

Thickened white patches on mucous membranes, on the lips, in the mouth and on the genitals. Painless

SYMPTOMS & SIGNS

- Thickened, possibly hardened, white patches which cannot be removed
- May disappear themselves, leaving a red area

> NOTE
> Associated with Syphilis, pre-cancerous changes, AIDs, smoking, drinking, sepsis and sharp teeth. If this condition is suspected, medical help should be sought.

Lice

Infestations of lice, which can be found in the hair, the body or in the genital area. They are spread by contact with another affected individual, and do not reflect the hygiene of the individual or their family in any way, although pubic lice may be spread sexually.

SYMPTOMS & SIGNS

- Extreme itchiness where the infestation occurs
- Eggs may be seen in the hair, although the lice themselves are often not apparent
- May affect any hairy area, including the eyelids and eyebrows and the genitals

> NOTE
> Treatment is available.

CROSS-REFERENCED UNDER:

Nits; Headlice

Lichen Planus

Irregularly shaped, shiny patches on the skin, which may be found all over the body, but usually on the legs and wrists. Can affect mouth and genitals. Usually an autoimmune condition, occasionally occurs as a drug reaction.

SYMPTOMS & SIGNS

- Small, shiny skin changes
- Fine white lines and small white spots on the lips and in the mouth
- May be associated ulcers between the lines and spots
- Ulcers may form
- Nails may be involved, and become shaped like spoons, lined, flaky and may even be destroyed
- Intense itch or pain as spots ulcerate

> NOTE
> Most likely in those over 30 years in age.

Lichen Simplex

Thickening of the skin caused by continual scratching in one particular area.

SYMPTOMS & SIGNS

- Affected area develops thicker skin, which may be raised above the surrounding area
- Scratching only temporary relieves the itch, so the individual scratches again, and the cycle continues

Ligament Damage (Knee)

see LIGAMENTOUS TEAR (KNEE)

Ligamentous Tear (Knee)

Ligaments of the knee may be damaged or torn,

usually because of direct injury or severe trauma. The severity of the symptoms will depend on how bad the tear or damage is.

SYMPTOMS & SIGNS
- Pain at the site of injury
- Reduced movement and function
- Swelling, which may take some hours to develop
- Knee may lock or give way
- Bruising at site of injury

NOTE
If a tear is suspected, medical help should be sought. Once ligaments have been damaged, the knee may then become more susceptible to a similar injury.

CROSS-REFERENCED UNDER:
Ligament Damage (Knee)

Lipoma

Fatty lump (benign tumour), either superficial or which may grow into the skin, found anywhere there is fatty tissue.

SYMPTOMS & SIGNS
- A soft slightly mobile smooth lump develops under the skin
- Painless, unless it becomes infected
- May be present for many years and may increase slowly in size
- Has no a central 'opening'
- Benign

NOTE
Does not normally need treatment unless very disfiguring, but medical help should be sought to exclude any underlying conditions such as cancer.

Little's Disease
see CEREBRAL PALSY

Liver Cancer
see CANCER OF THE LIVER

Liver Disease and Infection
see HEPATITIS

Livido Reticularis

Pattern of blue blood vessels just below the skin, caused by a disorder in the response to cold or to heat.

SYMPTOMS & SIGNS
- Pattern of fine blue lines on the skin

Lockjaw
see TETANUS

Longsightedness

Small pupils are normal in individuals who are long-sighted

SYMPTOMS & SIGNS
- Both pupils are small
- Both pupils react quickly and in unison in sudden changes to light and dark
- No other symptoms

NOTE
Eye test may be needed.

Loose Body in the Knee

Loose bodies can become trapped in the knee joint, often as result of Osteoarthritis or direct injury.

SYMPTOMS & SIGNS
- Pain, intense in nature and sudden in onset

- Leg cannot be straightened or may suddenly lock or give way
- Knee may become swollen
- Resolves by itself as the loose body is dislodged from the joint
- Loose body can be felt in the joint
- Recurs

NOTE
Medical help may be necessary.

Loud Noises

Prolonged long-term exposure to loud noises, such as very loud music or industrial processes, can damage the hearing. One-off or occasional exposure may result in temporary deafness and tinnitus, but this will usually resolve.

SYMPTOMS & SIGNS
- Deafness and hearing impairment
- Ringing in the ears (tinnitus)

NOTE
Prolonged exposure to loud noises or music should be avoided to reduce damage to the ear.

CROSS-REFERENCED UNDER:
Acoustic Trauma

Low Blood Pressure

Blood pressure becomes too low, associated with Shock, severe infections, heart disease, bleeding, and medication for high blood pressure.

SYMPTOMS & SIGNS
- Giddiness or dizziness or lightheadedness when rising to the feet from sitting
- Prolonged weakness and fatigue

- Possible that the individual may faint
- Attack lasts only a short time

NOTE
Most likely in the elderly. If persistent can lead to kidney failure and stroke. Medical attention should be sought.

CROSS-REFERENCED UNDER:
Hypotension; Blood Pressure, Low

Low Blood Sugar (hypoglyceamia)

Low blood sugar is caused by excess insulin with too little food, lack of hormones that work counter to insulin (steroid hormones) or with some medications including insulin and some diabetic tablets. It may affect any individual to some degree, but is of particular importance to diabetics because it can be severe and is more likely to recur. Diabetics should check their blood sugar before driving..

SYMPTOMS & SIGNS
- Drowsiness
- May be sudden weakness
- Problems thinking straight or concentrating
- Behaviour may become bizzare and irrational
- Irritability
- Sweating
- Feeling cold and clammy
- Individual looks pale
- Feeling of hunger
- Palpitations
- Often excessive hunger and craving for food

NOTE
Resolves when the individual eats.

CROSS-REFERENCED UNDER:
Hypoglycaemia

Low Sex Drive

see LOW OR ABSENT SEXUAL DRIVE

Low or Absent Sexual Drive

Interest in sex varies between individuals, and at different times, such as during a female's monthly cycle, after a woman has given birth, or if individuals are depressed, in a long-term relationship, or even just tired. It is rare for there to be anything physically wrong.

SYMPTOMS & SIGNS

- May feel that sex is dirty or feel guilty about sexual contact
- May not want to be touched or to have any physical contact
- May have been unpleasant or unwanted sexual experiences in the past
- May be tensions within a relationship

NOTE
Counsellors may be able to help with some problems, but an individual's level of interest in sex may be a personal thing and not be the sign of an underlying condition.

CROSS-REFERENCED UNDER:
Low Sex Drive; Frigidity

Lower Arm Bones (Radius, Ulna and wrist) Fracture

see BROKEN LOWER ARM BONES (RADIUS, ULNA AND WRIST)

Lower Leg (femur, tibia and fibula) Fractures

see FRACTURES OF THE LOWER LEG (FEMUR, TIBIA AND FIBULA)

Ludwig's Angina

Severe infection of the floor of the mouth, associated with infected teeth or gums and poor oral hygiene.

SYMPTOMS & SIGNS

- Severe pain
- May be swollen upper airways, causing difficulty breathing
- Pain when swallowing
- Fever
- Bad breath and unpleasant taste in mouth

NOTE
Medical help should be sought.

Lumbago

see BACK STRAIN

Lung Abscess

An abscess, filled with pus, may form in the lung, usually associated with severe infection. It may be caused by exposure to infective material, as a complication of Pneumonia, or the spread of an abscess from the liver, although this latter case is very unusual.

SYMPTOMS & SIGNS

- Pre-existing chest infection
- Chest pain, particularly severe when inhaling or exhaling (Pleurisy)
- Foul sputum and associated bad breath
- Fever
- Sweating and shivering

- Loss of appetite, weight loss
- Generally feeling unwell
- May be Horner's Syndrome: one pupil of the eye may be unusually small with drooping of the eyelid and a bulging eye

> NOTE
> Medical help should be sought.

Lung Cancer

Cancer of the lung. The tumour may narrow or block airways within the lung. The tumour either directly or through associated pneumonia can result in increasingly difficult in breathing. Often associated with a dry cough and chest pain.

SYMPTOMS & SIGNS

- Persistent dry cough, although there may also be the production of sputum
- Sputum streaked with blood: small tumours can produce fresh blood
- Voice may be hoarse due to pressure on the laryngeal nerve
- Shortness of breath: tumours can cause a lung or part of a lung to collapse
- Chest pain due to inflammation in the lung caused by the tumour
- Chest infections, which are persistent and do not resolve readily
- Generally feeling unwell
- Swollen lymph glands in the neck
- Loss of appetite and progressive weight loss
- Bad breath
- Obstruction of vena cava
- May be Horner's Syndrome: one pupil of the eye may be unusually small with drooping of the eyelid and a bulging eye

- Clubbing of end of fingers and finger nails
- May be muscle wasting
- May be high calcium
- May be polymyositis or neuropathy

> NOTE
> Risks of contracting lung cancer are massively increased by smoking, and more likely in the older individual.

CROSS-REFERENCED UNDER:
Cancer of the Lung

Lymphangitis

Infection from a wound, affecting the lymphatic system. The infection can spread up the lymph duct towards the lymph gland, and the wound itself may appear very minor.

SYMPTOMS & SIGNS

- A red line travels from the area of the wound towards the armpit
- Tender lymph nodes at the top of the affected limb
- Fever
- Headache
- Loss of appetite, feels ill

> NOTE
> May need antibiotics to resolve.

Lymphatic Obstruction of the Breast

Fluid drains from the breast and chest through the armpit. If this does not occur, one breast can become enlarged from the build up of fluid.

SYMPTOMS & SIGNS

- One breast becomes larger and firm to the touch

■ Arm may also be swollen

> NOTE
> May occur after radiotherapy to the chest or surgery affecting the lymph nodes in the armpit.

Lymphoedema

Failure of the drainage of lymph, which causes a build up of fluid, caused by congenital abnormalities, malignant disease or as a consequence of surgical removal of glands, parasite infection, or for no apparent reason.

Post-Phlebitic Limb is a condition following Deep Vein Thrombosis.

SYMPTOMS & SIGNS

■ Limb is swollen and tender: it does not vary in size
■ Skin becomes thickened, and sometimes has the texture of elephant skin
■ May be inflammation or infection

> NOTE
> Medical help should be sought.

CROSS-REFERENCED UNDER:

Post-Phlebitic Limb; Swollen Ankle

Lymphogranuloma Venerium

see CHANCROID

Lymphoma

Cancer of the lymphatic system, which may be benign or malignant, the cause of which remains unclear. There may be few symptoms.

SYMPTOMS & SIGNS

■ Lymph nodes become swollen (sometimes very

large and rubbery) but painless
■ May be extreme itchiness

If malignant, the following may also be present

■ Fever
■ Weight loss
■ Night sweats
■ Anaemia

> NOTE
> Medical help should be sought immediately as the earlier the condition is diagnosed the better the chance of a cure.

ME (Myalgic Encephalomyelitis)

see POST-VIRAL SYNDROME

Macular Degeneration

Deterioration in eyesight, caused by a problem with the most sensitive part of the retina (the part at the back of the eye where cells are light sensitive).

SYMPTOMS & SIGNS

■ Blurred vision
■ Loss of clarity of vision over time, which is not aided by wearing spectacles or contact lenses
■ This area may increase in size and blindness is progressive
■ Vision is not completely lost
■ Distortion of vision
■ Deterioration in vision may prevent driving

> NOTE
> Most likely in elderly people: it cannot be corrected by spectacles or contact lenses.

Malaria

Tropical disease caused by parasites that are

passed to humans by the bite of mosquitoes that carry the infection.

Symptoms & Signs
- Sweats
- Headache
- Aching muscles
- Fatigue
- Nausea, loss of appetite, vomiting
- Recurrent bouts of fever and rigors, every few days
- Enlarged spleen, felt as a mass under the left side of the rib cage. Enlarged liver
- Spontaneous and generalised bleeding, caused by failure of blood to clot
- Urine is dark and brown in colour, caused by red blood cells being broken down and excreted in urine (haemaglobinuria)
- Mepacrine, an antimalarial drug, can cause the skin to become yellow
- The disease may recur months after returning from abroad

Note
Individuals travelling to malarial areas should take medication to prevent Malaria: the course of medicine is started some time before the trip and continues after return. Parts of the world affected by malaria are Africa, India and the Far East and other tropical areas. If someone contracting a fever has not been taking preventative medication and fever occurs, medical help should be sought immediately. The disease kills hundreds of thousands of people every year.

Malignant Ascites

Retention of fluid in the abdominal cavity, caused by

cancers of a number of organs including bowel, ovaries, womb and kidneys.

Symptoms & Signs
- Swollen abdomen
- Swollen ankles
- May be prominent blood vessels in the abdomen
- May be difficulty in breathing because of pressure put on the diaphragm
- Usually wasting of muscles
- Loss of appetite

Note
Medical help should be sought immediately.

Cross-referenced under:
Ascites, Malignant

Mallet Finger and Thumb

Damage to tendons in the fingers, usually caused by injury or conditions such as Rheumatoid Arthritis.

Symptoms & Signs
- End digit of the finger cannot be straightened and is left bent

Note
Medical help should be sought as will need splinting or surgery.

Mallory-Weiss Tear

Small tear in the lining of the upper part of the stomach or gullet.

Symptoms & Signs
- Vomiting
- Fresh blood in vomit (haematemesis)
- Faeces like tar

> NOTE
> May resolve by itself but medical help should be sought, even if just to exclude more severe conditions.

Malnutrition

If a diet has insufficient protein and vitamins, this can lead to many problems. Malnutrition is associated with poverty, alcoholism, drug abuse, mental problems and with wasting diseases. Lack of sufficient iron in the diet can cause Anaemia.

SYMPTOMS & SIGNS
- Night blindness
- Difficulty in distinguishing colours
- Hair loss
- Change of skin tone
- Pallid skin
- Swollen ankles
- May be weight loss
- Easily fatigued and constantly tired

In children also:
- Failure to grow and thrive
- Swollen belly
- Mental impairment

> NOTE
> Eating a properly balanced diet with a mix of carbohydrates, protein, fat, vitamins and minerals should prevent malnutrition in otherwise healthy individuals.

CROSS-REFERENCED UNDER:
Poor Diet

Malnutrition

see KWASHIORKOR

Manic Depression

see DEPRESSION AND MANIC DEPRESSION

Marble Bones

see OSTEOPETROSIS

Mastitis

The breast becomes inflamed, usually as a result of an infection.

SYMPTOMS & SIGNS
- Tenderness around the nipple
- Pain in the breast
- Hard, very tender area develops
- An abscess may form

> NOTE
> Medical help should be sought as antibiotics may be needed.

Mastoiditis

Inflammation of the mastoid bone, which is found just behind the ears. Although rare, this is a potentially serious condition as the infection can spread to the brain.

SYMPTOMS & SIGNS
- Onset with an ear infection
- Pain behind the ear
- Mastoid bone becomes inflamed, the area red and tender
- Thick discharge from the ear, yellow in colour
- General feeling of ill health
- Fever

> NOTE
> Formerly more common, although now unusual with the advent of antibiotics.

Measles

Acute infectious, possibly serious, condition, caused by a virus. It often appears in epidemics.

SYMPTOMS & SIGNS
- Fever, feeling unwell
- Loss of appetite
- Runnig nose, cough
- Inflamed eyes, eyes are reddened
- In around four days a blotchy red rash appears, which first appears on the forehead and by the ears then spreads down over the chest and abdomen during one week to other parts of the body
- White spots in the mouth, beside the molars, small in size and surrounded by a reddened area
- Rarely, may be Pneumonia or Encephalitis

> NOTE
> There is a routine vaccination.

Measles, German

see RUBELLA

Meckel's Diverticulum

A pouch may form in the small intestine, the remnant of the duct which connected the yoke sac in embryos. This can become inflamed and can bleed, although this is very unusual.

SYMPTOMS & SIGNS
- Change of bowel habit
- Colicky or persistent abdominal pain
- Swollen abdomen
- Faeces may contain blood, either bright red or dark and tarry, or blood may be passed from the rectum

- May be diarrhoea

If badly inflamed:
- Fever
- Anaemia
- Severe pain
- Tender area in the abdomen
- Intestinal obstruction

> NOTE
> May appear to be Appendicitis as symptoms are very similar.

Melanoma, Malignant

see CANCER OF THE SKIN

Meniere's Disease

Condition of the inner ear, affecting both hearing and balance, caused by an infection. It is often difficult to treat, and there may be several recurrent attacks.

SYMPTOMS & SIGNS
- Deafness or hearing impairment
- Tinnitus
- Vertigo and loss of balance
- May be severe enough to cause nausea and vomiting

> NOTE
> Medical help should be sought as there are medications which may help the condition.

Meningitis

Inflammation of the membranes (lining) of the brain and spinal cord, caused by viral, bacterial or rarely fungal infections. It should always be taken seriously, especially in babies, children, teenagers and young adults as it can be life-threatening.

SYMPTOMS & SIGNS

- Neck stiffness: it is not possible to bend the head forward and bending the neck exacerbates the headache
- Headache, usually severe in intensity and generalised
- Vomiting
- General feeling of being ill and unusually irritable (this may be a significant symptom in a baby or child)
- Fever
- Purple rash
- Exposure to light is extremely painful (photophobia)
- May be double vision
- Consciousness impaired, drowsiness and confusion
- May be painful, swollen and protruding eyes with restricted movement caused by blood clots in the tissues behind the eyes
- Progressive drowsiness
- May be convulsions
- May unconsciousness and coma

In children or babies also:

- May be red flecks in the whites of the eyes
- May be bulging in the baby's head, caused by increased pressure in the head forcing its way through the soft parts of a baby's skull
- Infant is extremely irritable and does not want to be touched
- May be convulsions
- May cause permanent deafness

NOTE
Medical help should be sought immediately. It is particularly severe in children and young adults, and can develop extremely quickly, possibly leading to collapse and death. A vaccination is available for the most common type of Meningitis.

CROSS-REFERENCED UNDER:
Encephalitis

Meninogococcal Septicaemia

Sudden development of a purple rash along with fever, severe illness and collapse. The condition can develop very quickly, is extremely serious and can be rapidly fatal. Also *see* Meningitis.

SYMPTOMS & SIGNS

- Fever
- Nausea, vomiting, headache
- Severely aching muscles
- Very quick onset of a purple rash, which may cover large areas of the body or may only affect a small area. Typically on the trunk
- General feeling of progressive ill health
- May be accompanied by Meningitis
- Shock, collapse and even death

NOTE
May be life threatening, and particularly severe in infants and pre-school children. If this condition is suspected, or the individual has been in contact with another with this condition, medical help should be sought immediately as collapse and death can occur within hours of onset.

Menopause

The normal processes of stopping of ovulation and menstruation, known as the 'change of life' which occurs in all women with ageing. Symptoms and their severity are dependent on the individual, and are caused by changes in hormone levels.

- Menstruation becomes erratic and lighter and eventually stops
- Skin of the vagina becomes drier, there is less lubrication, and sexual intercourse may be painful: rarely there they may be a watery discharge with blood from the vagina (this will usually be pink rather than red)
- Skin changes texture
- Hot flushes – often severe and prolonged
- Heavy sweats especially at night
- Headaches of varying intensity
- Hair may lose some of its life, lustre and texture, and become thinner
- Increased or excessive amount of body hair, including on the face
- May be loss of sexual interest
- Mood change including depression and irritability
- Greater risk of Osteoporosis as bone mineral falls in the years after menopause, which may be reduced by Hormone Replacement Therapy (HRT): although this has some small risks itself

> NOTE
>
> Usually occurs in women between 45 and 55 years of age, and signs or symptoms can last for years. If there is a discharge of blood years after menstruation has stopped, medical help should be sought to exclude disease or cancer.

Menstruation

Menstruation is an entirely normal and healthy function in post-adolescent and pre-menopausal women. Although in no way a disease, various problems can arise from periods, typically mild, occasionally serious. It is usual for most girls to have started menstruating by the age of 16, although there is great variation. If onset of periods is delayed beyond 16 medical advice should be sought.

SYMPTOMS & SIGNS

- Most girls have started menstruating by the age of 16, but some are later. If development of sexual characteristics, such as breasts and pubic hair, is otherwise normal, this is not usually anything to worry about, especially if there is a similar family history. In a very few cases, late menstruation may be because of some underlying physical problem such as a membrane blocking menstrual flow, hormonal disorders, eating disorders, excessive exercise, or genetic or congenital disorders
- Periods may be irregular, particularly in younger women who have only recently begun menstruating. If these are otherwise normal for the individual, there are probably no underlying problems, but if they are heavy and painful, or there is bleeding between periods, medical help should be sought to exclude underlying problems
- May be light bleeding between periods, but as above, if this persists medical help should be sought

Periods can cause a range of symptoms, but the severity will vary greatly from individual to individual:

- May be headache of varying intensity, linked to a woman's hormone cycle
- Breasts may noticeably change in size during the cycle and may be tender to touch
- May be fluid retention, starting a few days before menstruation, causing several parts of the body,

such as the ankles, breasts and abdomen, to become swollen. This should only last for a couple of days

- May be Carpal Tunnel Syndrome, caused by fluid retention affecting the nerves in the wrist
- Hands may look swollen for the same reason
- May be mood changes such as Depression and irritability
- May be fatigue
- May be abdominal and back pain, linked to a woman's hormone cycle, either associated with periods (dysmenorrhoea) or with ovulation (mittelschmerz). Pain, varying in severity from individual to individual, starts around a day before menstruation begins, and is often worse in younger women. The pain lasts a couple of days

Heavy periods, although again what constitutes a heavy period varies from individual to individual, may be a problem, although there may be no obvious underlying cause:

- Large amount of blood which floods
- May last for more than a week
- May be clots of blood
- May be Anaemia from loss of blood, signs including pallor, fatigue and lethargy
- If combined with symptoms such as a missed period, tender breasts, nausea, lower abdominal pain and heavy bleeding with jelly-like material, this may be a miscarriage

Foreign Body in Vagina – it is possible that a tampon or other item may get lodged inside the vagina, or it is possible that a tampon is used for too long:

- Discharge from the vagina, yellow or green in colour, which becomes more copious
- Unpleasant smell

- May be fever
- In extreme cases, may be Toxic Shock Syndrome, with a very high fever, low blood pressure, a rash, eye infection, diarrhoea, aching muscles, and problems with the kidneys. In a few cases, it may be fatal. This is usually caused by not changing a tampon soon enough, so care should be taken

> NOTE
> Some women my need to seek medical help for various problems with periods, such as heavy bleeding, miscarriage or irregular periods; and especially with Toxic Shock Syndrome.

CROSS-REFERENCED UNDER:
Periods; Toxic Shock Syndrome

Mesenteric Adenitis

Glands in the stomach become swollen, caused in most cases by a virus. May be confused with Appendicitis, especially in children.

SYMPTOMS & SIGNS

- Symptoms of the Common Cold
- Fever
- Nausea and vomiting
- Pain experienced in the lower part of the abdomen on the right side, along with tenderness to the touch
- May be pain throughout the abdomen

NOTE
Will probably resolve itself, but often confused with appendicitis in children. This may only be discovered after surgery.

Mesenteric Vascular Occlusion

Blood supply to part of the intestine is interrupted, caused by a blockage in a blood vessel.

SYMPTOMS & SIGNS

- Severe, persistent pain in the abdomen, with a sudden onset
- Peritonitis
- Abdomen may be swollen
- Blood in faeces
- Vomiting
- Shock
- Drowsiness

NOTE
Medical help should be sought immediately, typically requires surgery.

Metastasis

Secondary cancers, result from spread of a primary cancerous tumour. They may be located anywhere in the body but commonly in the liver, lungs and bones. Normally the cancer will already be obvious before secondary cancers appear.

SYMPTOMS & SIGNS

- May appear as hard fleshy nodules in the skin
- May be hard to the touch
- May appear singly or in groups
- Bone pain due to spread to the bones
- Jaundice due to spread to and damage to the liver
- Cough and shortness of breath due to spread to lungs
- Headache, personality change and paralysis if spread to the brain

NOTE
Medical help should be sought immediately.

CROSS-REFERENCED UNDER:
Secondary Cancer

Methyl Alcohol

Methyl Alcohol is sometimes consumed rather than normal drink. This is far more dangerous than ordinary alcohol, and may cause many problems including blindness.

SYMPTOMS & SIGNS

- Blindness in one or both eyes
- Sudden onset
- May be permanent
- Other problems

NOTE
Methyl Alcohol should simply not be consumed.

Middle Ear Infection

see EAR INFECTION

Migraine

Migraines are headaches that typically affect one side of the head (but sometimes both). They are characterised by a range of symptoms such as visual disturbance and sensitivity to light, tingling in parts of the body and vomiting. The cause is not clear, although fluctuations in the blood flow in the small blood vessels around the brain are included. Triggers may be bright light, cold, low blood sugar, stress or certain foods such as chocolate, cheese, yoghurt, meat, yeast extracts or red wine.

SYMPTOMS & SIGNS

- Visual disturbance at onset of migraine, usually

only in one eye, including flashing or flickering lights, bright area or patch of light, or patchy loss of the field of vision
- May be blindness on one side
- Reversible numbness, tingling or weakness in one limb or lip, localised to one side of the body
- May be slurred speech
- These symptoms will usually resolve relatively quickly, then
- Pain, possibly very severe, originally localised to one side of the head, although may be experienced more widely as migraine progresses
- May be severe vomiting
- May be facial pain, only affecting one side of the face and severe in nature.
- Desire to avoid bright light

NOTE
Onset of migraines is often in adolescence. Migraines will normally last up to 12 hours, although they can last for some days. Medication is available to prevent or alleviate the symptoms.

Miscarriage
see PREGNANCY

Mitral Stenosis
see MITRAL VALVE DISEASE

Mitral Valve Disease

Mitral valves in the heart do not function properly either because they become thickened and narrow or they become leaky. The body tissues become short of oxygen. The condition may be caused by Rheumatic Fever, which is not common in developed countries, or develops in old age. Mitral Stenosis may lead to Heart Failure if left untreated.

SYMPTOMS & SIGNS
- Shortness of breath, especially when lying flat
- Irregular heart beat
- Face looks red and flushed, particularly below the eyes, where there will be dilated veins
- May be purple flush over the cheek bones
- Progressive heart failure
- Heart murmur
- Lungs become congested
- Ankles become swollen
- May cough up blood
- May be Bronchitis

NOTE
Medical help should be sought immediately. A history of Rheumatic Fever increases the likelihood of Mitral Stenosis.

CROSS-REFERENCED UNDER:
Mitral Stenosis

Mole

Moles and freckles are small pigmented areas, which can be either black or brown in colour, found anywhere on the body including very unusually on the whites of the eyes. It is also common for them to have hairs growing from them. Moles do not change darkness if exposed to sunlight, while freckles will become darker.

SYMPTOMS & SIGNS
- Small areas of the skin which are pigmented, and either brown or black in colour
- Freckles may become darker if exposed to sunlight and appear in groups
- Some individuals, particularly those with red hair, may have many, many freckles and they

can cover the whole of the body

- Cafe-Au-Lait Spots are like large freckles, and again they may be found singly or in groups. These may be associated with Neurofibromatosis.

> NOTE
> Not usually a cause for concern, although Skin Cancer is an increasing problem. Single moles that become inflamed or bleed or suddenly start growing should receive medical attention.

CROSS-REFERENCED UNDER:
Freckles; Cafe-Au-Lait Spots

Molluscum Contagiosum

Numerous lumps on the skin, caused by a virus, which are harmless, but contagious.

SYMPTOMS & SIGNS
- Groups of small lumps, pink in colour, with a small depression in the middle
- Most likely on the trunk or face but can be on the limbs

> NOTE
> Will usually resolve without treatment.

Mongolian Blue Spot

Blue or black areas on the skin.

SYMPTOMS & SIGNS
- A blue or black area of skin, sometimes very small

> NOTE
> Most usually found in Asian children.

CROSS-REFERENCED UNDER:
Blue Naevus

Morphoea

Autoimmune problem in the body.

SYMPTOMS & SIGNS
- Localised or widespread patches of thickened skin, which are well defined
- Skin is hard and smooth on these areas
- Hair may be lost from the affected area
- May be ulceration of affected area

> NOTE
> Medical help should be sought.

Morton's Metatarsalgia

Pain in the forefoot, caused by problems with a nerve.

SYMPTOMS & SIGNS
- Pain in the foot, exacerbated by squeezing it
- Pain also in the toes

> NOTE
> Most likely in older individuals, and may require surgery.

Motion Sickness

see TRAVEL SICKNESS

Motor Neurone Disease

Typically, rapidly progressive nervous condition with increasing muscle wasting and weakness. The onset may be heralded by problems with the muscles in the hands, but eventually affects speech, swallowing and breathing. This is a particularly unpleasant and unrelenting condition.

SYMPTOMS & SIGNS
- Slow but persistent muscle bulk loss and reduction in strength and stamina resulting in paralysis
- Rippling contractions of muscles even when at rest
- Face may become paralysed because of muscle weakness
- Swallowing difficulties caused by poor control of the tongue and may appear to be too much saliva
- May inhale food or liquid into the lungs
- Speech may be slurred or unclear
- Slow but persistent weight loss

NOTE
Medical help should be sought although there is no cure.

Mountain Sickness

Potentially severe condition caused by being at an altitude of 8,000 feet or higher, where the air is thinner. Acclimatisation is likely over time, but rapid ascent is particularly risky, even for the fit and healthy. This condition is impossible to develop at low altitudes, while it is highly likely at high ones.

SYMPTOMS & SIGNS
- Headache
- Poor sleep
- Fatigue, even with slight exertion
- May be nausea, vomiting and loss of appetite
- Breathlessness, which is exacerbated by over breathing: steady relaxed breathing may help
- May be confusion

- May develop into coma and even cause death

NOTE
This condition will be helped by descending as quickly as possible, and over time the body will become acclimatised.

CROSS-REFERENCED UNDER:
Soroche; Altitude Sickness

Mouth Breathing

Constant breathing through the mouth, rather than through the nose, can dry out the saliva in the mouth and cause bad breath. Several conditions can cause mouth breathing, including Hay Fever, Nasal Polyps, a broken nose or even snoring.

SYMPTOMS & SIGNS
- Bad breath
- Difficulty breathing through the nose
- No other symptoms

NOTE
Not usually a cause for concern unless there is an injury such as a broken nose.

Mouth Ulcer
see APHTHOUS ULCER

Mucocele

One of the small glands on the inner lip can become blocked.

SYMPTOMS & SIGNS
- Lump appears on the lip with a sudden onset
- Lump is bluish and translucent
- No pain

> **NOTE**
> May resolve suddenly and does not usually last more than a couple of days.

CROSS-REFERENCED UNDER:
Retention Cyst

Multiple Sclerosis

Typically, but not invariably, progressive, at times severe, condition in which the nerves degenerate because of inflammation. The cause is not known. Typically neurological problems wax and wane. A large range of symptoms can be present, including weakness, unsteadiness, problems with urination, double or impaired vision, altered sensation in limbs or body, and progressive weight loss.

SYMPTOMS & SIGNS
- Impaired, blurred, loss of, or double vision
- May be blindness in one eye, with a rapid onset, as well as pain
- Eyes may have twitching movements in advanced cases of the disease
- Limbs may have altered sensation with weakness, numbness, tingling, heaviness or spasms
- Unsteady on feet
- Tremor
- Slow but increasing paralysis
- May be Horner's Syndrome: one pupil of the eye may be unusually small with drooping of the eyelid and a bulging eye
- Problems with urinating: incontinence or retention or urine are both possible, along with hesitancy in beginning urination or increased frequency
- Speech may be unclear or slurred

- Difficulty when swallowing and may appear to be too much saliva
- May regurgitate food into chest
- May be ulcerated or infected feet
- Slow but persistent weight loss

> **NOTE**
> Most likely to develop in young adults between the teens and the middle 30s. There is no cure, but symptoms may be alleviated.

Mumps

Inflammation of the parotid glands (salivary glands located in front of and below the ear), which is caused by a virus.

SYMPTOMS & SIGNS
- Fever with chills and rigors
- Headache, muscle aches and loss of appetite
- Within about two days, both parotid glands are swollen (the lymph glands can be mistaken for these glands)
- May be difficult to open the mouth because of the swelling
- In adults, the pancreas and testes may also be affected
- Testicles, either one or both, may become swollen and sore (orchitis). This may affect fertility
- Other complications may be inflammation of the ovary, breast, pancreas, brain and Meningitis
- Rarely Mumps may cause deafness

> **NOTE**
> The condition will usually resolve within one to two weeks, although there is no cure. There is a routine vaccination.

CROSS-REFERENCED UNDER:
Infectious Parotitis

Muscle Cramp

Spasm in a muscle, causing it to become hard and extremely painful, usually occurring during sleep or excessive exercise.

SYMPTOMS & SIGNS
- Spasm or cramp in muscle, usually the calf muscle, making it a hard mass
- Pain may be severe
- Resolves but is helped by massage and stretching
- May be some residual ache and pain

> NOTE
> Not usually a sign of an underlying disease.

CROSS-REFERENCED UNDER:
Cramp

Muscle Damage
see MUSCLE INJURY

Muscle Injury

When an individual damages a joint or muscle, causing pain, inflammation or bruising, it is difficult or impossible to move that part of the body. Muscle loss, wastage and reduction in stamina can occur remarkably quickly when parts of the body are not exercised. If an injury is incapacitating, it is necessary to do as much exercise as possible without aggravating any injury.

SYMPTOMS & SIGNS
- Damage to a joint or muscle, making movement difficult or impossible

- Pain
- Similar action or movement which caused the injury aggravates it further
- If incapacitated for any length of time, related muscles lose strength, stamina and bulk within a week or so

> NOTE
> Most injuries will resolve with time.

CROSS-REFERENCED UNDER:
Muscle Damage

Muscular Dystrophy

Genetic conditions which are characterised by progressive muscle disease and wasting, probably as a result of a fault in the chemistry within the muscle. Some forms are very severe and are life threatening at a young age.

SYMPTOMS & SIGNS
- Wasting of muscles
- Reduction in strength and stamina
- Onset is in the back and pelvis
- Waddling gait
- Degeneration is progressive and relentless, causing immobility, incapacitation and deformity
- Different types range in severity, and the earlier the symptoms develop the more severe will be the illness
- Curvation of spine.

> NOTE
> Medical help should be sought although there is no cure. The most severe type, Duchenne's Dystrophy, only affects boys, but may be passed on to their children by girls.

305

CROSS-REFERENCED UNDER:
Duchenne's Dystrophy

Myasthenia Gravis

Severe condition characterised by progressive muscle fatigue and weakness with continued use of muscles especially affecting the eyelids, eyes and limbs.

SYMPTOMS & SIGNS
- Muscle fatigue and weakness that progresses with use of muscles
- Double vision
- Both eyes or eyelids are affected
- Eyelids droop
- Weak and hoarse voice
- Swallowing difficulties
- May be accompanied by weight loss
- Progressive weakness of limb muscles

> NOTE
> The condition may be treated but tests need to be undertaken to confirm a diagnosis.

Myelofibrosis

Fibrous tissue forms within the cavity where bone marrow is formed. It interferes with the creation of white blood cells, and may be associated with other conditions such as leukaemia and cancer.

SYMPTOMS & SIGNS
- Anaemia
- Weakness and severe fatigue
- Night sweats
- Gout
- Spleen is very enlarged and is felt as a mass below the rib cage on the left hand side of the abdomen.
- Liver usually very enlarged
- Severe bone and joint pain

> NOTE
> Medical help should be sought.

Myeloid Leukaemia

see LEUKAEMIA

Myocarditis

Serious conditions characterised by inflammation of the heart muscle usually caused by infections and viral infections including viral and bacterial infections. Occasionally associated with diseases causing vasculitis including systemic lupus erythematosis.

SYMPTOMS & SIGNS
- Feverish illness with sudden onset
- Breathlessness, especially when lying flat
- Ankles swollen
- Fatigue
- Altered heart rhythm including fast heart rate (tacycarda)
- May compromise heart function leading to heart failure and shock

> NOTE
> Tests will be needed to confirm a diagnosis.

Myxoedema

Generalised swelling of the body especially around the face and eyes and limbs, including the hands. Caused by underactive thyroid gland (Hypothyroidism).

SYMPTOMS SIGNS AND CONDITIONS

SYMPTOMS & SIGNS
- Generalised swelling of body – especially face and limbs
- Skin hs a pale waxy appearance
- Limbs and eyes are swollen, and skin looks puffy about these areas.
- Dry skin
- Features of hypothyroidism including: low body temperature
- Very gruff and deep voice
- Movements are slow
- Slow mentally
- May be Carpal Tunnel Syndrome
- Progressive tiredness

NOTE
Medical help should be sought.

Narcolepsy

Rare inherited condition where the individual suddenly becomes very drowsy and falls into a deep sleep without warning. In rare cases, this has been mistaken for death.

SYMPTOMS & SIGNS
- Sudden onset of drowsiness
- Individual falls into a deep sleep
- Cannot be woken

NOTE
The condition runs in families and can be managed with amphetamines.

Narcotics
see ALCOHOL OR NARCOTICS

Nasal Polyps

Fleshy growths in the nose, which are usually benign, and may be visible. They have been linked to allergies, and those individuals who suffer from Allergic Rhinitis may be particularly prone to polyps.

SYMPTOMS & SIGNS
- May cause an obstruction in the nose, and the nose will feel as if it is constantly blocked
- May be production of clear discharge from nose
- Loss of smell
- Speech may be muffled or nasal
- May be nosebleeds

NOTE
Surgery may be needed to remove the polyp should it become a problem, although they can recur even after removal.

CROSS-REFERENCED UNDER:
Benign Tumours of the Nose

Nasal Septal Necrosis

Damage to the cartilage in the nose (nasal septum). One cause is the inhalation of cocaine over long periods.

SYMPTOMS & SIGNS
- Pain at the end of the nose
- End of the nose is wider
- Reduced or absent sensation on the skin of the nose
- Headache
- Cartilage deteriorates over time: bridge flattens and a hole develops that links the two nostrils

NOTE
Medical help should be sought.

Nephritic Cancer

see CANCER OF THE KIDNEY

Nephritis

see KIDNEY DISEASE OR FAILURE

Nephrotic Syndrome

Build up of fluid throughout the body, caused by Kidney problems in which excessive amounts of protein leak from damaged kidneys. Associated with many forms of kidney inflammation (glomerulonephritis) or occaionally with other conditions such as diabetes mellitus

SYMPTOMS & SIGNS

- Gradual onset and progresive
- Parts of the body become swollen with fluid, including the ankles, face and abdomen
- Breathlessness

NOTE
Medical help should be sought immediately. Most likely in male infants around two years of age.

Nerve Disease

see NERVE INJURY

Nerve Injury

Damage or injury to nerves can occur. One common example is pressure neuropathy, where pressure is put upon a nerve when sleeping in an awkward position. Nerves often affected are those of the upper arm, elbow and by the knee.

SYMPTOMS & SIGNS
When waking:

- Numbness in affected area
- Loss of movement or function in affected area

Then:

- Sensation returns
- Tingling, then pins and needles and pain
- Normal function and movement returns

Long-term nerve injury:

- Muscle wastage and reduction in strength and stamina

NOTE
Pressure neuropathy will usually resolve within a short time, but it may take some time for full function to return.

CROSS-REFERENCED UNDER:
Nerve Disease; Pressure Neuropathy

Nerve Irritation in Chest

Nerves can become irritated between the ribs and cause a considerable amount of pain.

SYMPTOMS & SIGNS

- Stabbing pain in the chest, which goes round from the back to the front
- Moving exacerbates pain
- No associated breathless or sweating (except from the sharp pain)
- Pain comes and goes
- May be tenderness at a site on the chest
- No other symptoms

NOTE
Although this condition may be distressing, it is usually not a sign of any underlying problem and will resolve with rest and painkillers. Investigations may be necessary, however, to exclude and other problem.

Nerve Palsies of the Eye

Paralysis of certain nerves controlling the eyes can result in problems with the eye, including double vision, inability to move an eye in some or all directions and can result in squint.

SYMPTOMS & SIGNS
- Double vision
- Squint appears, eye most commonly points down and out but can be turned inwards
- Typically sudden onset
- Eyelid may droop
- Size of the pupil of the eye may change

NOTE
Medical help should be sought.

Neuralgia, Trigeminal

see TRIGEMINAL NEURALGIA

Nicotine

see CIGARETTES

Nits

see LICE

Nodular Prurigo

Areas of warts, which may have been spread by scratching.

SYMPTOMS & SIGNS
- Areas of groups of warts
- Areas are extremely itchy

NOTE
Warts may be treated although they are harmless.

Non-Specific Urethritis (NSU)

Inflammation of urethra (tube which takes urine from the bladder), usually caused an infection from sexual contact and the organism Chlamydia. Although there may be no or few symptoms, this can be especially serious in women, causing infection in the womb and Fallopian tubes, and even infertility.

SYMPTOMS & SIGNS
In women:
- May be no symptoms
- Burning pain when urinating
- May be discharge from the vagina
- Can infect the womb (uterus) and Fallopian tubes, and even cause infertility
In men:
- May be no symptoms
- Pain, discomfort or itchiness when urinating
- Creamy or yellow discharge from the penis

NOTE
Medical help should be sought. Both partners should seek treatment, even if one of them shows no symptoms.

Non-Specific Urethritis (NSU)

also see CHLAMYDIA

Non-Specific Urethritis (NSU)

also see URINARY TRACT INFECTION

Nose Cancer

see CANCER OF THE NOSE

Nose Picking

see PICKING NOSE

Nystagmus

Twitching movement of the eyes, which may have no obvious cause, although it can be caused by conditions such as damage to the balance centre (cerebellum) through Alcoholism, Multiple Sclerosis, Brain Tumours, or occur as a result of Congenital Blindness or Poor Vision, particularly if the latter is left uncorrected.

SYMPTOMS & SIGNS
■ Twitching movement of the eyes usually from side to side but occasionally in an up and down direction

NOTE
Can be a sign of a serious disease.

Obstruction of the Intestine

see INTESTINAL OBSTRUCTION

Occupational Asthma

see ASTHMA

Ochronosis

Discoloration of cartilage beneath the skin, which can appear blue or blackish-blue. It can affect the whites of the eyes, and is caused by an abnormality in body chemistry.

SYMPTOMS & SIGNS
■ Any area of the body where cartilage is found can appear blue or blackish-blue
■ Whites of the eyes may be discoloured

NOTE
Not serious. Does not do any harm.

Oesophageal Cancer

see CANCER OF THE OESOPHAGUS

Oesophageal Spasm

Spasm of the muscles of the gullet, which may be caused by eating or by some kind of shock or emotional trauma.

SYMPTOMS & SIGNS
■ Difficulty when swallowing
■ Pain may be mild or very severe, is felt in chest and may radiate to back or elsewhere

NOTE
Will usually resolve, although tests may be needed to exclude any problems.

Oesophageal Stricture

see PEPTIC OR OESOPHAGEAL STRICTURE

Oesophageal Varices

Distended veins at the lower end of the oesophagus. This can cause vomiting of blood, and loss of blood can be so serious that the condition can be fatal. It may be associated with Cirrhosis of the Liver.

SYMPTOMS & SIGNS
■ Vomiting, with fresh bright red blood or old blood which may look like coffee grounds
■ May be blood coming from the rectum or faeces may be very dark and tar-like, caused by blood

NOTE
Medical help should be sought immediately.

Oesophagitis

Acid and stomach contents are regurgitated into the gullet, throat and mouth. Associated pain, including heartburn may be mistaken for a heart attack.

SYMPTOMS & SIGNS

- Burning pain when swallowing, often behind the breast bone
- Heartburn
- Pain in the centre of the chest, either at the front or back, and occasionally down the arms (this is more common however with angina, heart pain)
- Stomach contents regurgitated into the throat and mouth
- Acid or bitter taste in the mouth
- Made worse when hot or spicy foods, such as curries, are eaten or when alcohol is consumed
- May be vomiting, with blood, if severe
- May be blood in faeces, making them dark and tar-like
- May be anaemia because of blood loss
- May be long-term weight loss

NOTE
Relieved by antacids, although if persists help should be sought. If a heart attack is suspected, however, medical help should be sought immediately.

Optic Neuritis

Inflammation of the optic nerve, which may be associated with Multiple Sclerosis, although other causes may be Syphilis, Diabetes or deficiency in Vitamin B.

SYMPTOMS & SIGNS

- Blindness in one eye, although this usually does not affect peripheral vision
- Sudden onset
- Pain in or around the eye

NOTE
Most common in adolescents and young adults. Will usually resolve after several days. Requires medical attention.

Orbital Cellulitis

Progressive infection around the eyelid.

SYMPTOMS & SIGNS

- Only affects one eye
- May be centred around a Stye or scratch
- Eyelid becomes extremely swollen, making it impossible to open the affected eye
- Eyelid is red and tender
- May be fever and general feeling of ill-health

NOTE
Medical help should be sought immediately to prevent it spreading further. Treatment is with antibiotics.

Orchitis

Testicle becomes swollen and inflamed, caused by infection, injury or as a complication of Mumps.

SYMPTOMS & SIGNS

- Starts with an ache, but severity of pain builds up over time
- Scrotum may also become swollen

NOTE
Medical help should be sought as soon as possible.

Osgood Schlatter's Disease

see UPPER TIBIAL EPIPHYSIS AND APOPHYSIS

Osteitis Deformans

see PAGET'S DISEASE

Osteoarthritis

Deterioration of joints caused by normal wear and tear, often affecting the weight-bearing joints, such as the lower spine, hips and knee, but any joint can be affected.

SYMPTOMS & SIGNS
- Bone and joint pain, usually mild in nature, but often very progressive
- Movement of the joint is restricted
- Swollen joints with nodules, such as the joints between the fingers becoming large and knobbly (Heberden's nodes)
- Using the joint, such as during exercise, exacerbates the pain
- Loose bodies in the joint
- Often subsides with rest, although not always, and eventually may be pain at all times, even disturbing sleep

> NOTE
> Most likely in older individuals. Painkillers and physiotherapy can reduce symptoms. If severely limits activities osteoarthritis of hip or knee may require joint replacement

CROSS-REFERENCED UNDER:
Arthritis (Osteoarthritis)

Osteogenesis Imperfecta Congenita

see BRITTLE BONE DISEASE

Osteogenesis Imperfecta Tarda

see BRITTLE BONE DISEASE

Osteomalacia

see VITAMIN D (CALCIFEROL) DEFICIENCY

Osteomyelitis

Infection of bone, usually caused by spread from elsewhere in the body.

SYMPTOMS & SIGNS
- Bone pain and inflammation, although the latter may not be obvious
- Pain exacerbated by movement
- Swelling and redness of associated soft tissues
- Sudden chills and shivering
- Severe fever
- General feeling of ill health
- Affected bone can collapse or fracture

If not treated or where caused by penetrating trauma and bone injury:
- Bone becomes thicker
- Pain and inflammation at wound
- Pus

> NOTE
> Medical help should be sought immediately.

Osteopetrosis

Bones become hard and brittle, increasing the chance of breaks and fractures. It is caused by an inherited disorder.

SYMPTOMS & SIGNS
- Bones are prone to fractures and breaks
- Growth may be affected

CROSS-REFERENCED UNDER:
Marble Bones

Osteoporosis

Thinning and weakening of bone, usually as the individual gets older, that leads to increased risk of fracture (breaking) because the bones are more fragile. Can affect any bone; when present usually affects all bones. The occurrence of a fracture, most commonly of the wrist, may be the first sign that osteoporosis is present.

SYMPTOMS & SIGNS

- Bones more likely to break or fracture; any bone can be affected
- Most serious, common break, usually caused by a fall, is of the neck of the thigh bone (femur), causing pain, inability to put weight on the affected leg, and the foot being turned outwards
- Individual may become shorter over time as the spine compacts due to fracture of vertebrae in the spine (kyphosis)
- Bone pain or chronic back pain
- Fracture of bone associated with higher risk of having other fractures at other sites

NOTE
Most likely in post-menopausal women especially if the menopause occurs early. Hormone Replacement Therapy (HRT) may prevent the condition. Associated with hormone deficiency in men. Commoner in people treated with steroids and with a range of other conditions including Coelic disease, Overactive Thyroid, Rheumatoid Arthritis and Inflammatory Bowel Disease. Low trauma fractures in women and men over 50 years should stimulate medical assessment for osteoporosis.

Otitis Externa

Dermatitis within the ear canal: this part of the body is as prone to this condition as any other. It may be triggered by chlorine or other chemicals from swimming pools, and things being thrust into the ear, such as cotton buds or pencils. The condition can be made much worse by opportunistic infection such as a fungus.

SYMPTOMS & SIGNS

- Inside of ear is itchy
- Feeling of pressure in the ear
- Skin of the ear is inflamed and flaky
- Thin discharge from ear, watery in viscosity, but persistent
- If the ear becomes infected, the discharge is much thicker and there may be black spores

NOTE
May resolve, but if infection occurs may need medication such as antifungal preparations.

CROSS-REFERENCED UNDER:
Fungal Infection of the Ear

Otitis Media
see EAR INFECTION

Otosclerosis

Problems with the bones in the ear.

SYMPTOMS & SIGNS

- Progressive hearing impairment and deafness
- Ringing in ears (tinnitus)
- Giddiness and vertigo

Ovarian Cancer

see CANCER OF THE OVARIES

Ovarian Cyst

A cyst, sometimes very large in size, may form on an ovary.

SYMPTOMS & SIGNS

- Swollen abdomen if cyst is very large
- May be prominent blood vessels in the abdomen
- Heavy periods and bleeding

NOTE

Typically benign but can be associated with increased risk of cancer. Will require tests to confirm and will probably need surgery. Can appear to be Appendicitis if it is a cyst on the right ovary.

Overactive Thyroid Gland

see HYPERTHYROIDISM

Over Breathing

see HYPERVENTILATION

PKU (Phenylketonuria)

see PHENYLKETONURIA (PKU)

Paget's Disease

Condition of bone in which the normal preocesses of removal of older bone and replacement with newer bone occur excessively and in an uncoordinated way.

Can affect single or multiple bones. Bones can be enlarged but are often weaker and may bend; they are more likely to fracture.

SYMPTOMS & SIGNS

- May be no symptoms
- If long bones in limbs are affected these may bend and become deformed. Sometimes if excessive the deformity can be crippling
- Pain at affected sites, often at night
- Head may enlarge if the skull is affected
- Collapse of vertebrae leading to height loss or rarely spinal cord compression
- Prone to fractures and breaks
- Problems with the nervous system due to pressure on nerves or occasionally the spinal cord
- May be hearing loss, deafness and ringing in the ears, particularly in later life, caused by enlarged bone pressing on the nerve associated with hearing
- May be blindness, caused by bones pressing on the optic nerve
- Very rarely sarcoma of the affected bones
- If severe and affecting many bones, can lead to heart failure

NOTE

Medical help should be sought if causes symptoms. Tests may be needed to confirm a diagnosis.

CROSS-REFERENCED UNDER:

Osteitis Deformans

Paget's Disease of the Nipple

Inflammation and redness of the nipple or the pink

area surrounding it (areola), which appears to be similar to Dermatitis.

SYMPTOMS & SIGNS

- Nipple and areola are inflamed and red
- Skin of the nipple and areola can be scaly
- A lump may be felt
- Bloody discharge from the nipple

> NOTE
> Often a sign of breast cancer, although it may be entirely innocent. Medical help should be sought immediately to exclude cancer.

Painful Arc Syndrome (Shoulder)

Pain and restricted movement in the shoulder as it is being rotated.

SYMPTOMS & SIGNS

- Pain, which comes and goes, at the tip of the shoulder, often worse during the night
- Tender area localised to one area of the shoulder
- Pain exacerbated by rotating the shoulder through moving the arm: usually one part of the arc causes possibly very severe pain when reached
- Restricted shoulder movement

> NOTE
> Most likely in older individuals. Exercise to strengthen muscles and physiotherapy may help.

Pancreatic Cancer

see CANCER OF THE PANCREAS

Pancreatitis

Inflammation of the pancreas. The pancreas can produce enzymes which can digest other organs and tissues. Although the condition can be mild, it can also be severe and even life threatening. A cyst, sometimes large and detectable, can form on the pancreas.

SYMPTOMS & SIGNS

- Persistent pain in the middle of the abdomen, which may be also be felt round the back. This may have a sudden onset, and may resemble heartburn. Pain may be exacerbated by eating and drinking. This pain may also radiate into the chest and back
- Vomiting, usually of undigested food
- Faeces may be pale, loose and copious, as well as being greasy or fatty. This latter sign is caused because of poor digestion caused by a lack of enzymes from the pancreas
- May be prominent blood vessels in the abdomen
- Generally feeling ill
- May be slight jaundice, which becomes apparent after a couple of days, along with pale faeces and dark urine
- May be extreme itchiness
- May be bruising or discoloration around the tummy button (umbilicus)
- May be fever
- May be collapse
- Mass may be discernible in the middle of the abdomen as a large cyst can form on the pancreas

If chronic:

- Weight loss: progressive and persistent
- Diabetes will develop, as insulin from the pancreas is no longer produced
- Severe, chronic or recurrent abdominal and back pain

> NOTE
> Individuals at risk include those who drink excessive amounts of alcohol or have a history of problems with their gall bladder and gallstones. Medical help should be sought immediately as it is potentially fatal.

Papilloma

see WARTS

Paraphimosis

Foreskin becomes stuck after being rolled back.

SYMPTOMS & SIGNS
- Pain
- Foreskin cannot roll back over the end of the penis

> NOTE
> Medical help should be sought as surgery may be needed.

Paratyphoid

see TYPHOID FEVER

Parkinson's Disease

Progressive neurological condition which is characterised by a loss of facial expression, a shuffling walk, trembling limbs, and 'pill-rolling' movements of the fingers.

SYMPTOMS & SIGNS
- Shaking and trembling particularly at rest; hands have a characteristic 'pill-rolling' tremor in the hands
- Muscle stiffness with difficulty starting movement
- Face may appear to be expressionless
- Handwriting may become progressively smaller
- Stooped posture and stiff gait: may have trouble walking
- Speech may be muffled or unclear
- Difficulty in starting to swallow
- May be occasional choking and may appear to be too much saliva
- Weight loss
- May be fainting when rising to the feet, caused by a drop in blood pressure (postural hypotension)

> NOTE
> Usually a condition which affects older people, but may affect younger people, and may be caused by certain drugs used for psychiatric disorders. The disease may be controlled, but not cured, by drugs.

Paronychia

see INJURY TO THE NAILS

Paroxysmal Tachycardia

Rapid heart rate with no obvious disease of the heart.

SYMPTOMS & SIGNS
- Quick onset of rapid heart rate
- Rhythm of the heart usually remains regular
- Extremely rapid heart rate, which may cause feelings of light-headedness or may cause fainting
- May stop as suddenly as it began
  If the person is prone to angina, Paroxysmal Tachycardia may proke it
- If the attack is prolonged, may cause breathlessness as the muscle of the heart

becomes exhausted. This may require medical or surgical intervention

> NOTE
> May cause anxiety and distress, and often will need investigation to confirm there is no underlying illness.

Pellagra

see VITAMIN B3 (NIACIN) DEFICIENCY

Pelvic Infection

see PELVIC INFLAMMATORY DISEASE

Pelvic Inflammatory Disease

Infection of the genital tract in women, which may have been caused by a sexually transmitted infection or a coil (an intra-uterine contraceptive coil (IUCD)).

SYMPTOMS & SIGNS
- Abdominal and low back pain, which can range in severity from mild to excruciating
- May be no pain
- Sexual intercourse may be painful
- Heavy and painful menstruation
- Discharge from the vagina, which can be yellow, green or even brown in colour
- Discharge may smell unpleasant
- Itchiness, tenderness and pain
- May be fever
- May be vomiting
- May be infertility

> NOTE
> Medical help should be sought as leaving the condition untreated may lead to infertility.

CROSS-REFERENCED UNDER:
Pelvic Infection

Pelvic Injury

see INJURY TO THE LOWER CHEST OR PELVIS

Pemphigus Vulgaris

Skin disease with resultant blistering and possible secondary infections.

SYMPTOMS & SIGNS
- Fluid-filled blisters on the skin around the face, scalp and chest or in the mouth, which blister and can leave large raw and red areas.
- The blister can burst, even if only subjected to small amounts of force, and then crust over and form scabs
- Pain is present wuth the blister but usually lessens when the blister bursts
- The ulcers left after the blisters burst can become infected

> NOTE
> Most likely in older people, between the ages of 40 and 60. Treatment by steroids and antibiotics should improve the condition without curing it.

Peptic Ulcer

An ulcer, either in the stomach or, more commonly, the duodenum. Symptoms may vary from person to person. For example, many individuals loss their appetite for food, while others may actually eat more to reduce discomfort from stomach acid.

SYMPTOMS & SIGNS
- Pain, intermittent in nature but recurrent usually in middle of upper abdomen or behind lower

chest. Occasionally felt also in the back. May last several days or even a couple of weeks.

■ Pain may be eased or exacerbated by eating: certain foods may make things considerably worse. May also be bad at night, sufficiently so to wake from sleeping

■ May be heartburn

■ Vomiting. May start with normal partly or undigested food, but later will become greener, less viscous with mucous and slime. Blood may also be present, appearing as brown staining or 'coffee grounds': should this be the case medical help should be sought immediately

■ If bleeding is persistent, can cause anaemia

■ May be black and tarry faeces (blood turns black by the action of the gastrointestinal tract) if the ulcer is bleeding

■ May be collapse caused by severe blood loss

■ Weight loss with loss of appetite

NOTE
Most likely in smokers and those habitually using painkillers such as aspirin, although family history also plays a part. Ulcers can be treated with antacids and increasingly with antibiotics.

CROSS-REFERENCED UNDER:
Stomach Ulcer; Ulcer, Peptic

Peptic or Oesophageal Stricture

Gullet becomes narrower because of persistent reflux Oesophagitis.

SYMPTOMS & SIGNS
■ Heartburn
■ Food regurgitated along with stomach contents
■ Food sticks on swallowing especially solids. May

be associated chest pain
■ Associated with weight loss if persists
■ Also associated with Chest Infections
■ May be associated with Hiatus Hernia

NOTE
The sufferer may have a long history of reflux oesophagitis. It can also be caused by the swallowing of toxic chemicals, either accidentally or deliberately. Requires medical attention.

CROSS-REFERENCED UNDER:
Oesophageal Stricture

Perforated Viscus

If gastrointestinal organs (stomach, bowel, colon or appendix) are damaged or inflamed, they can burst and leak stomach or bowel contents into the abdominal cavity. These bowel contents are full of bacteria which can cause inflammation of the abdominal cavity (peritonitis). Stomach ulcers, the appendix and diverticula can all rupture.

SYMPTOMS & SIGNS
■ Sudden and severe pain
■ Fever
■ Abdomen is very tender to the touch
■ Abdominal wall muscles may appear rigid
■ Face may be pale and sweaty
■ Swollen abdomen may develop from the leakage of stomach and bowel contents
■ Shock

NOTE
Medical help should be sought immediately as may be fatal without an operation.

Pericardial Effusion

see PERICARDITIS

Pericarditis

Fluid collects around the heart after its lining becomes inflamed. May be caused by a Heart Attack, infection, tumours, Kidney Failure, injury, or auto-immune conditions – or there may be no obvious cause.

SYMPTOMS & SIGNS

- Shortness of breath when lying flat
- Prominent symmetrical veins in the neck
- Chest feels tight, although this varies with movement
- Progressive breathlessness as fluid collects
- Rapid and irregular heart beat
- Fever if the condition is caused by infection
- General feeling of being ill with loss of appetite
- Pain which is central in the chest and sharp in nature may be caused by initial Pericarditis: this can last for days
- Pain radiates to the shoulders
- Swelling of both legs

NOTE
Difficult to confirm without several tests, but if suspected, medical help should be sought immediately. The condition can usually be treated.

CROSS-REFERENCED UNDER:
Pericardial Effusion

Perichondritis

Inflammation of the outer ear, which may be caused by injury or a blow, or even by cold weather.

SYMPTOMS & SIGNS

- Severe pain in the outer ear
- Skin of the ear is red

NOTE
Will usually resolve by itself, but may need antibiotics in severe cases.

Periods

see MENSTRUATION

Peripheral Vascular Disease

Arteries harden and become progressively furred up and blocked. This causes Arteriosclerosis and reduced blood supply to parts of the body, especially the legs.

SYMPTOMS & SIGNS

- Limbs feel cold, especially the legs, and may become rapidly pale if lifted in the air
- Cramps and pain in calf muscles develop on walking (the more rapid onset of pain, the greater is the severity of the vascular disease). Resolves if individual rests
- Pain in feet at night – usually relieved by dangling leg from bed
- Altered sensation and numbness
- May be difficult to detect a pulse in some areas
- Ulcerated or infected feet

In severe cases an artery to a limb, usually the legs, can become completely blocked (medical help should be sought immediately or it may not be possible to save the limb and it may need amputated):

- Severe pain with sudden onset
- Limb quickly goes pale then blue
- Limb is paralysed

■ Limbs feels cold to the touch

> NOTE
> Most likely in older individuals and those who smoke. Medical help should be sought.

CROSS-REFERENCED UNDER:
Atheriosclerosis; Arterial Disease

Peritonitis

The peritoneum, a membrane which lines the abdomen, may become inflamed and irritated, caused by infection, injury and conditions such as Appendicitis, Pancreatitis, Diverticulitis, and a perforated Duodenal Ulcer.

SYMPTOMS & SIGNS
■ Severe abdominal pain
■ Abdomen feels rigid
■ Later, vomiting as the bowel ceases to move food down it
■ May develop serious illness and Shock if not treated

> NOTE
> Medical help should be sought immediately, and most individuals make a recovery.

Peritonsillar Abscess

Acute inflammation of the tonsil, and surrounding area, with the formation of an abscess. Symptoms are similar to Tonsillitis except there is also pain when opening the mouth.

SYMPTOMS & SIGNS
■ Pain when opening mouth caused by the abscess
■ Enlarged and inflamed tonsil, or more unusually tonsils
■ Reddened throat
■ Inflamed and tender lymph nodes in neck
■ May be difficult to open the mouth because of the swelling
■ Pain when swallowing
■ May appear to be too much saliva
■ Fever
■ May be an associated cough

> NOTE
> Will require surgical drainage.

CROSS-REFERENCED UNDER:
Quinsy

Pernicious Anaemia

Failure of the stomach to produce a certain substance to allow the absorption of vitamin B12. Vitamin B12 (cyanocobalamin) is responsible for the development of mature red blood cells, so deficiency leads to Anaemia. This condition may develop over a very long time, and not be noticed until severe. Can run in families. Can be associated with thyroid disorders.

SYMPTOMS & SIGNS
■ Progressive anaemia, perhaps over a long period
■ Pallor
■ Fatigue and easily tired and out of breath with any exercise
■ Feeling dizzy
■ Palpitations
■ Sore tongue
■ Mild jaundice
■ Tingling or numbness in limbs
■ Progressive weakness oflegs

- May be Heart Failure in some cases
- Poor memory, leading to dementia

> NOTE
> Medical help should be sought. Most likely in middle and old age. Although the condition cannot be reversed, it can be treated by giving (life-long) injections of the vitamin or a factor which allows the absorption of the vitamin.

CROSS-REFERENCED UNDER:
Anaemia, Pernicious

Perthes' Disease

Pain and restricted movement in the hip, caused by a loss of blood supply to the top of the thigh bone.

SYMPTOMS & SIGNS
- Pain or discomfort in hip, which comes and goes
- Restricted movement and limp during episodes of pain

> NOTE
> Most likely in children around seven years old. Medical help should be sought.

Pertussis

see WHOOPING COUGH

Pes Cavus

Arch of the foot is unusually raised, caused by problems with imbalance in strength of muscles and associated with Claw Toes. It is associated with Spina Bifida, Cerebral Palsy and Poliomyelitis.

SYMPTOMS & SIGNS
- Claw or curled toes
- Arch of foot is unusually high

- Hardened skin on weight-bearing areas
- Pain in the foot

CROSS-REFERENCED UNDER:
Claw Toes

Peyronie's Disease

Penis becomes curved because of a band of tissue forms on the shaft.

SYMPTOMS & SIGNS
- Erect penis is curved
- Pain

> NOTE
> Most likely in older men. There is no easy treatment, and it may resolve by itself.

Phaeochromocytoma

Excess secretion of adrenaline and related hormones, caused usually by a tumour of one or both adrenal glands or associated structures. Symptoms are caused by the over production of adrenaline and other associated hormones. Occasionally phaeochromocytoma can run in familes and can be associated with problems in other glands.

SYMPTOMS & SIGNS
- High blood pressure which can be intermittent. Occasionally the blood pressure cann be low particularly when steady
- Anxiety with sudden and severe onset
- Heavy sweating
- Palpitations
- Diarrhoea and abdominal pain
- Face looks pallid or flushed

■ Headache

> **NOTE**
> Medical help should be sought immediately as the tumour will require removal by surgery.

Pharyngeal Pouch

Pouch may develop on one side of the upper gullet. Food may gather in this pouch and it is the swelling that results or the emptying of its contents that lead to awareness of this.

SYMPTOMS & SIGNS
■ May cause difficulty when swallowing
■ Food can be regurgitated
■ Not painful but can become uncomfortable
■ May vary in size
■ Gets bigger during eating or drinking
■ May gurgle as it empties
■ May be emptied by putting pressure on the pouch

> **NOTE**
> Medical help should be sought.

Pharyngitis

Inflammation of the pharynx. The pharynx is a cavity in the mouth behind the tonsils and above the larynx (voice box) and oesophagus (gullet). Similar to Tonsillitis (but not affecting the tonsils). Commoner in smokers.

SYMPTOMS & SIGNS
■ Pain when swallowing
■ Back of throat reddened
■ Bad breath and unpleasant taste in mouth
■ May be enlarged lymph nodes

■ May be an increased production of saliva in the mouth
■ May be headache
■ May be fever

> **NOTE**
> Pharyngitis may result from an infection in those who have had their tonsils removed.

Phenylketonuria (PKU)

Accumulation of the harmful chemical, phenytatinine in the brain caused by an inherited error of metabolism.

SYMPTOMS & SIGNS
■ Blond hair
■ Blue eyes
■ Fair skin
■ Individual can be aggressive and suffer from progressive and severe mental deficiency, if not treated

> **NOTE**
> Babies are screened at birth, and those affected need to avoid food containing phenylalanine.

CROSS-REFERENCED UNDER:
PKU (Phenylketonuria)

Phimosis

Foreskin of the penis cannot be pulled back from the end of the penis. In young boys this is normal, and it should not be possible to do so, nor should it be attempted, until the age of five.

SYMPTOMS & SIGNS
It is possible this will be associated with:
■ Infection of the foreskin with pain and discharge

- Inflammation of the foreskin when urinating

> **NOTE**
> Medical help should be sought as treatment may be needed.

Phlegmasia Cerula Dolens

Condition caused by gross swelling of the legs due to blockage of the veins by which thrombosis; the swelling leads to compression of the arteries and reduces the blood flow to the limbs.

SYMPTOMS & SIGNS
- General feeling of ill-health
- Pain in the thigh and extending into the groin
- Leg becomes progressively swollen
- The affected legs looks pale and feels cold to the touch

> **NOTE**
> Very rare. Usually found in those individuals who have been extremely inactive, such as individuals who have been bedridden. Needs medical attention urgently.

Picking Nose

Picking the nose may cause nosebleeds as the fingernail damages the inside of the nose.

SYMPTOMS & SIGNS
- Nosebleeds
- May be copious bleeding
- No other symptoms

> **NOTE**
> Most likely in children. Nosebleeds will usually resolve by applying pressure to the nose.

CROSS-REFERENCED UNDER:
Nose Picking

Pickwickian Syndrome

see SLEEP APNOEA SYNDROME

Piles

Dilated and protruding veins in or about the anus and rectum, which can be internal or external. Causes of piles include constipation because of too little roughage in the diet and pregnancy.

SYMPTOMS & SIGNS
- Bright red blood issuing from the anus after passing faeces
- Itchy anus
- Usually no pain, but can be very painful particularly if they remain protruding
- Lumps can be felt around the anus. These will usually go back inside the anus after defecation, but may remain protruding

> **NOTE**
> Very common condition. May be resolved by increasing roughage in diet in most cases, but may need surgery or other treatment. Creams are available.

CROSS-REFERENCED UNDER:
Haemorrhoids

Pilonidal Sinus

Small hole can occur between the buttocks, believed to be caused by in-turned hair growing under the skin.

SYMPTOMS & SIGNS
- Itching anus or between the buttocks

- The itchy area may be inflamed and infected

NOTE
Medical help may be needed.

Pinquecula

Yellow-coloured patches in the eye.

SYMPTOMS & SIGNS
- Lumps, yellow in colour and triangular in shape, which form on the white of the eye

NOTE
Most likely in elderly individuals.

Pituitary Gland Disease
see Excess of Prolactin

Pituitary Gland Disease
see Hypopituitarism

Pituitary Tumour

The pituitary gland is located in the brain and controls the function of many hormone-producing glands. Most growths in the pituitary are benign and are called 'adrnomas'. These may themselves produce hormones in excess or they may compromise normal hormone secretion and may press on nearby structures. Rarely cancers can arise in or around the pituitary or can spread to the pituitary (metastasis). Cancers are likely to compromise hormone production or cause local pressure effects because they tend to grow rapidly.

SYMPTOMS & SIGNS
- Excessive hormone production. Excess growth hormone, prolactin, thyroid hormone, steroid hormones.

- May alternatively lead to lack of the above hormones, also testosterone or oestrogen deficiency (hypogonadism)
- Loss of peripheral vision, affecting both eyes
- Mild headache
- May lead to double vision if nerves beside pituitary are affected

NOTE
Medical help should be sought immediately.

Pityriasis Rosea

Itchy blotchy rash, which may be caused by a viral infection.

SYMPTOMS & SIGNS
- Onset is a single red patch which is very itchy. This can develop on any area of the body, and is known as the 'herald patch'
- Within a few days other pink patches develop, which are raised above the surrounding skin. Usually they will be found on the skin of the ribs
- Occasionally the rash is preceded by headache and malaise

NOTE
Most likely in younger people. Will normally resolve by itself after about three weeks, although antihistimines may be needed.

Plague

Infectious disease due to a bacterium that is spread by fleas on rats.

SYMPTOMS & SIGNS
- Sudden onset of high fever and chills
- Weakness. Headache

- Confusion and delirium
- Swollen and tender lymph nodes in the groin and elsewhere
- Nausea, vomiting, abdominal pain
- Low blood pressure and collapse

> NOTE
> Rare in developed parts of the world, but possible in Africa, India, the Far East and South America. Medical help should be sought if suspected.

Plantar Fasciitis

Inflammation of membrane (fascia) of the sole of the foot.

SYMPTOMS & SIGNS
- Pain beneath the heel, exacerbated by walking or running

> NOTE
> Most likely in individuals over 40 years of age and in those who have occupations involving long periods on their feet.

Pleurisy

Inflammation of the membranes (pleurae) which encloses the lungs, caused by conditions such as viral or bacterial infections. Often accompanies a Chest Infection but can be due to other conditions including trauma and pulmonary embolism.

SYMPTOMS & SIGNS
- Sharp, stabbing pain in part of the chest
- Pain exacerbated by inhaling breath
- Breathlessness, caused by avoiding deep breaths

> NOTE
> Medical help should be sought immediately and may be managed with antibiotics.

Pneumoconiosis

Conditions characterised by fibrosis and stiffening of the tissue of the lung, caused by long-term exposure to and inhalation of harmful dust, usually in heavy industrial environments such as coal mining or formerly the production of or work with asbestos. Types of this condition include silicosis and asbestosis, although Pneumoconiosis can also be linked to rheumatic disease.

SYMPTOMS & SIGNS
- May take a long time to develop
- Progressive and increasing difficulty breathing and shortness of breath, first when exercising but eventually even when at rest
- Intermittent cough which may be dry in nature rather than productive
- Bronchitis
- Blue tinge to the lips, ear lobes, under the fingernails and elsewhere caused by a lack of oxygen reaching tissues (cyanosis)
- Finger clubbing
- Respiratory failure
- Heart failure

> NOTE
> These are severe conditions, although modern precautions are limiting the risk of contracting them, at least in developed countries.

CROSS-REFERENCED UNDER:
Silicosis; Asbestosis

Pneumonia

Group of conditions which produce breathing difficulties, usually associated with a severe Chest Infection, bacterial, fungal or viral infections, and from inhaling foreign particles.

SYMPTOMS & SIGNS
- Severe fever
- Painful cough and pain over the affected part of the lung
- Rapid breathing and breathlessness
- Production of sputum, which may contain blood and be rust coloured (rather than look particularly red)
- Sweats, which may be severe and particularly bad at night
- Fatigue and aching all over
- Blue tinge to the lips, ear lobes, under the fingernails and elsewhere caused by a lack of oxygen reaching tissues (cyanosis)
- May be irregular and rapid heart rate, which should resolve as the individual recovers
- Tiredness, fever
- Confusion may be present

NOTE
Most likely and severe in the elderly and the very young, as well as individuals with heart conditions, Bronchitis and Diabetes. Medical help should be sought immediately. The condition may be treated with antibiotics, but will need a chest X-ray to confirm a diagnosis.

Pneumothorax

Collapse of part or whole of a lung which reduces the ability of the lungs to function.

SYMPTOMS & SIGNS
- Severe chest pain, cutting or stabbing in nature
- Feeling of pressure in lungs
- Pain exacerbated by inhaling breath
- Pain is usually centred to the side of the chest rather than the middle
- Breathlessness, which becomes progressively worse over some minutes
- May be collapse due to lack of oxygen (cyanosis)
- Occasionally can recur

NOTE
Medical help should be sought immediately.

Poisoning

Many compounds and drugs can damage different body systems. Some of them are listed below (*also see* separate entry for ADVERSE DRUG REACTIONS or for other substances):

SYMPTOMS & SIGNS
Poisoning or inhalation of toxic substances may cause the following:
- Breathing difficulties, coughing and wheezing
- Headache
- Nausea and vomiting
- Clammy skin
- May look flushed
- Fever
- Confusion
- Unconsciousness

Also may be:
- Problems with, or inability to, urinate, caused by kidney failure. May be result of poisoning by mercury, lead, bismuth or arsenic
- Discoloured areas on the mouth and lips
- May be bad breath: many poisons have

characteristic smells

- Problems with vision such as blind spots and loss of vision can be caused by poisoning by lead, tobacco and Ethyl Alcohol
- Strychnine poisoning has similar signs to Tetanus (see separate entry) except there is no wound or cut as the entry point for infection. It may also be fatal
- Exposure to many toxic fumes and substances can cause headache and drowsiness. These can include carbon monoxide, dry-cleaning agents, diesel and tar. Even people who have been exposed to agents over a long period can develop intolerance to them
- Difficulty in distinguishing colour can be caused by alcohol and tobacco, although in very large quantities
- Coughing with no other signs of illness usually indicates a dry and dusty atmosphere, particularly where the symptoms resolve in fresh air. If this is a long-term problem, the atmosphere should be investigated as there may be a more serious underlying cause than just dust

NOTE

If poisoning is suspected, medical help should be sought, and if toxic chemicals are suspected, the Fire Service should be called. Retain, with care, any suspected substance, syringe or associated packaging, or even vomit. Care should be taken with contaminated material, clothing, or even touching the poisoned individual. The individual should not be made to vomit, as this may cause further problems, especially with caustic substances, not should they be given anything to drink or eat.

CROSS-REFERENCED UNDER:
Toxic Chemicals; Irritant Atmosphere

Polio

Infectious illness, caused by a virus which acts on the brain and spinal cord

SYMPTOMS & SIGNS

- Onset with mild symptoms such as muscle aches, diarrhoea and sore throat
- Develops into Meningitis-type disease
- Paralysis of the leg and shoulder muscles
- The nerves of the face can be involved, causing symptoms similar to Bell's Palsy
- High foot arch (Pes Cavus) and claw toes
- May be permanent paralysis

NOTE

No longer common as children may be immunised against the virus. Symptoms will eventually resolve, but there may be permanent paralysis or muscle wasting.

CROSS-REFERENCED UNDER:
Poliomyelitis

Poliomyelitis
see POLIO

Polycystic Ovaries

Ovaries develop cysts and produce slightly higher than usual levels of male hormones (androgens). Common.

SYMPTOMS & SIGNS

- Ovaries have multiple cysts, impairing their function
- Periods may be absent or irregular

- Acne
- Excessive hairiness of face and elsewhere
- Individual is overweight or obese
- Because of the irregular periods this can be associated with increased risk of infertility

> NOTE
>
> Most likely in young women. Tests would be needed to confirm diagnosis, and treatment is available.

CROSS-REFERENCED UNDER:
Stein-Leventhal Syndrome

Polycythaemia

Blood is too concentrated (in contrast to Anaemia), usually in association with lung problems such as Bronchitis and Emphysema. Commoner in smokers.

SYMPTOMS & SIGNS
- Red complexion
- Headache
- Skin is itchy
- Ringing in the ears
- Tiredness
- Shortness of breath

> NOTE
>
> Medical help should be sought immediately to treat the underlying cause.

Polymyalgia Rheumatica

Generalised pain and stiffness in muscles and joints.

SYMPTOMS & SIGNS
- Aching and stiffness of muscles around shoulders, hips, neck or trunk

- Tender arteries on the temples (if temporal arteritis also present)
- Fever
- General feeling of ill health with tiredness, loss of appetite and weight loss
- Some have sore joints and some have swelling of hands and feet

> NOTE
>
> Most likely in elderly women. Treatment is available in the form of steriods although this may be required long term.

Polymyositis

Inflammation and pain in the muscles, associated with connective tissue diseases such as systemic lups erythematosis and with some cancers especially lung.

SYMPTOMS & SIGNS
- Inflamed and painful muscles, which become progressively worse and weaker especially involves the muscles of the upper arms and thighs
- Exacerbated by exercise or use of affected muscles
- Difficulty climbing stairs and in lifting
- Muscle tenderness
- Fever
- General feeling of ill health
- May be associated with a skin rash
- Occasionally difficulty swallowing

> NOTE
>
> May resolve but then recur.

Polyp in Ear

see EAR POLYP

Poor Diet

see MALNUTRITION

Poor Eyesight

Many people are born with poor eyesight, and this is not normally a problem except where vision problems are left undiagnosed in childhood or when undertaking activities such as driving, particularly at night. Visual problems can occur as the individual gets older, so regular eye tests should be taken. This is also important to diagnose any possibility of Glaucoma.

SYMPTOMS & SIGNS
- Blurred vision
- Severe short-sightedness can cause the production of many Floaters
- Children with poor eyesight may have twitching movement in their eyes (Nystagmus)
- Night vision is usually worse

NOTE
An eye test will be necessary to determine the nature of poor eyesight.

Poor Oral Hygiene

Failure to brush teeth properly can lead to the increased likelihood of cavities and gum disease as well as cause bad breath as food residue decays.

SYMPTOMS & SIGNS
- Bad breath (halitosis), particularly on waking
- Teeth become stained
- Staining may be irregular across teeth (right-handed people find it easier to brush their teeth

on the left side and vice versa)

NOTE
Good oral hygiene also requires regular visits to the dentist.

Porphyria

Metabolic disease which causes changes in nervous and muscular tissues. May be inherited. Attacks can be provoked by a number of prescription and other medication.

SYMPTOMS & SIGNS
- Intermittent severe abdominal pain
- Vomiting
- Constipation
- Fever
- Racing pulse, high blood pressure
- Other nervous and muscular problems including 'wrist droop' with floppiness of the hands at the wrists

NOTE
Medical help should be sought.

Porphyria Cutanea Tarda

Condition caused by liver damage, usually because the individual consumes too much alcohol.

SYMPTOMS & SIGNS
- Widespread rash with blisters on sun exposed areas. Leads to scarring and even areas of pigmented skin
- May be excessive hair growth on the face

NOTE
For the condition to improve, among other things, the individual will need to stop drinking.

Port Wine Stain

see SALMON PATCH NAEVUS

Post-Gastrectomy Syndrome

The surgical removal of the stomach, leaving only a small part, may mean that even light meals or snacks produce a feeling of being full.

SYMPTOMS & SIGNS
- Feeling full when only eating a small amount
- Vomiting, usually thin and green fluid with mucous

Within a few hours of eating, the following may occur:
- May be diarrhoea
- Abdomen may be swollen
- Faintness and weakness
- Palpitations
- Sweating

> NOTE
> The removal of the stomach because of stomach ulcers is now much less common than formerly due to improved treatment with drugs and antibiotics.

CROSS-REFERENCED UNDER:
Gastrectomy

Post-Herpetic Neuralgia

An attack of Shingles can leave a chronic burning pain at the site of the rash.

SYMPTOMS & SIGNS
- Pain is very severe
- Touching the area affected by shingles may precipitate the pain

> NOTE
> Most likely in elderly individuals.

Post-Phlebitic Limb

see LYMPHOEDEMA

Post-Viral Fatigue

see POST-VIRAL SYNDROME

Post-Viral Syndrome

Condition or syndrome, where fatigue and even exhaustion is a common feature, precipitated by a viral infection such as Glandular Fever or Flu. Symptoms vary from individual to individual, but other possible symptoms include Depression, Anxiety, bowel problems, intolerance to certain foods, photophobia, muscle ache, headache and swollen lymph nodes. This can become a long-term problem in previously fit individuals. It should also be pointed out that deconditioning from prolonged bed rest can cause problems in itself.

SYMPTOMS & SIGNS
- Fatigue, tiredness, weakness and exhaustion following an infection
- May be Depression and Anxiety
- May be headache
- May be muscle ache
- May be swollen lymph nodes
- May be bowel problems
- May be range of other symptoms

> NOTE
> There is no general agreement on the best way of managing this condition. Antidepressants may help, as can remaining as active as possible, both physically and mentally, without overdoing it: this balance may be very difficult to achieve.

CROSS-REFERENCED UNDER:
Post-Viral Fatigue; ME (Myalgic Encephalomyelitis)

Potassium Deficiency

Too little potassium in the body can cause a range of problems. Usually caused by prolonged used of diuretics or chronic disease with diarrhoea. Also a feature of aldosteronism.

SYMPTOMS & SIGNS
- Excessive thirst
- Excessive urination
- Muscle weakness
- General tiredness and lethargy
- Constipation

NOTE
Medical help should be sought.

CROSS-REFERENCED UNDER:
Deficiency in Potassium

Potato Nose

see RHINOPHYMA

Pregnancy

Although pregnancy can in no way be thought of as an illness, some women will experience morning sickness during early pregnancy, piles, and other conditions including indigestion.

It should be mentioned that sadly one in eight pregnancies (or possibly more) end in a miscarriage.

The fertilised egg may also implant in the Fallopian tube, causing an ectopic pregnancy ion which the egg has too little room to grow, and causes severe pain on one side of the abdomen. Medical help should be sought immediately, as this can be a life-threatening condition.

Bleeding from the vagina is also possible during pregnancy and can be a feature of miscarriage. vaginal bleeding during pregnancy should always be investigated and medical help sought urgently.

Pregnancy and birth can be traumatic, physically, mentally and emotionally. Depression can be a problem during pregnancy, and more often post-natal, when it can be severe.

SYMPTOMS & SIGNS
- Breasts become tender or ache. This may be the first sign of pregnancy
- Tiredness may be an early sign
- Absence of menstruation (periods)
- Weight gain and increase in appetite
- More easily fatigued
- Heart rate will be increased by about ten beats per minute to cope with extra demands from the developing baby
- May be vomiting on waking from sleep (morning sickness) especially in the first four months of pregnancy
- May be heartburn and excessive stomach acid
- May be piles as pressure is put on the veins around the rectum. These may bleed, producing bright red blood
- The nipples, genitalia and a line down the middle of the abdomen can become darker in colour. The face can also become browner due to increased pigmentation
- May be constipation, caused by either pressure on the intestine by the enlarged womb and growing child, or because of decreased movement (peristalsis) in the intestine
- May be breathlessness as the womb becomes larger and exerts pressure on the diaphragm at

the bottom of the lungs

- May be tendency to faint: this is not uncommon during pregnancy
- May be extreme itchiness, particularly in the last months of pregnancy: Thrush as a cause should be checked
- Rarely may be pale faeces, associated with jaundice of pregnancy
- Hair may became thinner and finer in texture during pregnancy, and some women can also suffer from hair loss, especially after giving birth. In most cases, this hair should grow back
- May be Carpal Tunnel Syndrome, caused by fluid retention affecting the nerves in the wrist
- May be swollen hands for the same reason
- Breasts will become larger
- May be milky discharge from the nipple or nipples before giving birth - this is normal
- Menstruation is usually still abscent or might recur and be irregular during breast feeding: this does not mean that pregnancy cannot occur. It is possible to get pregnant when breast feeding and usual contraception should be used to avoid unwanted pregnancy

Miscarriage:

- May appear to be a heavy period
- Bleeding with jelly-like material
- Lower abdominal pain
- Tender breasts
- Nausea

Ectopic Pregnancy (medical help should be sought immediately):

- Severe pain on one side of the abdomen
- Bleeding
- May pass out and may be collapse
- May occur in women using the contraceptive coil

Problems in late pregnancy (medical help should be sought immediately):

- Bleeding
- May be pain
- Convulsions, caused by extremely high blood pressure, with swollen feet and hands, headache and flashing lights

Pre-Eclampsia, caused by fluid retention in late pregnancy. Medical help should be sought immediately is suspected as it may develop into a dramatic rise in blood pressure, endangering both the mother and baby:

- Swollen fingers and feet
- Rapid weight gain over a few days
- Dizziness and headaches
- Nausea
- May be epileptic fits

NOTE

If in any doubt about whether pregnant or not, pregnancy tests are widely available and extremely accurate.

CROSS-REFERENCED UNDER:
Childbirth; Miscarriage

Premature Ejaculation

The man ejaculates before intended, either before penetration or shortly afterwards. How much this is a problem is very much up to the couple, and it is a more common condition in young men. This is most usually a psychological problem, which can be helped by counselling and certain techniques.

SYMPTOMS & SIGNS

- Ejaculation before intended

NOTE
If this becomes a long-term problem then help should be sought from a psychosexual therapist.

Presbyacusis

Hearing loss, usually for high tones, as individuals get older, ranging in severity from individual to individual.

SYMPTOMS & SIGNS
- Progressive deafness in both ears
- No pain
- No other symptoms

NOTE
Most likely in those individuals more than 60 years old.

Pressure Neuropathy
see NERVE INJURY

Primary Aldosteronism
see ALDOSTERONISM

Prolapse of the Bladder

Bladder can prolapse and be felt as a lump in the vagina.

SYMPTOMS & SIGNS
- Protrusion felt at the front of the vagina
- May be urinary incontinence when laughing or coughing

NOTE
Surgery may be needed.

Prolapse of the Rectum

Rectum can prolapse and can project out through the anus. Can occur in men and women.

SYMPTOMS & SIGNS
- Protrusion felt at the back of the vagina
- Pain in and around back passage
- Deep red bowel projects from anus
- In women the rectum can prolapse forward and can be felt as a lump in the vagina

NOTE
Medical attention should be sought. Surgery may be needed.

Prolapse of the Womb
see WOMB PROLAPSE

Prolapsed Cervical Disc

Degeneration in the cervical (neck) vertebral discs.

SYMPTOMS & SIGNS
- Neck pain and stiffness
- Spasm in the neck and upper back
- Sudden occurrence of symptoms, although they may appear to resolve but then recur
- Pain may extend to the arms, which may also have altered feeling
- Sometimes the prolapsed disc can press on nerves or even the spinal cord causing arm and occasionally leg weakness

NOTE
Medical help should be sought, and may require physiotherapy or the services of a Chiropractor.

Prolapsed Intervertebral Disc
see SLIPPED DISC

333

Prostatitis

Inflammation and infection of the prostate gland, which is located at the base of the bladder (but only found in men).

SYMPTOMS & SIGNS
- Pain in the rectal area behind the groin or low backache
- Problems with urinating because of pressure put on the urethra by the inflamed prostate
- Burning sensation when urinating as if urine is scalding
- Fever
- May be blood in urine, either making it red, pink or cloudy
- May be urinary incontinence such as a dribble of urine after finishing

> NOTE
> Medical help should be sought as this condition may require antibiotics.

Psoriasis

Common skin condition, although the cause is not certain, which can affect any part of the body, although most severely the knees, elbows and scalp.

SYMPTOMS & SIGNS
- Widespread painless, nonitchy but scaly red rash, with spots that can vary in size
- Scaly skin covering these affected areas: the scales are silver in colour
- If the scales come away or are scraped off, the underlying skin will bleed
- In some cases, blisters with crusting can occur, forming scabs
- Hair loss may occur from affecting areas

- May be joint pain and inflammation, most often affecting the joints of the fingers
- Occasionally this arthritis can result in joint destruction and deformity
- Pitting of fingernails and nails come away from the nail bed

> NOTE
> Medical help should be sought.

CROSS-REFERENCED UNDER:
Pustular Psoriasis

Pterygium

Discoloured area on the eye, caused by an area of blood vessels and tissue.

SYMPTOMS & SIGNS
- Wing-shaped area of white tissue and blood vessels which grows over the eyeball

> NOTE
> Most likely in older individuals. Not usually a cause for concern and doesn't do any damage although can be unsightly.

Pulmonary Embolism

Blood clot spreads from veins, usually in the legs, to the lungs and blocks the blood supply to part of the lungs.

SYMPTOMS & SIGNS
- Sudden onset difficulty breathing or shortness of breath
- Sudden cutting or stabbing chest pain
- Frothy sputum which may be pink or red with blood
- Heart rate and rhythm may vary from regular to

irregular

- May be suffocation and breathlessness
- Blue tinge to the lips, ear lobes, under the fingernails and elsewhere caused by a lack of oxygen reaching tissues (cyanosis)
- Collapse
- May be swelling of one or both legs (site of original blood clot)

> NOTE
> Medical help should be sought immediately. Usually is a complication of a thrombosis in the leg (particularly where the calf muscle looks swollen and feels painful) (deep vein thrombosis) that occurs after bed rest, surgery or other illness.

Pulmonary Oedema

Retention of fluid in the lungs, usually caused by heart failure due to damaged heart muscle or heart valves.

SYMPTOMS & SIGNS

- Difficulty breathing or shortness of breath during even relatively mild exercise or exertion
- Shortness of breath when lying down
- Shortness of breath at night, often results in need to get up
- Frothy sputum which may be pink or red with blood
- Blue tinge to the lips, ear lobes, under the fingernails and elsewhere caused by a lack of oxygen reaching tissues (cyanosis)
- Heart beat may be irregular and pulse may be weak
- Swollen ankles or other area because of the retention of fluid

> NOTE
> Medical help should be sought immediately.

Pustular Psoriasis

see PSORIASIS

Pyelonephritis

see KIDNEY DISEASE OR FAILURE

Pyloric Stenosis

Outlet from the stomach becomes narrower or even blocked.

SYMPTOMS & SIGNS

- Vomiting of undigested food, typically the vomiting is projectile
- Rapid weight loss

> NOTE
> Most likely in infants of about six months in age or older individuals with a history of duodenal ulcers. Requires medical attention and usually needs an operation.

Pyogenic Granuloma

Benign growth on the skin, which may be caused by injury.

SYMPTOMS & SIGNS

- Lump is fleshy and soft, and is red in colour
- May bleed if touched or injured
- Most likely to be near a fingernail or toenail

> NOTE
> Not usually a cause for concern.

Pyorrhoea Alveolaris

Severe type of gum disease also affecting the

sockets of the teeth.

SYMPTOMS & SIGNS
- Teeth become loose and gums recede
- Toothache and gum pain
- Bad breath
- Pus can leak out from between the gums and teeth
- May be headache

> NOTE
> Dentist should be visited immediately.

Q Fever

Rare infection, carried by tics and associated with cattle and sheep.

SYMPTOMS & SIGNS
- Takes up to three weeks to incubate
- High fever
- Aching muscles
- Severe headache
- Pneumonia-like illness with dry cough
- Pleuritic chest pain
- Nausea, vomiting, diarrheoa
- Occasionally causes encephalitis or confusion or can affect the heart
- Occasionally occurs as a chronic disease typically as an infection of the heart valves. Often associated with finger clubbing, enlarged liver and spleen.

> NOTE
> Tests will need to be done to confirm a diagnosis and recovery usually takes many weeks.

Quinsy

see PERITONSILLAR ABSCESS

Rabies

Viral disease, which affects the nervous system, and is often transmitted by animal bites, usually dogs. The incubation period between bite and disease ranges between a few days and three months, occasionally longer. It is very rare in Europe, and there have been no cases in Britain for many years. It is, however, usually fatal.

SYMPTOMS & SIGNS
- Onset is usually a dog or animal bite, but the virus may get into the body through any cut or scratch
- Itching, pain or tingling at the site of the animal bite
- General feeling of ill health, headache
- Fever, chills
- Muscular pain
- Sore throat
- Restlessness and inability to sleep, depression
- Later: hydrophobia. The individual has a craving for water, but when presented with water will become terrified and develop throat spasms. Such spasms can lead to convulsions and violent spasms
- Spasms and convulsions develop, and become progressively worse
- May seem to resolve, but them become worse again
- Some develop a rapidly progressive paralysis that spreads from the bitten limb
- Death occurs in around two weeks

> NOTE
> Medical help should be sought immediately. Vaccination is available, although there is no cure.

Raised Intracranial Pressure

Raised pressure within the skull, caused by a tumour, infection, haemorrhage or by increased pressure in the fluid around the brain (cerebraspinal fluid). Haemorrhage can be caused by trauma or head injury.

SYMPTOMS & SIGNS
- Headache typically worse if lying, bending or coughing
- Vomiting
- Drowsiness leading to coma

In babies under 18 months of age
- Bulging fontanelles, the soft areas in a baby's skull before the bones have fused.

> NOTE
> Medical help should be sought immediately.

Ramsey-Hunt Syndrome

Shingles affecting nerves of face and throat.

SYMPTOMS & SIGNS
- Pain localised to the throat and ear on one side of the body
- Hearing very sensitive
- Loss of taste on side affected
- Blistering spots that ulcerate in the ear and throat emerge after seven days or so. Spots form crusts.
- May cause weakness of facial muscles on the affected side

Raynaud's Disease

see RAYNAUD'S PHENOMENON

Raynaud's Phenomenon

Circulation in the fingers and toes reacts severely and goes into spasm in response to low ambient temperature. There may be no obvious cause, although it is associated with beta-blockers (drugs taken for high blood pressure), connective tissue disorders, Rheumatoid Arthritis, or working with shaking or vibrating machinery.

SYMPTOMS & SIGNS
- Fingers and less usually toes are usually cold to the touch
- Fingers look white or even bluish when it is cold
- Pain and fingers go red as they warm up
- May be ulcerated or infected fingers and toes if severe

> NOTE
> Not usually a cause for concern, but may need investigations in some cases.

CROSS-REFERENCED UNDER:
Raynaud's Disease; White Finger

Rectocele

see STRESS INCONTINENCE

Reddened Eyes

Can result from a wide range of causes inlcuding trauma, inflammation, infection or allergy. Painless red eyes with impared vision require medical attention. Commonly red eyes can result from allergy, which is less serious. Allergies can cause a range of symptoms, including reddened eyes. This can be caused by allergens such as pollen, dust, smoke, air pollution and cosmetics. Contact lenses, or lenses' solutions, may also be responsible.

SYMPTOMS & SIGNS

- Eyes become reddened and itchy
- Eyelid may be affected and inflamed
- Any discharge is white or clear
- May be worse at different times or seasons of the year: if so, will often by accompanied by sneezing and a running nose
- May be a feeling as if something is in the eye and eyes may very sensitive to bright light

> NOTE
>
> Symptoms may resolve by removal from the precipitating allergen, although obviously this is not always possible. There are several anti-allergy therapies.

Reiter's Disease

A form of athritis that occurs as a reaction to urethritis – an infection of the outlet from the bladder to the penis or some form of infectious diarrhoea or gastroenteritis.

SYMPTOMS & SIGNS

- Inflammation of the outlet of the bladder to the penis (Urethritis) or diarrhoea (gastroenteritis) Genital ulcers
- Some weeks later painful red eyes due to conjunctivitis or uveitis
- Some weeks later mild arthritis usually of knees, ankles and feet

> NOTE
>
> Medical help should be sought. Most likely in young men.

Relapsing Fever

Infectious disease, spread by tics or lice.

SYMPTOMS & SIGNS

- Sudden onset of very high fever shaking (rigors)
- Initial stage then resolves and health improves
- Fever recurs after 1–2 weeks, and may do so several times
- Liver and spleen are enlarged
- Headache, stiffness, aching joints and muscles
- Confusion or coma may result
- Meningitis and nerve damage can occur occasionally

> NOTE
>
> Most likely in parts of the Mediterranean, Africa, India and South America. The condition may be treated.

Repetitive Strain (Wrist)

see CARPAL TUNNEL SYNDROME

Retention Cyst

see MUCOCELE

Retinitis Pigmentosa

Dark pigment develops over the retina, usually as result of an inherited condition. This causes problems with vision, and is progressive in nature.

SYMPTOMS & SIGNS

- Onset is a gradual but persistent loss of peripheral vision
- Eventually tunnel vision
- Night blindness

> NOTE
>
> Onset is in adolescence or young adulthood, and the individual may be totally blind by the age of 50 years.

Retracted Nipple

see RETRACTION OF THE NIPPLE

Retractile Testicle

Testicle gets pulled up into the groin, a normal reflex to the cold, fear or other emotion. This can also happen during sexual activity.

SYMPTOMS & SIGNS

- Testicle inside the groin rather than the scrotum during periods of cold or fear
- In the scrotum at other times

> NOTE
> Usually not important or serious.

CROSS-REFERENCED UNDER:
Testicle, Retractile

Retraction of the Nipple

Nipples of the breast can be sunken (retracted). This is a normal variation and present from birth.

SYMPTOMS & SIGNS

- Retracted nipple or nipples from birth
- No other signs
- If a normal nipple becomes retracted this may be a sign of breast disease including breast cancer (*see below*).

> NOTE
> Retracted nipple may cause problems breast feeding. It may be a sign of breast cancer, particularly when the nipple has formerly protruded. If the latter is suspected, medical help should be sought, although often a lump in the breast and discharge from the nipple will also be present.

CROSS-REFERENCED UNDER:
Sunken Nipple; Retracted Nipple

Retrobulbar Neuritis

Inflammation of the optic nerve, which can cause blindness and pain in the affected eye, and often associated with Multiple Sclerosis.

SYMPTOMS & SIGNS

- Blindness or loss of vision in one eye
- Rapid onset
- Pain when the eye is moved

> NOTE
> Medical help should be sought.

Rheumatic Carditis

see RHEUMATIC FEVER

Rheumatic Fever

A condition which is a delayed complication of Streptococcus, a specific form of sore throat caused by bacteria. Typically occurs in children.

SYMPTOMS & SIGNS
Onset
- Sore throat
Then (two to four weeks later):
- General feeling of ill health
- Fever
- Fatigue
- Loss of appetite and weight
- Rash with a red line enclosing a paler area of skin
- Joint pain and inflammation (arthritis), although typically this moves from joint to joint
- Firm painless nodules over bones or tendons

- Movements of the body may become jerky and may be uncontrolled (St Vitus's Dance)
- Inflammation of the heart and its valves that can lead to long-term heart problems. Typically this can leave heart valves narrowed or leaky and can eventually lead to heart failure.

> NOTE
> Most likely in young individuals, although only some people are susceptible. This is now a rare condition in the West and more prosperous parts of the world. It is still a serious problem in the developing world.

CROSS-REFERENCED UNDER:
Rheumatic Carditis

Rheumatoid Arthritis

Inflammation of connective tissue associated with joints, often accompanied by crippling pain and sometimes by general ill health. It is often an inherited condition, and Still's Disease is a form of the condition which affects children and adolescents.

SYMPTOMS & SIGNS
- Joint swelling, often tender, especially of hands and feet (but any joint can be altered)
- Pain, often severe in joints
- Stiffness of joints in morning especially
- Range of movement of joints is reduced
- Joints may become deformed and the joints larger and more prominent
- May be weakness, then wasting, in muscles as well as sensory changes
- May be lumps (or nodules) near joints and over pressure points

- General feeling of ill health and anaemia
- Skin may be pale and there may be skin rashes
- May be Carpal Tunnel Syndrome
- Can be associated with Osteoporosis
- May be persistent fever lasting for several weeks
- May be associated with pleurisy (chest pain), nerve damage and Sjogren's Syndrome

> NOTE
> Most likely in young women, and may appear to resolve then reoccur.

CROSS-REFERENCED UNDER:
Arthritis, Rheumatoid; Still's Disease

Rhinitis

Inflammation of the mucous membranes in the nose. It usually produces a lot of phlegm, often precipitated by, probably as a reaction to, environmental factors such as a change in temperature or humidity, or by allergies such as pollen, dust mites, cats and other animals.

SYMPTOMS & SIGNS
- Production of phlegm, usually clear and runny, which may collect in the throat
- Difficulty breathing through nose
- Sneezing, wheezing and watery eyes
- Eyes may be reddened and there may be a feeling as if something is in the eye
- May be bad breath and unpleasant taste in mouth
- May be dry cough which produces no phlegm
- Caused by irritants in the environment

> NOTE
> The apparent increase in rhinitis may be linked to modern housing with central heating and double glazing. Allergic rhinitis is associated with a family history of Asthma, Dermatitis and Hay Fever.

CROSS-REFERENCED UNDER:
Allergic Rhinitis; Vasomotor Rhinitis

Rhinophyma

Large, purple and bulbous nose, caused by a problem with a sebaceous glands in the nose.

SYMPTOMS & SIGNS
- Nose is large and bulbous, and purple in colour
- Surface of the nose is pitted

> NOTE
> Surgical treatment may be necessary.

CROSS-REFERENCED UNDER:
Potato Nose; Bottle Nose

Riboflavine Deficiency
see VITAMIN B2 (RIBOFLAVINE) DEFICIENCY

Rickets
see VITAMIN D (CALCIFEROL) DEFICIENCY

Ringworm

Infection of the scalp by a fungus, which grows outward in a ring, hence the name.

SYMPTOMS & SIGNS
- Round patches of baldness
- Raised red patches with a definite margin and a paler middle
- Stumps of hair remain

- Skin becomes scaly
- Patches become larger over several days

> NOTE
> Treatment is by anti-fungal preparations.

CROSS-REFERENCED UNDER:
Tinea Capitis

Rodent Ulcer

Small cancerous sore, often found on the face, such as the orbit of the eye or by the nose, or on or in the ears. The cancer almost never spreads beyond the sore and usually cured by removal.

SYMPTOMS & SIGNS
- Begins as a small pink lump, which grows over time. Usually painless
- Becomes ulcerated after some time, weeks to months
- May crust and bleed
- May spread into the underlying tissues if not treated

> NOTE
> Most likely found in older individuals. The ulcer can be removed by surgery and medical help should be sought immediately.

CROSS-REFERENCED UNDER:
Basal Cell Carcinoma

Roseola

Mild viral infection which is similar, although not so serious, as Measles.

SYMPTOMS & SIGNS
- High fever, which lasts for a few days

■ Widespread rash develops over the body

> NOTE
>
> Resolves itself within a few days, although medical help should be sought to exclude other infections.

Ross River Fever

Rare infectious disease, found only in parts of Australia and the Pacific, carried by mosquitoes.

SYMPTOMS & SIGNS
■ Takes up to two weeks to incubate
■ Fever
■ Enlarged lymph nodes
■ Pain in the joints
■ Tingling in hands and feet
■ Rash

> NOTE
>
> Recovery may take around four weeks.

Rotator Cuff Tear (Shoulder)

Damage to or rupture of the tendons of the shoulder, possibly caused by trauma from a fall or lifting.

SYMPTOMS & SIGNS
■ Sudden onset
■ Pain
■ Restricted movement of arm outwards

> NOTE
>
> Medical help should be sought immediately. Most likely in older individuals.

Roundworms

Infestation of roundworm (nematodes), of which there are several types. Eggs are passed in faeces, and can be ingested from contaminated food, or some types may be passed by blood-sucking insects. The worms can migrate through the tissues of the body before returning to the bowel as mature worms (they can be coughed up: both terrifying and extremely unpleasant). They may be the cause of serious illness, such as river blindness and elephantiasis.

SYMPTOMS & SIGNS
■ May be no symptoms
■ Worms may be seen in faeces
■ May be abdominal pain, or even Intestinal Obstruction or Appendicitis
■ May be lung inflammation and infection, as well as Pneumonia
■ May cause a urticarial skin infection

> NOTE
>
> Medical help should be sought as need to be treated with drugs, although this kind of worm is very rare in Britain and Europe.

Rubella

Acute, infectious and potentially serious condition, caused by a virus. If it is contracted during the first few months of pregnancy, the disease can cause deafness, heart disease, cataracts and mental problems in the unborn infant.

SYMPTOMS & SIGNS
■ Painful joints
■ Fever
■ Within a couple of days, red or brown rash, often

very faint, appearing anywhere on the body, Usually starts on the face then spreads down the body

- Lymph nodes in the head and neck are enlarged and tender, especially at the back of the head
- Runny nose, sore eyes and cough
- Reddened eyes
- The blistering of the rash can leave scarring or pitting of the skin
- Rarely it may cause permanent deafness

If contracted during the first few months of pregnancy, the infant may develop:

- Heart problems
- Deafness
- Cataracts
- Mental deficiency

> **NOTE**
> There is a routine vaccination for German Measles.

CROSS-REFERENCED UNDER:
German Measles; Measles, German

Ruptured Biceps Tendon

Tendon of the large muscle at the front of the upper arm (biceps) can become damaged or ruptured, associated with wear and tear.

SYMPTOMS & SIGNS
- Pain at the tip of the shoulder
- Upper end of the biceps becomes bunched

> **NOTE**
> Medical help should be sought immediately.

Ruptured Eardrum

Trauma to the head can lead to the rupture of the eardrum, as can Injury to the Head.

SYMPTOMS & SIGNS
- Deafness, which may be complete or partial
- Ringing in ears
- Discharge from ear
- Bleeding from ear

> **NOTE**
> Medical help should be sought immediately.

CROSS-REFERENCED UNDER:
Eardrum, Ruptured

Salivary Gland Calculus

Major salivary glands can become blocked by stones (calculus), reducing the amount of saliva in the mouth.

SYMPTOMS & SIGNS
- Swollen area over the gland on one side, which is uncomfortable and more swollen when eating (or thinking about eating)
- Mouth dry, particularly noticeable on the side of the mouth on which the duct is blocked
- Swelling may suddenly reduce as the stone allows saliva passed or it is displaced

> **NOTE**
> Stones may resolve by themselves although surgery may be necessary.

Salmon Patch Naevus

Two types of birth mark. Salmon Patch Naevus will usually (but not always) fade and disappear over several years, while Port Wine Stain is permanent.

SYMPTOMS & SIGNS

Salmon Patch Naevus

- Pink birth mark, which can be found anywhere, but usually on the neck

Port Wine Stain

- Purple birth mark, caused by an underlying abnormality of blood vessels below the skin

> NOTE
>
> Port Wine Stains are permanent but can be disguised with cosmetics or tattooing.

CROSS-REFERENCED UNDER:

Port Wine Stain; Strawberry Naevus

Salpingitis

Inflammation of the Fallopian tubes (the tubes that take eggs from the ovaries to the womb), caused by a bacterial infection.

SYMPTOMS & SIGNS

- Pain low in the abdomen and backache, also experienced on both sides
- Discharge from the vagina, which is thick in consistency and smells
- Sexual intercourse is very painful
- General feeling of ill health
- May be fever
- May be vomiting
- May be no symptoms except infertility

> NOTE
>
> Medical help should be sought immediately. May sometimes be confused with an Ectopic Pregnancy.

CROSS-REFERENCED UNDER:

Chronic Pelvic Inflammatory Disease

Sarcoidosis

Condition which can affect may organs, although most likely the lymph nodes, skin and bones of the hands. Resembles tuberculosis.

SYMPTOMS & SIGNS

- Skin rash of raised red plaques often with discomfort, usually on legs
- Swollen lymph nodes
- May lead to chronic lung disease – with associated shortness of breath
- Voice may be hoarse because may affect the larynx
- Signs of excessive calcium in the blood, such as lack of appetite, nausea, vomiting, thirst, frequent urination, muscle fatigue and constipation
- Can affect any organ, often many simultaneosly

> NOTE
>
> Medical help should be sought.

Sarcoma

Malignant cancers, fleshy in nature, which may develop anywhere in the body but usually in muscle or bone. Kaposi's Sarcoma, which are purple lumps, are usually associated with AIDS.

SYMPTOMS & SIGNS

- Fleshy swellings within muscle or bone especially
- Pain at site of sarcoma

NOTE
Medical help should be sought immediately. The tumour can often be surgically removed. More likely in younger individuals. Commoner in Paget's disease of bone.

Scabies

Skin condition which is caused by infestation of the scabies mite (tiny insects) or 'crabs'. The latter can be passed sexually.

SYMPTOMS & SIGNS

- Affected area is intensely itchy, and may or may not have a rash. The need to scratch may be so pressing that bleeding results
- Short and fine red lines appear on the skin where the mites have burrowed into the skin, often between the fingers or on the front of the wrists, but also found the nipples, elbow, penis, scrotum, ankles and feet
- Later reddened areas and rash, raised above the surrounding skin, develop widely over the body
- These can develop scabs

NOTE
Will need medical treatment.

CROSS-REFERENCED UNDER:
Crab Lice

Scalded Skin Syndrome

Potentially life-threatening skin condition, caused by adverse drug reactions – viral or bacterial infections.

SYMPTOMS & SIGNS

- Widespread red and angry rash with many blisters
- Large blisters can form on areas of the skin, which can then peel off
- Swift onset of condition and general feeling of ill health
- Raised temperature and fever

NOTE
If this condition is suspected, help should be sought immediately as it can prove to be fatal.

Scarlatina

see SCARLET FEVER

Scarlet Fever

Condition with a very bright red rash, caused by a bacterial infection.

SYMPTOMS & SIGNS

- Onset usually preceded by throat infection, Tonsillitis or a sore throat
- May be fever
- Bright red rash appears within a couple of days, and lasts for about two to three days. Most likely to be most prominent at the armpits, elbow and groin
- Tongue is coated and sore
- The area around the mouth is not affected and consequently looks very pale against the rash
- May develop inflammation of the middle ear with possibly hearing damage
- Rarely may cause Rheumatic Fever or Kidney Disease
- Large areas of skin may peel off as the rash resolves
- Nausea, vomiting
- Abdominal pain

NOTE
Most likely in children and will require antibiotics.

CROSS-REFERENCED UNDER:
Scarlatina

Schistomiasis

see BILHARZIA

Schizophrenia

Acute or chronic mental illness, with fluctuating level of consciousness or disorientation, with altered concentration and perception. Alteration of perception often features hallucinations in which imaginary objects, sounds or even smells are regarded as very real experoences. The individual may hold bizarre or damaging beliefs or ideas, about themselves, others of the world. Diagnosis is not always easy, as it shares features with other mental illnesses such as Anxiety and Depression.

SYMPTOMS & SIGNS
- The condition may appear to happen spontaneously, or it may take a long time to develop
- Anxiety
- Delusions about reality and mania
- Hallucinations
- Paranoia
- Lack of interest and neglect
- Individual may be apathetic
- May appear to be unemotional and unresponsive

NOTE
Common mental illness, believed to affect about one in a hundred of the general population. Many drug treatments are available for those diagnosed with this condition.

Sciatica

Pain and altered sensation caused by pressure of the Sciatic Nerve in the lower back. It is often associated with back pain and strain or a Slipped Disc.

SYMPTOMS & SIGNS
- Pain in the lower back and into the buttock
- Also pain into the leg and down to the foot
- Limb may have tingling and altered sensation
- Pain and tingling may be exacerbated by moving the leg
- All or some of leg may be weak. Feet may be dragged
- In some cases may be urinary and faecal incontinence

NOTE
If pain persists for a long time, it should be investigated as it may be an indication for a serious underlying condition.

Scleroderma

Hardening of the skin with ulceration, atrophy and deformity. Unusually it can also spread more widely, causing immobility of the face and contraction of the fingers. The condition is caused by autoimmune problems in the body.

SYMPTOMS & SIGNS
- Skin is smooth, shiny and hard to the touch
- Contraction of the skin of the fingers caused by stiffness
- Mouth is difficult to open due to skin changes
- As muscles of the face become immobile, face may appear expressionless
- Iche

- Damage to blood vessels causing Raynaud's Phenomenon
- Difficulty swallowing
- Slow but persistent weight loss
- Also associated with gastrointestinal tract, cardiac, kidney and pulmonary problems

NOTE
Medical help should be sought. Most likely to be found in women in their 30s and 40s.

Sclerosing Cholangitis (Adult)

Inflammation of the bile ducts which become fibrous and hardened. Associated with inflammatory bowel disease.

SYMPTOMS & SIGNS
- Often no symptoms initially
- Fatigue, chills
- Itching
- Progressive jaundice with pale faeces
- Leads to liver failure

NOTE
Medical help should be sought immediately.

Scoliosis

Deformity of the spine, associated with disease (children or adults) or as an inherited problem (from birth). Associated with curvature from left to right.

SYMPTOMS & SIGNS
- Spine curves in more than one direction, most noticeable if viewed from behind
- Back pain

NOTE
Medical help should be sought.

Scurvy
see VITAMIN C (ASCORBIC ACID) DEFICIENCY

Sebaceous Cyst

Swelling of a sebaceous gland (which produces an oily substance) in the skin, causing a painless lump.

SYMPTOMS & SIGNS
- Painless, unless it becomes infected
- May be present for many years and may increase slowly in size
- Has a central 'opening', which is the blocked area
- Smooth to the touch
- May range in size

NOTE
Not usually a cause for concern.

Secondary Cancer
see METASTASIS

Self Harm

Cuts, burns or scratches which have no obvious cause may be inflicted by the individual. Damage is most usually inflicted around the wrists.

SYMPTOMS & SIGNS
- Unexplained scars on the body, for which there is no obvious explanation

NOTE
If injuries are severe, medical help should be sought, and psychiatric or psychological help may be needed.

Senile Confusion
see DEMENTIA

Senile Purpura

Blotchy areas may develop, especially on the limbs – in particular around the hands – caused by bleeding under the skin. Not serious or important.

SYMPTOMS & SIGNS
- Purple patches on the limbs, blotchy in nature
- No other symptoms

> NOTE
> Most likely in elderly people, and doesn't need treatment.

Septal Deviation

Blockage or one or both nostrils, either partially or completely, caused by injury or as a birth defect in children

SYMPTOMS & SIGNS
- Speech is nasal or muffled
- Nose may partially or completely blocked
- Breathing through mouth

> NOTE
> Medical help should be sought, particularly if the result of trauma or injury.

Septicaemia

Potentially severe and even life-threatening condition, characterised by an infection of the blood and affecting the whole body. It can lead to Shock. May start as a localised infection in a cut, but the infection may progress rapidly and become more deep rooted and serious.

SYMPTOMS & SIGNS
- Fever
- Chills and rigors
- Severe illness, loss of appetite
- Confusion or reduced conscious level
- Collapse and may be coma
- Shock
- Generalised bleeding as blood does not clot as normal
- May cause problems or inability to urinate because of acute kidney failure
- May be death

> NOTE
> Medical help should be sought as this is a potentially life-threatening problem.

CROSS-REFERENCED UNDER:
Blood Poisoning

Sexual Abuse

Young girls who have unusual discharges from the vagina may be being sexually abused, although this is obviously a very delicate and potentially damaging accusation.

SYMPTOMS & SIGNS
- Discharge from the vagina
- Vagina or anus are bruised
- Changes in mood or behaviour

> NOTE
> This is a difficult subject as child abuse can damage the children for the rest of their lives. Mistaken accusations can also be very damaging, however, especially for parents and for others. If there is any question of this, it may be necessary to seek professional advice.

CROSS-REFERENCED UNDER:
Child Abuse

Shingles

Viral infection characterised by pain and ulcers and fluid-filled spots or blisters (vesicles). Usually found on one half of the body most typically in a strip corresponding to an area of skin served by a single nerve. Occasionally can affect the forehead and eye. It is caused by the same viral infection which is responsible for chicken pox. This may lie dormant for years before reappearing.

SYMPTOMS & SIGNS
- Blisters and sores in the mouth, throat or gullet which can appear as a red rash. These blisters and sores can crust and then form scabs.
- May affect facial nerve, causing paralysis and symptoms similar to Bell's Palsy (Ramsey-Hunt Syndrome)
- Severe pain associated with the vesicles or rash, which may be experienced before their eruption
- May be localised to one side of the body
- The eyes can become infected, causing Keratitis
- In extreme cases, fever and general ill health

NOTE
Most likely in the ill or elderly individuals. Shingles will normally resolve in a couple of weeks, but occasionally the pain can last a long time, even for years. If the eye becomes affected, medical help should be sought immediately as anti-viral medication and pain relief may be needed.

CROSS-REFERENCED UNDER:
Herpes Zoster

Shock

Potentially severe and life-threatening condition, caused by a dramatic fall in blood pressure due to blood loss, heart attack or serious infection. Sustained low blood pressure leads to organ failure, including the kidneys and the brain.

SYMPTOMS & SIGNS
- May look very pale or white
- Skin is clammy
- Sweating and tremor
- Rapid pulse which becomes progressively weaker
- Rapid, but often shallow, breathing
- May be blue tinge to the lips, ear lobes, under the fingernails and elsewhere caused by a lack of oxygen reaching tissues (cyanosis)
- May be nausea and vomiting
- Confusion, Anxiety and mental confusion
- Collapse
- May be problems or inability to urinate as kidneys fail to produce urine

NOTE
Medical help should be sought as soon as possible. If possible, staunch bleeding but firmly pressing a hand on a wound, or cool burns. The individual's clothing should be loosened, they should be kept warm, but they should not be given anything to drink or eat.

Shoulder Dislocation

Upper arm bone (humerus) can be knocked out of the shoulder joint, usually by violent contact.

SYMPTOMS & SIGNS
- Pain when moving arm

- Shape of the shoulder changes and upper arm droops at the shoulder. The arm is held out from the body at the elbow
- Top of upper arm may be felt below the outer part of the collar bone

NOTE
Often caused by trauma from playing contact sports such as rugby or judo. Medical help should be sought immediately.

CROSS-REFERENCED UNDER:
Dislocation of the Shoulder

Sick Sinus Syndrome

The rate and rhythm of the heart beat is controlled by the sino-atrial trigger located within the heart and which acts as the pacemaker for the heart. This can be damaged as a result of arterial disease, heart attack or inflammation of the heart muscle. Associated with marked fluctuation in rate and rhythm of the heart beat – typically from very slow beat (bradycardia) to very fast, at times irregular beat (tachycardia). Commoner in older people.

SYMPTOMS & SIGNS
- Heart rate may be too fast or too slow, and may appear not to be linked to exercise, exertion or being at rest
- May be no other symptoms
- May be symptoms such as fainting, dizziness, fatigue and loss of consciousness

NOTE
Treatment is usually by fitting a pacemaker to regulate the heart rate.

Sickle Cell Anaemia

Red blood cells are shaped like sickles, rather than the normal disc shape, caused by a genetic abnormality. This causes a range of problems from the blood not being able to carry so much oxygen, to blood vessels being blocked. Blockage of vessels leads to painful episodes (sickle cell crisis).

SYMPTOMS & SIGNS
- Anaemia
- Joint pain
- Fever
- Increased risk of infections including pneumonia and meningitis
- Jaundice and abdominal pain
- May be prolonged and unwanted erections
- Growth failure in children. Late puberty
- Stroke with paralysis

NOTE
Found in individuals whose ancestors came from Africa (the sickle cells provide some protection against Malaria). There is no treatment although symptoms may be alleviated.

Silicosis
see PNEUMOCONIOSIS

Singer's Nodules
see VOCAL NODULES

Sinus Arrhythmia

Change in pulse rate, depending whether the individual is inhaling or exhaling. This is a normal reaction to breathing, although it can be more noticeable in some individuals than others, and may cause them worry.

SYMPTOMS & SIGNS

- Heart rate changes during breathing: speeding up when inhaling, slowing down when exhaling (around about ten beats per minute)
- No other signs or symptoms

NOTE
Not usually a cause for concern.

Sinusitis

Inflamed nasal sinuses (passages in the front of the skull), usually caused by an infection, which may be temporary or chronic.

SYMPTOMS & SIGNS

- Headache and pain in inflamed sinuses, in the cheeks or forehead. Pain may be persistent and throbbing, although not of the most severe intensity
- May be production of yellow or green phlegm, either out of the nose or into the back of the throat. This may provoke a dry cough though, where little phlegm is produced
- May be fever and general feeling of ill health
- May be nosebleeds, blocked nostrils and loss of sense of smell
- Bad breath
- Speech may sound nasal or muffled
- Loss of sense of smell

NOTE
Will usually resolve by itself, but it maybe necessary to seek medical help and advice.

Sjogren's Syndrome

Inflamation and destruction of the secretory glands in the mouth causing dry mouth and of the tear producting lacrimal glands causing dryness of the eyes. The syndrome is caused by an autoimmune process. May occur in isolation or in association with rheumatoid arthritis, systemic lupus erythematosis and other autoimmune diseases.

SYMPTOMS & SIGNS

- Dry, gritty and sore eyes
- Dry mouth and bad breath
- Hoarse voice
- Salivary glands become swollen
- Dry nose
- Dry cough

NOTE
Commoner in women. Investigations will be needed to confirm a diagnosis.

CROSS-REFERENCED UNDER:
Keratoconjuctivitis Sicca

Skin Cancer
see CANCER OF THE SKIN

Skull Fracture
see HEAD INJURY

Sleep Apnoea Syndrome

Rasping breathing and snoring during sleeping, which will cause the sleeper to wake, as if they are being partially suffocated. It is often associated with lungs conditions such as Bronchitis and Emphysema.

SYMPTOMS & SIGNS

- During sleep, the individual snores
- Because they are not getting enough oxygen, they briefly awaken and snort to clear their airways, then return to sleep

- Individual may be obese
- Tiredness and drowsiness during the day
- Blood can thicken (polycythaemia)

> NOTE
> Needs medical assessment, losing weight will help, and the individual may need to wear an oxygen mask while sleeping.

CROSS-REFERENCED UNDER:
Pickwickian Syndrome

Sleeping Sickness

Infectious disease (Trypanosomiasis) due to spread of trypanusoner (parasite) by the bite of the tsetse fly.

SYMPTOMS & SIGNS
- Area of bite becomes ulcerated, painful and swollen
- Fever which comes and goes
- Enlarged lymph nodes

Long-term, months to years later can be associated with:
- Headache
- Personality change
- Lethargy and apathy
- Drowsiness
- Confusion
- Tremor
- Fits
- Damage to the nervous system

> NOTE
> Medical help should be sought. Most likely in tropical Africa: there is no vaccine and no cure.

CROSS-REFERENCED UNDER:
Trypanosomiasis

Slipped Disc

The vertebrae, the bones of the spine, have discs between them. With age or injury, these can be damaged and the jelly-like cetre can be forced out of itsnormal position and can press upon the spinal cord and nerves that run out from the spinal cord.

SYMPTOMS & SIGNS
- May be episodes of mild but recurrent localised back pain
- Very severe pain experienced after bending the spine: the actual movement may not have been very large
- Sciatica: pain and/or tingling and altered sensation either extensively from buttock and radiating into the leg and foot or more localised to smaller areas such as the lower leg
- Straining or movement exacerbates the pain
- May walk with stooped posture
- Very rarely may cause urine retention: if this is the case, medical help should be sought immediately

> NOTE
> Medical help should be sought. Most likely in older individuals, although direct injury can also cause the condition. Symptoms will usually resolve spontaneously, although may recur.

CROSS-REFERENCED UNDER:
Prolapsed Intervertebral Disc

Slipped Epiphysis

Part of the upper part of the thigh bone slips from the main part.

Symptoms & Signs
- Discomfort or pain in the hip
- Restricted movement
- Leg is shorter and may be limp
- Foot points outwards
- May be delayed sexual development or the individual may be obese

NOTE
Medical help should be sought. Most likely in boys around 12 years of age.

Small Testicles

see Damage to Testicles

Smoking

Smoking cigarettes or other tobacco products increases the chances of serious illness including Lung Cancer and other cancers including stomach and gullet, Heart Disease, respiratory infections and Bronchitis.

Symptoms & Signs
- Loss of sense of smell
- Bad breath
- Suppression of appetite
- Production of excessive or extra saliva, caused by nicotine
- Heavy or regular smokers will probably also have stained teeth and tar staining of fingers
- Greater risk of developing many serious illnesses
- Cough productive of phlegm especially in morning

NOTE
Smoking is associated with many severe illnesses, and there are many aids to giving up. It has also been shown that cigarette smoke affects the health of non-smokers who are exposed to a smoky atmosphere (passive smoking).

Snoring

General
Snoring is caused by air passing across the soft palate and making it vibrate. Although snoring can be extremely irritating for anyone sharing a bed with an individual so afflicted, it is not usually a sign of serious underlying disease. Snoring is associated with sleeping on the back and alcohol excess, and being overweight. Sleep Apnoea Syndrome, however, can be associated with snoring and needs medical assessment.

Symptoms & Signs
- Snoring sounds while asleep
- Breathing returns to normal when awake
- No other symptoms

NOTE
There are many different remedies and approaches for those who snore, including changing positions in bed and rearranging pillows. Often, however, these will simply not work.

Soroche

see Mountain Sickness

Spasmodic Torticollis

Neck twitches to one side with jerking movements.

Symptoms & Signs
- Neck is jerked to one side spasmodically
- No other symptoms

353

> NOTE
>
> Most likely in older individuals and not usually a sign of underlying disease.

Spider Naevi

Small red spots comprising networks of blood vessels (capillaries) that radiate from a central artery. The condition may be associated with liver disease. Small numbers occur in normal healthy people.

SYMPTOMS & SIGNS

- Small red spots with vessels emanating from them

> NOTE
>
> May be found in adults and children.

Spina Bifida

Congenital abnormality in the development of the nervous system that leaves a bulge in the spinal cord. The bones that protect the spinal cord are defective and are horse-shoe shaped as a consequence. The contents of the spinal canal including the nerves may lie exposed from the spine. However severe nerve damage and disability can result, depending on how far up the spine the opening occurs. The concequences are variable and range in severity from having no or few symptoms to some who have serious problems.

SYMPTOMS & SIGNS

- May be deformity of the legs and may not be able to walk. Legs fail to develop normally because of disuse
- May be club-feet: high foot arch (Pes Cavus) and claw toes

- May be hump-back
- May be swelling over lower back
- May be urinary incontinence
- May be incontinence of faeces

> NOTE
>
> Risk of having a child with Spina Bifida may be reduced by the mother taking folic acid.

Spinal Cord Injury

Spinal cord may become damaged due to trauma and injury, possibly severe.

SYMPTOMS & SIGNS

- May be pain at the site of the injury
- Spine may look deformed or be unusually shaped
- Limbs are weak or are paralysed below the site of the trauma or injury
- May be no feelings or senses below the site of the trauma or injury, or may be altered sensation
- May be loss of bladder control, although often this means that urine is retained and it is not possible to urinate
- May be loss of other body functions
- May be difficulty breathing

> NOTE
>
> Medical emergency if spinal cord injury is suspected, then medial help should be sought immediately. Great care must also be taken when moving someone suspected of suffering from trauma, and *generally they should not be moved* until expert medical help arrives unless their life is in danger. *Movement can exacerbate any spinal cord injury.*

CROSS-REFERENCED UNDER:
Spinal Injury; Injury to the Spine

Spinal Cord Tumours

Tumours can develop on the spinal cord, either as a primary cancer or (more usually) as the result of the spread of cancer from elsewhere in the body.

SYMPTOMS & SIGNS

- Symptoms will be progressively severe
- Feeling different in limbs with local or generalised numbness
- Weakness in limbs (often asymmetric) but typically progressive
- Muscle wasting
- May be difficulty in urinating
- Back pain

> NOTE
> Medical help should be sought immediately.

CROSS-REFERENCED UNDER:
Cancer of the Spinal Cord

Spinal Injury
see SPINAL CORD INJURY

Sprain of Wrist
see WRIST SPRAIN

Sprained Ankle
see Injury to the Ankle

Sprue

Diarrhoea often associated with malabsorption of food. Often associated with prolonged stays in the Tropics.

SYMPTOMS & SIGNS

- Persistent diarrhoea with faeces which are pale, greasy and copious and difficult to flush
- Progressive weight loss
- Anaemia, fatigue and weakness
- Swelling of parts of the body (oedema)
- Inflammation of the tongue (glossitis)

> NOTE
> Medical help should be sought as antibiotics will be required.

Squamous Cell Carcinoma

Malignant growth of cells lining organs – including including the skin itself or mouth or in other sites including the lungs.

SYMPTOMS & SIGNS

- Lump, often irregular in shape
- May bleed and ulcerate
- Lymph nodes in the area of the lump may be hard, enlarged, but often painless
- Most likely on the head and neck

> NOTE
> Medical help should be sought immediately. Most likely in the elderly.

Squint

Eyes look in different directions, caused by being out of alignment due to muscle strength inequality or because one eye is considerably weaker than the other (or is blind).

SYMPTOMS & SIGNS

- Eyes looking in different directions, particularly noticeable when the individual is tired

NOTE
If this condition is suspected in a child, help should be sought as leaving a squint untreated may lead to damage of the child's eyesight.

Staphylococcal Infection of the Nose

Swelling of hair follicles in the nose, caused by an infection

SYMPTOMS & SIGNS
- Part of nose looks swollen and red, and feels hot
- Severe localised pain

NOTE
May need antibiotics to resolve.

Stein-Leventhal Syndrome

see POLYCYSTIC OVARIES

Sternomastoid Tumour

Growth in the middle of the muscle at the side of the neck.

SYMPTOMS & SIGNS
- Lump in the muscle at the side of the neck
- Face is turned away from the side where the lump is

NOTE
Medical help should be sought.

Stevens-Johnson Syndrome

see ERYTHEMA MULTIFORME

Still's Disease

see RHEUMATOID ARTHRITIS

Sting, Insect

see BITE, INSECT

Stomach Cancer

see CANCER OF THE STOMACH

Stomach Ulcer

see PEPTIC ULCER

Stones in the Urinary System

see KIDNEY STONES

Strangulation

see SUFFOCATION

Strawberry Naevus

see SALMON PATCH NAEVUS

Stress Incontinence

Urinary incontinence, usually caused by the later after-effects of the stretching and trauma of giving birth; the vaginal wall is weakened, allowing the bladder (cystocele) or intestine (rectocele) to bulge into it. Occasionally associated with urinary tract infection.

SYMPTOMS & SIGNS
- Urinary incontinence with violent or spasmodic actions such as sneezing, coughing, laughing or straining
- Bulge may be felt in the vagina where the bladder or rectum press through a weakness in the vaginal wall

NOTE
Most likely in women who have recently given birth. May resolve itself although special exercises may help.

CROSS-REFERENCED UNDER:
Cystocele; Rectocele

Stress

see ANXIETY

Stroke

Brain damage due to vascular failure in the brain, because of blockage of blood vessels (thrombosis or embolism) or burst blood vessels (haemorrhage). The initial attack can lead to confusion, unconsciousness, coma and even death. Long-term damage done to the brain because of a stroke may leave paralysis or weakness on one side. Dementia can also follow if the individual suffers from several strokes which are mild.

SYMPTOMS & SIGNS

- Original onset will probably cause confusion or unconsciousness, and possibly coma, with associated problems breathing and incontinence. If in a deep coma, pupils may not respond to light
- No pain or may be sudden headache
- One limb or more commonly one side of the body and face may be paralysed or weakened and may lose sensation
- Speech may be slurred or impaired with difficulty producing words or in understanding others
- Vision may be lost or there may be blind spots in one or both eyes
- May be seizure
- May be urinary incontinence
- May be Dementia caused by multiple strokes, even although these are mild in nature

NOTE
Medical help should be sought immediately, even if symptoms appear to resolve. Most likely in older individuals, those with High Blood Pressure, Diabetes, high Cholesterol, and those who smoke, but possible at any age and in any individual. Sometimes stroke episodes can rapidly resolve (transient ischaemic attacks); these need medical attention as they can lead to major stroke.

Stye

Lump or swelling at the foot of one of the hairs around the eye, caused by an infection.

SYMPTOMS & SIGNS

- May be heralded by slight pain or discomfort
- Lump or swelling at the foot of an eyelash: swelling may spread to the whole of the eyelid
- May be a feeling as if something in the eye
- Discharge of pus

NOTE
Hair may need to be removed to aid draining of pus, and antibiotics may be needed.

Subarachnoid Haemorrhage

Leakage of blood (haemorrhage) from rupture of localised swellings (aneurysms) that are congenital abnormalities at the junctions of some blood vessels. Usually occurs in the brain. May be triggered by exercise or exertion.

SYMPTOMS & SIGNS

- Typically very sudden onset of headache, severe in intensity
- Headache may have a slower onset, but pain becomes progressively worse
- Vomiting
- Aversion to bright light
- Variable decline in conscious level from confusion to coma

357

- Stiff neck
- Limb weakness and difficulty speaking
- Convulsions
- May be paralysis

NOTE
Medical help should be sought immediately.

CROSS-REFERENCED UNDER:
Brain Haemorrhage

Subconjuctival Haemorrhage

Part of the white of the eye becomes red, caused by the rupture of a small blood vessel in the eye. There may be no obvious reason why it develops, or it may occur because of injury or trauma. If it is the latter, investigation may be needed to exclude more serious damage. Unsightly but not serious.

SYMPTOMS & SIGNS
- No pain
- Part of the white of the eye becomes red, not reaching the coloured part of the eye and fading away towards the outer part of the white of the eye

NOTE
Will normally resolve in a couple of weeks.

Subdural Haemorrhage

Blood leaking from vessels in the brain and collecting between the membranes around the brain. This causes increased pressure. It can be caused by a trauma to the head, although symptoms may take some days or even weeks to become noticeable. Commoner in elderly, in alcoholics and those on medication to thin the blood (anticoagulants).

SYMPTOMS & SIGNS
- Headache, although it may be fairly mild
- May drift in and out of consciousness or sleep
- Progressive confusion
- May be difficulty speaking
- May be convulsions

NOTE
Medical help should be sought immediately.

CROSS-REFERENCED UNDER:
Brain Haemorrhage

Subluxation of the Hip

Degeneration of the hip caused by problems with the cup-like socket (acetabulum) into which the top of the thigh bone (femur) goes.

SYMPTOMS & SIGNS
- Pain in groin, exacerbated by exercise
- Limp, which gets progressively worse

NOTE
Most likely in individuals around 20 years of age.

Submandibular Duct Stone

Stones can form in the ducts of the submandibular salivary glands that are located on each side of the jaw beneath the tongue.

SYMPTOMS & SIGNS
- Swelling on one side, just under the jaw bone (mandible) may also be felt below the tongue within the mouth
- Increases when eating, then reduces between meals
- No pain

> **NOTE**
> Medical help should be sought to exclude other conditions.

Submandibular Tumour

Tumour below the jaw, which may be malignant or benign.

SYMPTOMS & SIGNS
- Gland is swollen on one side below the jaw
- Gets larger over time and may become painful
- Lymph nodes may be involved

> **NOTE**
> Medical help should be sought.

Suffocation

The airway is constricted, stopping breathing. This is life threatening and is a medical emergency as suffocation may cause death.

SYMPTOMS & SIGNS
- Unconsciousness
- Difficulty breathing (if at all)
- Blue tinge to lips, finger nails and skin
- Bruising or other marks of strangulation around the neck
- Veins are prominent on face

> **NOTE**
> Medical help should be sought immediately. Anything preventing breathing should be removed immediately, check in mouth to ensure nothing is blocking the airway. The Heimlich manoeuvre (in which pressure is applied to upper abdomen of the suffocating individual) from behind, to expel the object from victim's airway.

CROSS-REFERENCED UNDER:
Hanging; Strangulation

Sun Stroke
see HEAT STROKE

Sunburn

Damage to the skin as a result of overexposure to the ultraviolet rays of the sun. Sun tans are not healthy, and pigmentation is the result of skin damage. If damage is persistent and the individual has fair or light-coloured skin or has red hair and freckles, there is a chance that they could develop Skin Cancer.

SYMPTOMS & SIGNS
- Skin is red, hot and angry where it has been exposed to the sun
- If damage is severe, skin can peel and flake
- May be an increased risk of developing Skin Cancer

> **NOTE**
> Over exposure to the sun should be avoided by covering up, not going out in the midday sun, and using sun-tan lotion to block out the sun's harmful rays. Overexposure to the sun can age the skin. Exposure to sunlight can help Psoriasis and Vitamin D Deficiency.

Sunken Nipple
see RETRACTION OF THE NIPPLE

Sweating
see EXERCISE

Swelling of the Larynx
see ALLERGIC REACTION, SEVERE

Swollen Ankle

see Lymphoedema

Syphilis

Sexually transmitted (or congenital) infection, which if untreated can be very severe. The primary stage is characterised by a sore or chancre (appearing about three to four weeks after sexual contact), the secondary stage (6 weeks to several months later) by skin eruptions, and the tertiary stage (some 15-30 years after initial infection) involves severe nervous and cardiovascular symptoms.

Symptoms & Signs
- Ulcer in mouth or on lips (chancre): single, shallow, painless and hard at the base. They do not bleed, and have a raised reddened margin. The genital chancre is often overlooked in women

Later (around six to 12 weeks):
- Skin eruptions (infectious)
- Genital warts like branching coral, particularly on the genitals or anus
- Faint copper-coloured rash, noticed on the trunk, hands, feet and the forehead
- Swollen painless lymph nodes
- Fever and general ill health
- Joint pain

Much later:
- Painless ulcerated skin or oral ulcers
- May be enlarged lymph nodes
- May be unsteady on feet
- Joints may be swollen and grossly disrupted but are painless
- Ulcerated or infected feet
- May be mental disturbance and Dementia
- Tunnel vision

- Deafness
- May be irregularly shaped pupils and drooping eyelids
- Cornea may become cloudy
- Severe bone pain in the limbs

> Note
>
> Although a severe illness historically, Syphilis may be treated with antibiotics, such as penicillin. Help, however, should be sought as soon as possible.

Cross-referenced under:
Chancre

Systemic Lupus Erythematosis (SLE) 'Lupus'

Progressive condition of connective tissues, due to an 'auto-immune' disorder, where the body acts against itself. Symptoms may be very vague at onset. Can affect any organ system and often affects many.

Symptoms & Signs
- Fever
- General fatigue and malaise, loss of appetite
- Joint pain or arthritis
- Rashes including 'butterfly rash' around the face
- Anaemia
- Raynaud's phenomenon
- Chest pain, breathlessness
- Pins and needles, epilepsy, stroke
- Some forms associated with increased risk of venous thrombosis and miscarriages

> NOTE
> Most likely in women in their 30s, 40s and 50s. Important that an early diagnosis is made as cardiac, kidney and brain involvement can be serious. Medical attention is necessary.

TB

see TUBERCULOSIS

Tapeworms

Infestation by tapeworms (cestodes): flat parasitic worms, which may grow up to 30 feet (9 metres) long. They may be caught from dog faeces or from contaminated meat. The worms can form cysts within organs in the body, such as the liver, and may cause serious illness; alternatively, there may no symptoms.

SYMPTOMS & SIGNS
- May be no symptoms, often incidental finding on X-ray
- Discomfort in the abdomen
- Increased appetite
- Occasionally cough
- Parts of the worms can be seen in faeces
- Large cysts can form in the abdomen

> NOTE
> Medical help should be sought.

CROSS-REFERENCED UNDER:
Hydatid Disease

Tea

see CAFFEINE

Teething Pain

The pain caused to an infant or adult when teeth erupt through the gums. In children teeth start erupting from around the age of six to ten months until about three years old. In adults the wisdom teeth also erupt through the gums (*also see* WISDOM TEETH).

SYMPTOMS & SIGNS
- Pain
- Excessive salivation
- Discomfort
- May be headache
- May earache, particularly when back teeth erupt

> NOTE
> Will normally resolve itself, although this will take some time.

Temporal Arteritis

Inflammation of the temporal artery, a vessel which runs along the side of the face. May be associated with inflammation of other arteries around the brain. It is associated with Polymyalgia Rheumatica. Can cause sudden blindness due to blockage of arteries to the rectina and similarly c an cause stroke

SYMPTOMS & SIGNS
- Headache or facial pain on one side of the face
- Blood vessels stand out prominently in the head
- Skin near the thickened artery is inflamed and sore to the touch
- Scalp may be sore on brushing or combing hair
- May develop jaw pain on chewing 'jaw claudication'

> NOTE
> Most likely in elderly men. Medical help should be sought *immediately* due to the risk of blindness. Steroids are used to treat the condition and may

be required for a number of years. Management is more effective the earlier treatment is begun.

Temporal Lobe Epilepsy

Epilepsy of the temporal lobe in the brain.

SYMPTOMS & SIGNS
- Altered feeling (aura) heralds an attack
- Smell becomes acute, as does taste: there may be hallucinations of smell and taste
- Visual disturbance
- Dizziness
- Drowsiness

> NOTE
> Medical help should be sought.

Tennis Elbow

Damage to the elbow joint, caused by repetitive and stressful actions, such as playing tennis or golf, or throwing the javelin.

SYMPTOMS & SIGNS
- Pain in the elbow
- Pain exacerbated by making similar to movements to that which caused the problem

> NOTE
> Most likely in older individuals. May resolve spontaneously through rest, but may need surgical or medical treatment.

Tension Headache

Headache where the pain is like a band around the head. It can be very severe in intensity, but is rarely a cause for concern, other than any underlying stresses or emotional distress.

SYMPTOMS & SIGNS
- Band-like pain around the head
- May be very severe in intensity
- May occur frequently in a series or intermittently, with periods without pain
- No other symptoms present

> NOTE
> Tension headaches will normally resolve by themselves as long as the underlying stresses are dealt with.

CROSS-REFERENCED UNDER:
Headache, Tension

Testicle, Ectopic
see ECTOPIC TESTICLE

Testicle, Retractile
see RETRACTILE TESTICLE

Testicle, Undescended
see UNDESCENDED TESTICLE

Tetanus

Infection with the organism Clostridium tetani, which causes spasms and muscle rigidity, hence its other name Lockjaw (trismus). The organism can be found in garden soil and manure, and can infect the individual through a small cut or abrasion, or from animal bites. This is a potentially severe condition and may cause death. It can take some time to incubate, usually around one week.

SYMPTOMS & SIGNS
- Onset may appear to be a mild feverish illness
- Muscular weakness around the cut or wound
- Muscular spasms
- Muscle rigidity, making it impossible to open the

mouth. This gives the individual an expression as if they were grinning, and hence 'Lockjaw'.

- Fever
- Rapid pulse with high or low blood pressure
- Saliva production
- Drenching sweats
- Spasm of swallowing muscles – may lead to aspiration pneumonia
- Weight loss
- Spasms may increase over time and eventually cause death

> NOTE
> Medical help should be sought immediately. Active immunity is gained by being immunised against the organism. It is necessary to get a booster every ten years.

CROSS-REFERENCED UNDER:
Lockjaw

Thalassaemia

see ANAEMIA

Third Nerve Palsy

The Third Nerve controls eye movements, and it can be damaged by inflammation of blood vessels (varculitis), as part of a stroke or by excessive pressure being applied by an underlying cause such as a brain tumour or an enlarged artery in the head.

SYMPTOMS & SIGNS
- Only one of the eyes is involved
- Eyelid drooping
- Pupil of the eye dilated and enlarged
- Eye turned outwards and downwards
- Sometimes only some of above are present, resulting in a partial third nreve palsy

> NOTE
> Medical help should be sought.

Threadworm

Infestation of the intestine by threadworms, a tiny white thread-like worm which lives and multiplies in the human bowel. The worm is found in soil.

SYMPTOMS & SIGNS
- Itchy anus, and may be itchy vagina
- White thread-like worms may be seen in faeces or on anus
- May stop children from sleeping as causes so much discomfort

> NOTE
> Most likely in children, from whom it can spread within families. Treatment needs to be taken by all family members, and may need to repeated as eggs of the worm are not necessarily affected.

Throat Cancer

see CANCER OF THE MOUTH

Thrush

see CANDIDIASIS

Thyroglossal Cyst

Benign cyst found in the middle of the front of the neck. A remnant left in the pathway that the thyroid gland follows during development as it grows down from the tongue to the neck.

SYMPTOMS & SIGNS
- Lump which moves up if the tongue is stuck out
- No pain
- No other symptoms

NOTE

Medical help should be sought and investigations undertaken, if only to exclude other conditions.

Tic Douloureux

see TRIGEMINAL NEURALGIA

Tinea Capitis

see RINGWORM

Tinea Versicolor

Appearance of brown areas on the skin, which later lose their pigmentation, forming pale or white areas. It is caused by a fungal infection.

SYMPTOMS & SIGNS

- Widespread rash, first brown in colour, found mostly on the upper body
- The areas of rash eventually lose pigmentation and the skin becomes pale or white

NOTE

May be managed using anti-fungal medication.

Tonsillitis

The tonsils, which are located at the back of the mouth on either side of the throat, may become infected and inflamed, caused by either a bacteria or virus.

SYMPTOMS & SIGNS

- Enlarged tonsils
- May be white spots on tonsils
- Reddened throat
- Inflamed and tender lymph nodes in neck
- Pain when swallowing
- Fever
- Lymph glands may be enlarged and tender
- May be an associated cough

- Increased production of saliva in mouth
- Bad breath and unpleasant taste in mouth
- May be difficult to open the mouth because of the pain or swelling
- May be headache
- May be earache, severe in intensity

NOTE

May need antibiotics to resolve. Smoking exacerbates symptoms and smokers may suffer from associated infections of the chest.

Tooth Decay and Abscess

Tooth decay is caused when tooth enamel is damaged and eaten away by bacteria. Regular brushing of teeth, with a fluoride toothpaste, and consuming as little sugary food and drink between meals as possible, may help prevent decay. A dental abscess can form very painful swelling around the infected tooth, in the jaw.

SYMPTOMS & SIGNS

- Teeth are sensitive, particularly when consuming particularly hot or cold food or drinks
- Bad breath
- A tooth or teeth is painful, sometimes severely so
- Earache, particularly if molar teeth are decayed
- May be difficult to open the mouth because of the pain or swelling

If an abscess has formed:

- Swollen area around the teeth, either upper or lower jaw
- May involve the whole side or cheek
- The abscess may increase in size over several days
- May be associated headache

May be fever, feeling of being unwell with loss of appetite

NOTE

Regular visits to the dentist may minimise tooth decay by dealing with problems as they arise. A dental abscess may require antibiotics before remedial treatment.

CROSS-REFERENCED UNDER:
Dental Caries; Toothache

Toothache

see TOOTH DECAY AND ABSCESS

Torn Medial Meniscus

see CARTILAGE TEAR (KNEE)

Torsion

The ducts and blood vessels that are attached to the testicles in the scrotum can become twisted.

SYMPTOMS & SIGNS
- Severe to excruciating pain in one testicle
- Testicle becomes inflamed and very tender to touch
- Nausea and vomiting
- Scrotum may become swollen

NOTE

Medical help should be sought as this condition will often require surgery. This is more likely in young men and boys than Epididymitis.

Torticollis

see WRYNECK

Tourette's Syndrome (or Giller de la Tourette's Syndrome)

Unusual condition which begins in childhood, but becomes most prominent in adolescence, usually to become more controlled in later life. It is best known for those affected to shout and swear at inappropriate times. This is, however, a very rare condition.

SYMPTOMS & SIGNS
- Multiple tics, twitching and gesturing
- Grunting
- Involuntary and repeated swearing and inappropriate comments
- Repeating what has been said

NOTE

There is no cure, but medications may be able to moderate behaviour.

Toxic Chemicals

see POISONING

Toxic Shock Syndrome

see MENSTRUATION

Toxoplasmosis

Infection by toxoplasma parasites, which occur widely in animals and man, although only about 20% of humans actually become ill. Can be caught by eating infected meat (especially if under cooked or raw), from cat faeces, and even from fruit and vegetable (especially if not washed). Pregnant women should take especial care, as infection of the unborn baby is particularly severe, and extra care should be taken with young infants. It may also be a severe condition in adults especially if their immunity is compromised.

Symptoms & Signs

- Fever
- General feeling of being unwell, fatigue, headache
- Lymph nodes in neck and elsewhere enlarged and may be tender
- In infants and the unborn, infection can result in convulsions, inflammation of the brain and nerve coverings, hydrocephalus, eye problems and even death
- In adults, can cause pneumonia, inflammation of the kidney, rashes and visual loss

Note
Medical help should be sought and diagnosis may be confirmed by a blood test.

Tracheitis

Inflammation of the main airway into the lungs (trachea), usually caused by an infection. It may develop into a chest infection.

Symptoms & Signs

- Similar signs to Laryngitis
- Raw pain from the lower neck and upper chest, often felt behind the breast bone
- May develop into a chest infection
- Recurrent barking cough

In particularly severe conditions:

- Inflammation may be so severe as to block the windpipe
- Laboured and forced breathing
- Bluish tinge to the skin, especially the lips, caused by a lack of oxygen (cyanosis)

Note
Medical help should be sought.

Trachoma

Acute or chronic infection of the conjunctivae. Swollen eyelids and progressive opacity of the cornea and eventual blindness; caused by an infection. Largely confined to developing countries.

Symptoms & Signs

- Eyelids swollen and under surface is grainy and red
- Cornea becomes progressive opaque
- May be blindness, partial or complete, caused by scarring of the cornea

Note
Most likely in developing countries; rare in developed countries. It can be treated, but is unfortunately a major cause of blindness in developing countries.

Travel Sickness

The movement or motion of a boat, car, aeroplane or train can make the individual feel unwell. The severity or presence of symptoms varies from individual to individual.

Symptoms & Signs

- May be dizziness
- May be nausea and vomiting
- May be headache
- May be pale skin
- May be drowsiness and yawning

> **NOTE**
> More likely in children. There are a wide range of medications available.

CROSS-REFERENCED UNDER:
Motion Sickness

Trench Mouth

see VINCENT'S ANGINA

Trichomonas

Infection and inflammation of the vagina (or penis) by a parasitic organism.

SYMPTOMS & SIGNS
- Discharge from the vagina, which is frothy and yellow or green in colour
- Discharge has an unpleasant smell
- Itchiness, tenderness and may be pain

> **NOTE**
> Medical help should be sought as treatment will be needed. Will affect about one in five of all women, and may also be found in some men.

CROSS-REFERENCED UNDER:
Vaginal Infection

Trigeminal Neuralgia

Severe unilateral facial pain associated with the Trigeminal nerve, triggered by touch, an attack of Shingles, occasionally as a manifestation of multiple sclerosis, or for no discernible reason. The Trigeminal nerve supplies the skin of the face, the eye, the teeth and the tongue.

SYMPTOMS & SIGNS
- Excruciating and spasmodic pain in the face, ear and nose
- May be triggered by causes such as the cold or by eating
- Tends to recur

> **NOTE**
> Help may be needed as the pain is so severe, although the condition itself is harmless.

CROSS-REFERENCED UNDER:
Neuralgia, Trigeminal; Tic Douloureux

Trigger Finger

As a result of inflammation of the tendons of joints of the fingers or thumb become locked in flexion, the bent position.

SYMPTOMS & SIGNS
- Digit cannot move, it is fixed in flexion
- May resolve spontaneously or may need surgical correction
- Small tender swollen area on the palm by the affected digit
- Area clicks when the digit is moved

> **NOTE**
> May resolve by itself, although surgical treatment may be needed.

Trypanosomiasis
see SLEEPING SICKNESS

Tuberculosis (TB)

Infectious disease caused by the organism Mycobacterium Tuberculosis, which can cause both pulmonary and other symptoms. Usually the lungs are affected but TB infection can be generalised and affect any organ system.

SYMPTOMS & SIGNS

- Cough, may be with sputum which includes or is streaked with blood
- Shortness of breath
- Chest pain
- Difficulty when swallowing
- Bad breath
- Fever which comes and goes
- Sweating, particularly bad at night
- Generally feeling unwell and fatigue
- Fatigue
- Loss of appetite
- Lymph nodes swollen although not tender
- Clubbing of end of fingers and finger nails

Tuberculosis may also affect other parts of the body:

- Weight loss, muscle wasting and reduction in strength and stamina
- Bone pain, mild at first but becoming more severe with time
- Painful swelling and destruction of bone including vertebrae in the spine

---

NOTE

Infection is most likely in those who are malnourished (commonly in alcoholics), live in poor housing, or are suffering from conditions with immunosuppression. Medical attention should be sought. Diagnosis can be made with blood or skin tests, or a biopsy of the lymph node. Treatment required.

CROSS-REFERENCED UNDER:

TB; Consumption

Tumour of the Eye

see CANCER OF THE EYE

Tumour of the Vagina

see CANCER OF THE VAGINA

Tumours of the Chest

see CANCER IN THE CHEST

Turner's Syndrome

Genetic condition of women characterised in which affected women have one X chromosome (XO) instead of two (normal is XX). Some affected women have milder variants of this condition.

SYMPTOMS & SIGNS

- Short in height and neck is very short
- Chest is broad with nipples spaced widely apart
- Deafness
- Excessive body hair
- May have lymphoedema swelling of hands and feet
- At higher risk of developing underactive thyroid, high blood pressure and diabetes
- No secondary sexual characteristics, failure of pubertal development and infertility
- Normal IQ
- Heart disease
- Osteoporosis

NOTE
Only found in women.

Typhoid Fever

Infectious disease, which is spread by contaminated food or water supply, and caused by a strain of salmonella. It may take around one to three weeks for the disease to incubate. Paratyphoid is a less serious illness which is similar to Typhoid.

SYMPTOMS & SIGNS

- Fever with chills, mild at first but becoming more severe: fever may appear to improve then becomes worse again
- Headache
- Cough

As it progresses:

- Abdominal pain
- Diarrhoea like pea soup
- Abdomen swollen
- Feeling generally very unwell
- Rose-coloured rash on the upper abdomen and on the back, typically around the end of the first week. This lasts for about three days
- Spontaneous and generalised bleeding caused by failure of the blood to clot
- Shock and unconciousness

NOTE

Some individuals may carry the infection without developing symptoms. It will usually take three weeks for the disease to resolve. Medical attention should be sought. Immunisation is available against Typhoid.

CROSS-REFERENCED UNDER:

Paratyphoid

Typhus Fever

A group of several infectious diseases (Rickettsia), spread by lice which are blood-sucking insects. These infections vary from mild to severe.

SYMPTOMS & SIGNS

- High fever increasing over several days, with chills
- Headache

- Red eyes
- Rash
- May be painful joints, painful muscles and abdominal pain
- Cough and shortness of breath
- Confusion, delirium, seizures and coma

NOTE

Medical help should be sought and investigations undertaken.

Ulcer, Mouth

see APHTHOUS ULCER

Ulcer, Peptic

see PEPTIC ULCER

Ulcerative Colitis

Inflammation and ulceration of the colon that may be restricted to rectum or affect variable lengths of colon up to and including the entire colon

SYMPTOMS & SIGNS

- Diarrhoea that may be mild to severe; often frequent by day and by night. Recurrent
- May be blood and mucous in faeces
- May be abdominal pain or pain experienced in the back
- May be mild fever
- Anaemia
- Abdomen may be swollen
- If severe, often weight loss, severe abdominal pain and croups, severe diarrhoea and high fever
- May be collapse in extreme cases

NOTE

Medical help should be sought, and investigation will be needed.

Ulnar Nerve Damage

Severe pain and altered sensation in the arm, caused by a knock or blow to the Ulnar Nerve in the elbow (commonly referred to as the 'funny bone').

Symptoms & Signs

- Severe pain down the forearm to the handsespecially in the little and ring fingers
- Tingling and altered sensation down the forearm to the hands in the little and ring fingers
- Weakness of grip and clumsiness of hand

Note
Should resolve within a short time.

Cross-referenced under:
Funny Bone

Undescended Testicle

In early childhood testicles should have descended into the scrotum. In a small number of boys, this is not the case.

Symptoms & Signs

- One or both testicles do not descend into the scrotum and may be felt as a lump(s) in the groin. Sometimes the testicles cannot be felt anywhere and may remain within the abdomen
- The person is otherwise normal
- If testicles do not descend this may reduce fertility and increase chances of malignant disease in testicles when older

Note
Medical help should be sought as the testicles will need to be brought down into the scrotum by surgery.

Cross-referenced under:
Testicle, Undescended

Upper Arm Bone (Humerus) Fracture
see Broken Upper Arm Bone (Humerus)

Upper Respiratory Tract Infections
see Cold, Common

Upper Tibial Epiphysis and Apophysitis

Injury sustained to the shin can damage to the tendons below the knee. Osgood Schlatter's Disease, most likely in young adults, has the same symptoms, although it does not occur as a result of trauma.

Symptoms & signs

- Swelling of the knee, most noticeable just below the kneecap
- Pain on weightbearing
- Raising a straight leg may be excruciatingly painful

Note
Medical help should be sought immediately.

Cross-referenced under:
Osgood Schlatter's Disease

Uraemia

Progressively larger amounts of urea collecting in the blood, caused by kidney failure

Symptoms & Signs

- Fatigue
- Breath smells of urine
- Tongue is dry and coated

- Skin can become progressively yellow and then brown in colour with a white tinge, and is dry.
- Hiccups
- Nausea and vomiting
- May be extreme itchiness
- Anaemia

> NOTE
> Medical help should be sought.

Urethral Cancer

see CANCER OF THE URETHRA

Urethral Caruncle

The urethra, which connects the bladder to the opening at the front of the vagina, can become inflamed.

SYMPTOMS & SIGNS
- Pain
- Pain from sexual intercourse or urinating
- Discharge of blood

> NOTE
> May require surgery.

Urethral Stricture

Narrowing of the urethra, the tube which takes and expels urine from the bladder. This can be cause by infections such as Gonorrhoea, as well as by damage from surgery, childbirth or inserting a catheter. Mild symptoms may be noticed to start with, but these may become progressively more severe. Similar symptoms can be caused by a tumour on the urethra, although this is more unlikely.

SYMPTOMS & SIGNS
- Little urine expelled and poor flow

- May be quite difficult and take some effort to empty the bladder
- In severe cases, it may not be possible to urinate at all. If this is the case, there will also be lower abdominal pain cause by a very full bladder.

> NOTE
> More likely in men than women, but can affect both.

Urethritis

see URINARY TRACT INFECTION

Urinary Tract Infection

Inflammation of the bladder or urethra (the tube which takes urine from the bladder), usually caused by bacterial infections.

SYMPTOMS & SIGNS
- Need to pass urine frequently, although not usually in very large amounts, and may continue overnight
- Urine may be dark, cloudy or stained with blood: this can be the colour of blood but may only appear to be slightly pinkish
- Passing urine causes searing or burning pain
- Very urgent feeling of needing to urinate or having a very full bladder but little urine actually produced
- Pain in the groin, front part of the abdomen and in the back
- May be discharge from the penis
- Fever, possibly severe, with chills and rigors
- Urinary incontinence, particularly in the elderly
- Vomiting and nausea
- Sweating

> NOTE
> More likely in females than males, and should always be investigated, if suspected in children. Serious infections will require antibiotics.

CROSS-REFERENCED UNDER:
Urethritis; Non-Specific Urethritis

Urticaria

Sudden development of single or large weal, caused by an allergic reaction to substances such as plants, chemicals, foods or drugs. The weals are usually very itchy. There are several different types.

SYMPTOMS & SIGNS
- Widespread rash with blotchy red swollen patches, which have paler areas in the centre of the patch
- Usually extremely itchy

> NOTE
> Will often resolve itself, but if persists medical help should be sought.

CROSS-REFERENCED UNDER:
Hives

Uterine Cancer

see CANCER OF THE WOMB

Vaginal Infection

see GARDNERELLA

Vaginal Infection

see TRICHOMONAS

Vaginal Polyp

see CERVICAL POLYP

Vaginal Spasm

see VAGINISMUS

Vaginismus

The vagina can go into spasm and the muscles around it contract, making it painful or impossible to have sexual intercourse. This is rarely a physical problem, although after childbirth a woman may be sore for some time; vaginismus is often a consequence of psychological problems.

SYMPTOMS & SIGNS
- Vagina contracts making it difficult or impossible to have penetrative sex, or even an investigation
- Pain if this is attempted
- No other physical symptoms
- May be a fear of penetration, pregnancy or some other psychological problem

> NOTE
> Although rarely a physical problem, investigations may be necessary to exclude underlying disease.

CROSS-REFERENCED UNDER:
Vaginal Spasm

Varicella

see CHICKENPOX

Varicocele

Enlarged veins may be felt behind the testicle. This is harmless except that it may damage fertility.

SYMPTOMS & SIGNS
- Swollen veins felt around the testicle in the scrotum
- Discomfort

- Greater risk of male infertility

> NOTE
> Most common in older men. Treatment is not usually needed.

Varicose Veins

Veins become prominent and enlarged, caused by damage to the valves in the veins. They are usually found in the lower leg, but they can also be present in the groin. The cause is not clear, but factors may include standing for long periods, injury, pregnancy, being overweight, and even Constipation.

SYMPTOMS & SIGNS

- Veins are visible as blue protuberances in the leg
- More prominent after standing, exercise or as the day progresses
- Veins become less prominent when the leg is raised and during the night
- Discomfort, although rarely painful
- Ankle may become swollen
- May be ulcers
- May be brown discoloration of the lower leg, ankle and feet

> NOTE
> Not usually a cause for concern. More common in females than males.

Vasomotor Rhinitis
see RHINITIS

Venous Thrombosis
see DEEP VEIN THROMBOSIS

Venous Ulceration

Ulcers in the skin due to chronic congestion of veins,

usually in legs and most often associated with varicose veins. Areas of skin with venous congestion are often fragile and pigmented and ulcerate easily with minor trauma. Very often slow to heal.

SYMPTOMS & SIGNS

- Ulceration, particularly on the outer part of the ankle
- Brown pigmentation of the lower legs

Verucca
see WARTS

Vestibulitis

Condition of the ears, affecting the part which controls balance, caused by a virus. It can occur in epidemics.

SYMPTOMS & SIGNS

- Dizziness or giddiness, usually with a sudden onset: it may be difficult or impossible to rise from seating or lying without falling over. Also with any movement of the head
- Nausea and vomiting, again particularly with any movement of the head
- Eyes may have twitching movements

> NOTE
> May be alarming symptoms, but the condition will normally resolve itself over time, taking about 14 days occasionally longer. It is possible that symptoms will recur.

Vincent's Acute Ulcerative Gingivitis
see VINCENT'S ANGINA

Vincent's Angina

General infection of all parts of the mouth, caused by

bacterial infection from the gums (Vincent's Acute Ulcerative Gingivitis) or from the tonsils (Vincent's Angina). The conditions are very contagious, and is known as Trench Mouth as it spread rapidly through soldiers in World War I.

SYMPTOMS & SIGNS

Vincent's Angina:

- Painful, bleeding gums
- Fever
- Pain and sore throat
- Lymph nodes swollen in neck
- Foul breath
- Often there is a membrane which can spread to the hard and soft palate
- Foul breath
- May be that only one tonsil is infected and ulcerated

Vincent's Acute Ulcerative Gingivitis:

- As above
- Ulcers on the gums

NOTE
Help should be sought immediately if these conditions are suspected, and they will need to be treated with antibiotics.

CROSS-REFERENCED UNDER:

Vincent's Acute Ulcerative Gingivitis; Trench Mouth

Viral Illness

see FLU

Vitamin A Deficiency

Caused by lack of the important Vitamin A, which is found in animal fat in foods such as liver, kidney, cheese, eggs, butter and fish liver oils (as well as margarine, to which it has been added) Carotene,

found in carrots, tomatoes, spinach, cabbage and other foods, may be converted into Vitamin A in the liver. Usually due to dietary deficiency or malabsorption.

SYMPTOMS & SIGNS

- Night blindness
- Problems with the eye, leading to inflammation and scarring of the cornea, and even blindness. Cornea looks thickened and course
- Whites of the eye become coloured
- Widespread rash: skin becomes dry and rough
- Reduced resistance to infection

NOTE
A normal diet will contain plenty of Vitamin A for most healthy people. In developing countries, however, this may be a serious problem. It is possible health problems may develop from taking too much of the vitamin, usually through supplements.

CROSS-REFERENCED UNDER:

Keratomalacia

Vitamin B1 (Thiamine) Deficiency

Deficiency of Vitamin B1, most likely in developing countries where the main diet is polished rice, although it is also common in alcoholics. Thiamine is found in whole-grain cereals and in liver.

SYMPTOMS & SIGNS

- Pins and needles in hands and feet
- Weakness of muscles
- Rapid pulse
- Heart failure with breathlessness and swollen ankles and legs
- Unsteady on feet due to loss of balance

- May be dementia, along with poor memory and feelings of disorientation
- Twitching movement of the eyes (nystagmus)

> **NOTE**
> Treatment is by correcting deficiency, although this needs to be done as soon as possible.

CROSS-REFERENCED UNDER:
Beri-Beri

Vitamin B2 (Riboflavine) Deficiency

Deficiency in vitamin B2 is likely to be part of overall malnutrition

SYMPTOMS & SIGNS
- Lips may be cracked and particularly red or sore looking, especially at the corners of the mouth

CROSS-REFERENCED UNDER:
Riboflavine Deficiency

Vitamin B3 (Niacin) Deficiency

Dietary deficiency of Niacin (Vitamin B3).

SYMPTOMS & SIGNS
- Dementia
- Severe diarrhoea
- Scaly skin, particularly where the skin is exposed to the air

CROSS-REFERENCED UNDER:
Pellagra

Vitamin B12 (Cyanocobalamin) Deficiency

Deficiency in Vitamin B12 causes problems with the development of mature red blood cells, and is rarely associated with Subacute Combined Degeneration of the Spinal Cord (SACD). B12 Deficiency is caused by Pernicious Anaemia, poor diet, some drugs, inability to absorb the vitamin due to malabsorption syndrome such as Coeliac Disease, and excessive drinking.

SYMPTOMS & SIGNS
- Tongue – smooth and shining
- Anaemia – pallor, skin may have lemon tinge
- Pins and needles in the feet and toes more than in the hands or fingers
- Unsteady when walking
- Muscle wasting and reduced strength in leg muscles
- General aches and pain
- May be slow developing paralysis
- Problems with position, balance and inability to feel vibrations
- Dementia

> **NOTE**
> Treatment is with Vitamin B12 or in the case of Pernicious Anaemia a factor which allows the absorption of the vitamin.

Vitamin C (Ascorbic Acid) Deficiency

Deficiency in Vitamin C causes fatigue and haemorrhage, particularly around hair follicles. Historically, mariners on long journeys suffered from the condition, as they had no fresh fruit or vegetables. Most Western diets should have enough vitamin C to prevent Scurvy, and it is found in foods such as potatoes, cabbage, cauliflower, blackcurrants, strawberries, as well as other fruits, and green and root vegetables.

SYMPTOMS & SIGNS

- Fatigue, feeling unwell, sore joints
- Haemorrhage and easily bruised
- Bleeding spots on the skin around hair follicles
- Bleeding gums
- Lips may be cracked and particularly red or sore looking, especially at the corners of the mouth

> NOTE
> Eating a well balanced diet should provide the body with plenty of Vitamin C.

CROSS-REFERENCED UNDER:

Scurvy

Vitamin D (Calciferol) Deficiency

Can lead to rickets (children) or osteomalacia (adults). Deformity of, and problems with, bones, caused by a lack of Vitamin D (Calciferol) in the diet or lack of sun exposure. Vitamin D is found in foods such as sardines, herring, cod liver oil, butter, milk and margarine and is produced in the skin when it is exposed to ultraviolet in sunlight. Vitamin D helps with the absorption of calcium from the diet.

SYMPTOMS & SIGNS

In children (Rickets):

- Bone deformity or problems, including the skull, joints such as the ankle and wrist, and the cartilage in the chest
- Misshapen bones in the leg, making the individual bowlegged
- May be curvature of the spine and back pain
- Hunched or stooped posture

In adults (osteomalacia):

- Dull, aching pain usually felt in bones, with associated tenderness especially in back and leg

- Muscle weakness and pain (can lead to waddling)
- Bones may break or fracture more easily
- May be shortening in stature due to the spine being compressed (vertebral fracture)
- Osteoporosis with fractures

> NOTE
> Sufficient Vitamin D in the diet will prevent this condition developing. It is possible to take too much Vitamin D, probably through supplements, and this will cause health problems.

CROSS-REFERENCED UNDER:

Rickets; Osteomalacia

Vitiligo

Painless destruction of cells which produce pigment in the skin causing lack of pigmentation. The areas are seen as patches of unusually white skin, particularly noticeable in sun exposed areas or those with black or dark skins. May be associated with conditions such as thyroid under- or over-activity and Addison's Disease.

SYMPTOMS & SIGNS

- Areas of white skin that do not darken with sun exposure

Vitreous Haemorrhage

Bleeding in the eye, usually associated with Diabetes or arterial disease. This bleeding may be mild or severe.

SYMPTOMS & SIGNS

If mild:

- Many floaters

If severe, also:
- Partial loss of vision in one eye
- No pain

> NOTE
> If this conditions is suspected, medical help should be sought immediately. Diagnosis needs to be confirmed by tests, although there is no direct treatment.

Vocal Nodules

Nodules can occur in the vocal region.

SYMPTOMS & SIGNS
- Voice may be hoarse and higher in timbre than normal

> NOTE
> Nodules may need to be removed by surgery.

CROSS-REFERENCED UNDER:
Singer's Nodules

Volkmann's Contracture

see ISCHAEMIC CONTRACTURE

Vomiting and Nausea

Vomiting and nausea is treated here as a condition - look under the relevant headings for conditions which produce vomiting as a sign or symptom.

SYMPTOMS & SIGNS
- Just before vomiting, the mouth feels as if it is full of very salty saliva

Warts

Warts are caused by viruses, and cause growths or lumps anywhere on the body, including on the eye and eyelid. There are several different kinds, and although they can be unsightly, they are usually harmless, although Veruccas (plantar warts) may cause pain as they are in weight bearing areas. They are, however, infectious and can pass from one individual to another. One type of wart which should be investigated is a type which looks like branching coral, and is found at sites of sexual contact. These warts are associated with Syphilis.

SYMPTOMS & SIGNS
- A small growth in the skin, raised above the surrounding area, with rough skin
- May spread over a wide area
- May be found singly or in groups

Seborrhoeic:
- Brown wart, which is slightly raised above the surrounding skin and flat in appearance
- There may many warts of this type
- Usually found in those who are middle-aged or older

Verucca (Plantar Wart):
- Often found on the soul of the feet
- May be painful if the wart presses into the skin while walking or running

> NOTE
> Warts or similar growths are unsightly but are rarely cause for concern. They may be removed if necessary.

CROSS-REFERENCED UNDER:
Papilloma; Verucca

Water on the Brain

see HYDROCEPHALUS

Weight Change

see ANOREXIA NERVOSA

Weil's Disease (Leplosprosis)

Infectious disease caught from water contaminated by rats or rodent urine. It takes about 10 days to incubate.

SYMPTOMS & SIGNS
- Sudden onset of high fever with rigors
- Headache and aching muscles
- Loss of appetite, nausea, vomiting, diarrhoea
- Occaionally sore joints, sore bones, abdominal pain
- Eyes are reddened
- May be jaundice, with enlarged liver
- May be spontaneous bleeding from the nose or mouth
- May be irritation of the lining of the brain
- In some cases, may be heart and kidney failure

NOTE
Most likely in people coming into contact with contaminated water, such as swimmers. Medical help should be sought. A test will be required to confirm a diagnosis, and treatment is with antibiotics.

CROSS-REFERENCED UNDER:
Leptospirosis

Wheat Intolerance

see COELIAC DISEASE

Whiplash Injury

Neck is injured or sprained by a violent or sudden movement, such as in a car accident when hit from behind or in front

SYMPTOMS & SIGNS
- Pain felt in both head and back, although it may take some time to develop after the injury
- Pain and stiffness may persist for a long time
- Movement of neck is constrained, reduced and difficult
- May be pain and weakness in the arms

NOTE
Medical help should be sought if the injury has been violent, although most injuries will resolve.

White Finger

see RAYNAUD'S PHENOMENON

Whitlow

see INJURY TO THE NAILS

Whooping Cough

Bacterial infection with a distinctive cough, a sudden intake of breath ('a whoop') following severe coughing. It is caused by inflammation of the lining of the lungs. Typically occurs in early childhood.

SYMPTOMS & SIGNS
- Onset is symptoms of a Cold that lasts about a week with mild fever, loss of appetite, non spesific respitory symptoms
- Severe and progressive coughing, causing extreme breathlessness and an intake of breath ('a whoop')

In severe coughing spasms:
- Vomiting after coughing spasm
- Face goes red or blue
- May stop breathing
- May be convulsions
- Thick sticky phlegm
- May lead to Pneumonia

■ May take months to resolve

> NOTE
> Possible in babies and young infants, although the condition is much rarer since the advent of immunisation. Anyone who has not been immunised or has not had the illness can contract it.

CROSS-REFERENCED UNDER:
Pertussis

Wilms' Tumour (Nephrabtastoma)

Malignant tumour growing on the kidney, that can occur in children.

SYMPTOMS & SIGNS
■ Swelling on one side of the abdomen
■ Blood in urine
■ Loss of appetite
■ Fever
■ Anaemia but occasionally blood count too high (polycythaemia)
■ Pain, although only in more advanced stages
■ Occasionally high blood pressure
■ Rarely causes low blood sugar

> NOTE
> Found in children. Early diagnosis is essential as highly malignant.

Wilson's Disease
see HEPATOLENTRICULAR DEGENERATION

Wind
see FLATULENCE

Wisdom Teeth

When a wisdom tooth erupts through the gum, it will cause pain and discomfort, particularly if it is impacted. An impacted tooth is blocked or prevented from erupting by other teeth: there may not be room for it. This tooth may need to be removed.

SYMPTOMS & SIGNS
■ Pain and discomfort at the back of the mouth
■ The area where the tooth is erupting may become infected
■ May be difficult to open the mouth because of the pain or swelling

> NOTE
> If this condition is suspected, seek advice and help from a dentist.

CROSS-REFERENCED UNDER:
Impacted Wisdom Teeth

Womb Prolapse

Prolapse or collapse of the womb (uterus), caused as a late after effect of the strain and trauma of giving birth, especially if a woman has had several babies; more common in older women.

SYMPTOMS & SIGNS
■ May be felt as a lump in the vagina as 'something coming down'
■ May bleed or an unusual discharge may occur
■ May be urinary incontinence
■ May be that the womb can be pushed back in, although it may recur with straining, sneezing or coughing

> NOTE
> Medical help should be sought.

CROSS-REFERENCED UNDER:
Prolapse of the Womb

Wrist Sprain

The wrist can be sprained by damage from a fall, or twisting or bending of the joint in which the ligaments supporting the joint are pulled/bruised.

SYMPTOMS & SIGNS
- Painful
- Range of joint movement not restricted, other than by the discomfort
- Local tenderness

> NOTE
> Will usually resolve within a few days.

CROSS-REFERENCED UNDER:
Sprain of Wrist

Wryneck

Head is drawn to one side because of the contraction of the sternomastoid muscle in the neck on that side. The face is rotated over the other shoulder.

SYMPTOMS & SIGNS
- Head drawn to one side, the face rotated over the other shoulder
- Neck movements are curtailed
- The sternomastoid muscle is a solid band
- Painless

> NOTE
> This condition may be present on waking up, but should resolve itself in a few days.

CROSS-REFERENCED UNDER:
Torticollis

Xanthelasma

see XANTHOMATA

Xanthomata

Deposit of fatty material just below the skin. The deposit is well defined, hard and yellowish in colour. Xanthomata can be a sign of underlying condition where there is excess fat in the blood. This may lead to arterial disease.

SYMPTOMS & SIGNS
- Small yellowish patches beneath the skin, most commonly beneath or above the corner of the eyes (known as xanthelasma), but also found on elbows, knees and hands.
- No pain associated with the lump
- May grow very slowly

CROSS-REFERENCED UNDER:
Xanthelasma

Yaws

Chronic infectious disease found in West and Central Africa and South America and Oceania, which has many symptoms similar to Syphilis, although it is not transmitted sexually.

SYMPTOMS & SIGNS
- Skin rash with ulcers, usually starts with single enlarging red, painful lump on the palms of the hands and souls of the feet
- Swollen lymph glands
- May be destruction of bone with bone pain
- Ulcerating lesions

> NOTE
> Medical help should be sought as soon as possible.

Yeast Infection

see CANDIDIASIS

Yellow Fever

Infectious feverish disease, which is caused by a virus spread by mosquitoes. Initial phase of non-specifica symptoms for 3–4 days, followed by improvement but progresses to a more serious phase of kidney and liver damage with bleeding.

SYMPTOMS & SIGNS

Initial stage of infection:

- Sudden onset of fever (often very high) with rigors
- Headache, photophobia (dislike of light), dizziness
- Pain in the abdomen and limbs
- Off food (anorexia), nausea, vomiting

Intoxication phase:

- Jaundice
- Progressive kidney failure with failure to produce urine
- Vomiting blood, nose bleeds, blood in urine and faeces
- Confusion, agitation, fits, coma

NOTE

Most likely in tropical western and southern parts of Africa and of South America, as well as parts of the Caribbean. An immunisation against Yellow Fever is available, although there is no cure. Life-long immunity is conferred following recovery. Medical help should be sought as soon as possible.